LWW's Foundations in
Pharmacology
for Pharmacy Technicians

LWW's Foundations in
Pharmacology
for Pharmacy Technicians

W. RENÉE ACOSTA, RPH, MS

University of Texas at Austin,
College of Pharmacy

Wolters Kluwer | Lippincott Williams & Wilkins
Health

Philadelphia · Baltimore · New York · London
Buenos Aires · Hong Kong · Sydney · Tokyo

Acquisitions Editor: David B. Troy
Product Manager: Renee Thomas
Art Director: Jennifer Clements
Vendor Manager: Kevin Johnson
Design Coordinator: Stephen Druding
Manufacturing Coordinator: Margie Orzech
Production Services/Compositor: Spearhead Global

First Edition

351 West Camden Street   530 Walnut Street
Baltimore, MD 21201   Philadelphia, PA 19106

Printed in China

9 8 7 6 5 4 3 2 1

Library of Congress Cataloging-in-Publication Data
Acosta, W. Renée.
  LWW's foundations in pharmacology for pharmacy technicians / W. Renée Acosta.
       p. ; cm.
  Includes bibliographical references and index.
  ISBN-13: 978-0-7817-6624-1
  ISBN-10: 0-7817-6624-9
1. Pharmacology. 2. Pharmacy technicians. I. Lippincott Williams & Wilkins. II. Title.
    III. Title: Foundations in pharmacology for pharmacy technicians.
  [DNLM: 1. Pharmaceutical Preparations. 2. Pharmacists' Aides. 3. Pharmacological Phenomena. QV 55 A185L 2010]
  RM301.A263 2010
  615'.1—dc22

                                                              2009028339

DISCLAIMER

Care has been taken to confirm the accuracy of the information present and to describe generally accepted practices. However, the authors, editors, and publisher are not responsible for errors or omissions or for any consequences from application of the information in this book and make no warranty, expressed or implied, with respect to the currency, completeness, or accuracy of the contents of the publication. Application of this information in a particular situation remains the professional responsibility of the practitioner; the clinical treatments described and recommended may not be considered absolute and universal recommendations.

The authors, editors, and publisher have exerted every effort to ensure that drug selection and dosage set forth in this text are in accordance with the current recommendations and practice at the time of publication. However, in view of ongoing research, changes in government regulations, and the constant flow of information relating to drug therapy and drug reactions, the reader is urged to check the package insert for each drug for any change in indications and dosage and for added warnings and precautions. This is particularly important when the recommended agent is a new or infrequently employed drug.

Some drugs and medical devices presented in this publication have Food and Drug Administration (FDA) clearance for limited use in restricted research settings. It is the responsibility of the health care provider to ascertain the FDA status of each drug or device planned for use in their clinical practice.

To purchase additional copies of this book, call our customer service department at (800) 638-3030 or fax orders to (301) 223-2320. International customers should call (301) 223-2300.

Visit Lippincott Williams & Wilkins on the Internet: http://www.lww.com. Lippincott Williams & Wilkins customer service representatives are available from 8:30 am to 6:00 pm, EST.

Preface

LWW's Foundations in Pharmacology for Pharmacy Technicians is the essential resource for pharmacy technician students and their instructors. The most relevant and focused book on the market, it has been developed specifically for pharmacy technician students and programs. Comprehensive yet concise, avoiding fluff or filler, the text is the right depth, the right length, the right choice. Pharmacy technician students who learn their pharmacology with this book will be knowledgeable, confident, and prepared for professional success.

LWW's Foundations in Pharmacology for Pharmacy Technicians is organized by drug class and by body system, which is ideal for students' understanding pharmacology concepts and absorbing drug information details. Throughout, the text maintains focus on the most essential information for pharmacy technicians: drugs and their actions, as opposed to the overemphasis on conditions and diseases common among other pharmacology texts. Each chapter contains information on how drugs circulate (pharmacokinetics), how drugs act (pharmacodynamics), how drugs are used (pharmacotherapeutics), and drug interactions. Special features highlight and reinforce key information, while the straightforward writing style engages students and pulls them into the material.

Features

Each chapter of *LWW's Foundations in Pharmacology for Pharmacy Technicians* includes the following features:

- **Chapter Objectives** prepare the student for each chapter's material by laying out the key topics.
- **Key Terms** set up students' understanding of the material while also providing handy lists for studying at the start of each chapter, including definitions. Terms are bolded and highlighted in color throughout the chapter for in-context reinforcement.
- **Tips** offer advice for remembering and applying the chapter's content.
- **At the Counter** relates drug facts to relevant scenarios with patients and poses application questions to students.

- **Proceed with Caution** pulls together in concise lists the possible adverse interactions for the most commonly-prescribed drugs.
- **How It Works** describes pharmacokinetics and pharmacodynamics in clear, easy-to-understand steps with illustrations where appropriate.
- **Drug Classification Tables** synthesize the basic information about all drugs covered in each chapter by drug class, generic name, and trade name.
- **Quick Quizzes** at the end of each chapter provide in-context self-study and review opportunities for students or assignment options for instructors. Questions are multiple choice, short answer, true-or-false, and matching. Answers are provided in the Appendix.

Additional Resources

LWW's Foundations in Pharmacology for Pharmacy Technicians includes additional resources for both instructors and students that are available on the book's companion website at *http://thePoint.lww.com/AcostaPharma.*

Approved adopting instructors will be given access to the following additional resources:

- Brownstone Test Generator
- PowerPoint Presentations
- Image Bank
- WebCT and Blackboard Ready Cartridge

Students who have purchased *LWW's Foundations in Pharmacology for Pharmacy Technicians* have access to an electronic Quiz Bank for independent study and review.

In addition, instructors and purchasers of the text can access the searchable Full Text Online by going to the *LWW's Foundations in Pharmacology for Pharmacy Technicians* website at *http://thePoint.lww.com/AcostaPharma.* See the inside front cover of this text for more details, including the passcode you will need to gain access to the website.

LWW's Foundations Series

Look for more titles in LWW's Foundations Series. This series is dedicated to providing pharmacy technician resources that are comprehensive, concise, and priced with the market in mind.

Reviewers

ANNE VUKADINOVIC
Centennial College
Toronto, Ontario

JANET McGREGOR LILES
Arkansas State University
Beebe, AR

KATHLEEN O'MALLEY
American Medical Careers
Flint, MI

CHRISTY BIVINS
North Georgia Technical College
Clarkesville, GA

MICHAEL C. MELVIN
Griffin Technical College
Griffin, GA

LARRY ALLEN
Arapahoe Community College
Littleton, CO

DENISE ANDERSON
International Education Corporation
Ontario, CA

Brief Contents

Contents

CHAPTER 1

Fundamentals of Pharmacology

CHAPTER OBJECTIVES

- Identify commonly used routes of administration and unique characteristics of each route
- Define pharmacokinetics, pharmacodynamics, and pharmacotherapeutics
- Describe the absorption process of a drug administered orally versus a drug infused intravenously
- List the factors that affect a drug's distribution
- Compare and contrast the different ways that drugs are metabolized
- Identify the different ways drugs are eliminated from the body
- Differentiate the ways an agonist, competitive antagonist, and noncompetitive antagonist affect a receptor
- Compare drug tolerance and drug dependence
- List potential drug interactions that commonly occur
- Describe common adverse drug reactions

KEY TERMS

active transport—diffusion that requires cellular energy to move the drug instead of spontaneous diffusion

additive effects—effects occurring when two drugs with similar actions are administered to a patient

adverse effect—see *adverse reaction*

adverse reaction—an undesirable drug effect; also known as an *adverse effect* or a *side effect*

agonist—a drug that binds with a receptor to produce a therapeutic response

alkaloid—a plant-derived drug formed from the most active component in plants that reacts with acids to form an easily dissolvable salt

anaphylactic reaction—a sudden, severe hypersensitivity reaction with symptoms that progress rapidly and may result in death if not treated

antagonist—a drug that joins with a receptor to prevent the action of an agonist at that receptor

antagonistic effect—an effect that occurs when the combined response of two drugs is less than the response produced by either drug alone

brand name—see *trade name*

buccal administration—a route of administration in which the drug is placed in the pouch between the cheek and gum of a patient's mouth

chemical name—a scientific name of a drug that precisely describes its atomic and molecular structure

competitive antagonist—an antagonist that competes with an agonist for receptor sites

dose-response curve—a graph used to represent the relationship between the dose of a drug and the response it produces

drug dependence—a physical or psychological need for a drug

drug tolerance—a patient's decreased response to a drug over time, requiring larger doses to produce the same response

enzymes—proteins produced by living cells that act as catalysts

expected therapeutic response—a drug's desired effect

fats—body fluids, usually fixed, obtained from animals as a drug source

first-pass effect—the metabolizing of a drug by the liver before it circulates to the rest of the body, including the site of action

gastric administration—a route of administration in which the drug is directly instilled into the gastrointestinal system

generic name—a drug's nonproprietary name

glycosides—drugs derived from active components found in plants that form sugars

gums—active components in plants that give products the ability to attract and hold water

hormone—chemical produced by glands in the body and released into the bloodstream

idiosyncratic response—unusual or abnormal drug response

intradermal administration—a route of administration in which substances are injected into the skin

intramuscular administration—a route of administration in which drugs are injected directly into various muscle groups

intravenous administration—a route of administration in which substances are injected directly into the bloodstream through a vein

margin of safety—see *therapeutic index*

natural sources—plants, animals, and minerals used for the derivation of drugs

noncompetitive antagonist—an antagonist that binds to receptor sites and blocks the effects of the agonist

oils—thick and greasy liquids used as a drug source, derived from either plants or animals

oral administration—a route of administration in which the drug is taken into the mouth and swallowed

passive transport—spontaneous diffusion of a substance across a membrane to equalize the concentration of the substance on both sides of the membrane

pharmacodynamics—the biochemical and physical effects of drugs and the mechanisms of drug actions

pharmacokinetics—the absorption, distribution, metabolism, and excretion of a drug

pharmacologic class—a group or family of drugs that share similar characteristics

pharmacotherapeutics—the use of drugs to prevent and treat diseases

potentiation—an effect that occurs when two drugs that produce the same effect are given together, and one drug enhances the effect of the other drug

prodrugs—inactive drugs that do not become active until they are metabolized

proprietary name—see *trade name*

rectal administration—a route of drug administration to treat local irritation or infection (suppositories, ointments, creams,

or gels), or for a systemic response (especially in situations where patients cannot take oral medications)

resin—naturally occurring viscous substance found in plants used as local irritants, laxatives, and caustic agents

respiratory administration—a route of drug administration requiring inhalation of gases, aerosols, and powders

side effect—see *adverse reaction*

subcutaneous administration—a route of administration in which the drug is injected under the skin

sublingual administration—a route of administration in which the drug is placed under the tongue where it is absorbed

synthetic drug—a drug developed through the use of traditional knowledge and chemical science without the impurities of natural substances

therapeutic class—drugs grouped together by similarities for the diseases they treat or by the effects they produce in the body

therapeutic index—the relationship between a drug's desired therapeutic effects and its adverse effects; also known as *margin of safety*

topical administration—drug delivery through the skin or a mucous membrane

trade name—a copyright-protected name selected by the drug company selling the product; also known as the *brand name* or *proprietary name*

translingual administration—a route of administration in which the drug is placed on the tongue and absorbed

vaccine—substance containing killed or weakened microorganisms for the purpose of creating resistance to a disease

vaginal administration—a route of drug administration used to treat local irritation or infection (suppositories, ointments, creams, or gels), and sometimes used for a systemic effect

---

In this chapter, you will be introduced to the fundamental principles of pharmacology. You will find basic information such as how drugs are named and how they're created. You will also learn about the different routes by which drugs can be administered.

This chapter also discusses what happens when a drug enters the body. This involves three main areas:

- **pharmacokinetics** (the absorption, distribution, metabolism, and excretion of a drug)
- **pharmacodynamics** (the biochemical and physical effects of drugs on the body and the mechanisms of drug actions)
- **pharmacotherapeutics** (the use of drugs to prevent and treat diseases)

In addition, this chapter provides an introduction to adverse drug reactions.

PHARMACOLOGY BASICS

Drugs can go by three different names:

- The **chemical name** is a scientific name that precisely describes the drug's atomic and molecular structure.

- The **generic name** is the drug's nonproprietary name.
- The **trade name** (also known as the **brand name** or **proprietary name**) is selected by the drug company selling the product. Trade names are protected by copyright. The symbol ® after the trade name indicates that the name is registered by and restricted to the drug manufacturer.

T I P Drugs have at least three names: a chemical name, a generic name, and a trade name. For example, Tylenol® is a trade name. The chemical name of this drug is N-(4-hydroxyphenyl) acetamide and the generic name is acetaminophen.

Prescribing patterns are likely to be very different depending on where you work as a pharmacy technician. In hospitals, most prescribers will use the generic name of the drug when writing a medication order. In community pharmacies, you will most likely encounter the trade name on prescriptions, especially for newer medications that do not have a generic form yet available. As a pharmacy technician, you should know both the trade and generic names readily.

In 1962, the federal government mandated the use of official names so that only one official name would represent each drug. The official names are listed in the *United States Pharmacopeia and National Formulary* (USP/NF). Most of these names are generic drug names.

Drugs that share similar characteristics are grouped together as a **pharmacologic class** (or family). Beta-adrenergic blockers are an example of a pharmacologic class.

The **therapeutic class** groups drugs by therapeutic use. Antihypertensives (drugs that are used to treat high blood pressure) are an example of a therapeutic class.

T I P Patients can become confused between brand and generic names. It's helpful if the patient knows the reason (symptom or condition) why he's taking the drug so that he can be certain to receive the right medication. If a patient is uncertain about the name of his medication, ask the pharmacist for help.

Drug Sources

Traditionally, drugs were derived from **natural** sources, such as plants, animals, and minerals. Today, however, laboratory researchers use traditional knowledge, along with chemical science, to develop **synthetic** drug sources. One advantage of chemically developed drugs is that they're free from the impurities found in natural substances.

In addition, researchers and developers can manipulate the molecular structure of substances such as antibiotics so that a slight change in the chemical structure makes the drug effective against different organisms. The first-, second-, third-, and fourth-generation cephalosporins are an example. (You'll learn more about cephalosporins in Chapter 9.)

Plant Sources

There are several types of active components found in plant sources and they vary in character and effect:

- **Alkaloids**, the most active components in plants, react with acids to form a salt that can dissolve more readily in body fluids. The names of alkaloids and their salts usually end in *-ine*. Examples include atropine, caffeine, and nicotine.
- **Glycosides** are also active components found in plants. Names of glycosides usually end in the letters *-in*, such as digoxin.
- **Gums** are another group of active components. Gums give products the ability to attract and hold water. Examples include seaweed extractions and seeds with starch.
- **Resins**, found primarily in pine tree sap, commonly act as local irritants or as laxatives and caustic agents.
- **Oils**, thick and sometimes greasy liquids, are classified as volatile or fixed. Examples of volatile oils, which readily evaporate, include peppermint, spearmint, and juniper. Fixed oils, which don't easily evaporate, include castor oil and olive oil.

Animal Sources

The body fluids or glands of animals can also be drug sources. The drugs obtained from animal sources include:

- **hormones**, such as insulin
- **oils** and **fats** (usually fixed), such as cod-liver oil
- **enzymes**, such as pancreatin and pepsin
- **vaccines**, which are suspensions of killed or weakened microorganisms, such as the influenza shot

Mineral Sources

Metallic and nonmetallic minerals provide various inorganic materials not available from plants or animals. The mineral sources are used as they occur in nature or are combined with other ingredients. Drugs that contain minerals include:

- iron
- iodine
- Epsom salts

Lab-Produced Drugs

Today, most drugs are produced in laboratories and can be natural (from animal, plant, or mineral sources) or synthetic. Examples of drugs produced in the laboratory include thyroid hormone (natural) and ranitidine (synthetic).

Recombinant deoxyribonucleic acid (rDNA) research has led to other chemical sources of organic compounds. For example, the reordering of genetic information has enabled scientists to develop bacteria that produce insulin for humans.

Drug Administration

A drug's administration route influences the amount given and the rate at which the drug is absorbed and distributed. These variables affect the drug's action and the patient's response. There are several different routes by which drugs can be administered:

- Certain drugs are given **buccally** (in the pouch between the cheek and the gum), **sublingually** (or SL, under the tongue), or **translingually** (on the tongue) to prevent their destruction or transformation in the stomach or small intestine.
- The **gastric** route of administration allows direct instillation of medication into the gastrointestinal (GI) system of patients who can't ingest the drug orally.
- Substances administered **intradermally** (ID) are injected into the skin (dermis). This route is used mainly for diagnostic purposes when testing for allergies or tuberculosis.
- The **intramuscular** (IM) route allows drugs to be injected directly into various muscle groups at varying tissue depths. It's used to give aqueous suspensions and solutions in oil and to give medications that aren't available in oral form.
- The **intravenous** (IV) route allows the injection of substances (drugs, fluids, blood or blood products, and diagnostic contrast agents) directly into the bloodstream through a vein. Administration can range from a single dose to an ongoing infusion delivered with great precision.

AT THE COUNTER

Ophthalmic or Otic?

You receive a prescription for tobramycin ophthalmic solution. You notice that the sig reads: "1–2 gtts au q 4 hours." Can this be correct?

Yes, ophthalmic drops may be used in the ear. In this situation, the prescriber wants a particular antibiotic that does not come in an ear drop form to be used in the ear. However, ear drops should never be used in the eye (they often contain alcohol and other ingredients that would irritate the eye). It's also important to note that ophthalmic medications must be sterile whereas otic preparations are not.

- **Oral** (PO) administration is usually the safest, most convenient, and least expensive route. Drugs are administered to patients who are conscious and can swallow.
- Suppositories, ointments, creams, or gels may be instilled **rectally** (PR) or **vaginally** (PV) to treat local irritation or infection. Some drugs applied to the mucosa of the rectum or vagina can be absorbed systemically.
- Drugs that are available as gases or powders can be administered into the **respiratory** system. Drugs given by inhalation are rapidly absorbed, and medications given by devices such as the metered-dose inhaler can be self-administered. Drugs can also be injected directly into the lungs through an endotracheal tube in emergency situations.
- With the **subcutaneous** (SubQ) route, small amounts of a drug are injected beneath the skin and into the subcutaneous tissue, usually in the patient's upper arm, thigh, or abdomen.

PROCEED WITH CAUTION

Check and Double-Check

Although drugs have usual routes of administration, sometimes they are administered differently. Always double-check the route of administration and do not make assumptions. For example:

- eye drops can be used in the ear, but ear drops cannot be used in the eye
- a liquid-filled capsule might be punctured and the liquid squirted under the tongue for sublingual absorption
- tablets and capsules can be used vaginally or rectally in certain circumstances

Make sure that the correct auxiliary label is applied in these situations!

- The **topical** route of administration is used to deliver a drug through the skin or a mucous membrane. It's used for most dermatologic, ophthalmic, otic, and nasal preparations.

Drugs may also be administered as specialized infusions given by a direct route to a specific site in the patient's body, such as an epidural infusion (the drug is injected into the epidural space), intrapleural infusion (the drug is injected into the pleural cavity), intraperitoneal infusion (the drug is injected into the peritoneal cavity), intraosseous infusion (the drug is injected into the rich vascular network of a long bone), and intra-articular infusion (the drug is injected into a joint).

PHARMACOKINETICS

Kinetics refers to movement. Pharmacokinetics deals with the body's action on a drug as the drug moves through the body. Therefore, pharmacokinetics discusses how a drug is:

- absorbed (taken into the body)
- distributed (moved into various tissues)
- metabolized (changed into a form that can be excreted)
- excreted (removed from the body)

This branch of pharmacology is also concerned with a drug's onset of action, peak concentration level, and duration of action.

TIP The acronym *ADME* describes how a drug moves through the body. It stands for absorption, distribution, metabolism, and excretion.

Absorption

Drug absorption covers a drug's progress from the time it's administered, through its passage to the tissues, until it becomes available for use by the body.

On a cellular level, drugs are absorbed by several means—primarily through active or passive transport.

- **Passive transport** does not require the cell to do any work to move the drug. When a drug is administered, it diffuses (moves from an area of high concentration to an area of low concentration) across a membrane to make the concentration of the drug equal on both sides of the membrane. Once the concentration is equalized, diffusion stops.
- **Active transport** needs the cell to provide energy to move the drug from an area of high concentration to one of low concentration. Active transport is used to absorb electrolytes, such as sodium and potassium, as well as some drugs such as levodopa.

Many factors influence the speed of a drug's absorption in the body. These factors are:

■ *Route of administration.* If only a few cells separate the active drug from the systemic circulation, absorption will occur rapidly, and the drug will quickly reach therapeutic levels in the body. Typically, absorption occurs within seconds or minutes of a drug's being administered sublingually, intravenously, or by inhalation. Absorption occurs at a slower rate when drugs are administered by the oral, intramuscular, or subcutaneous routes because the complex membrane systems of GI mucosal layers, muscle, and skin delay drug passage. At the slowest absorption rates, drugs can take several hours or days to reach peak concentration levels. A slow rate usually occurs with rectally administered or sustained-release drugs.

■ *Digestive tract.* Most absorption of oral drugs occurs in the small intestine. If a patient has had large sections of the small intestine surgically removed, drug absorption decreases because of the reduced surface area and the reduced time that the drug is in the intestine. Other GI factors that can affect drug absorption include the presence of food in the digestive tract, antacids, and slower motility.

■ *Solubility.* A drug that is administered in liquid form will be absorbed more quickly because it has already been broken down into a solution. A tablet, on the other hand, must first be dissolved (in the stomach, for instance) before being absorbed, a process that takes longer.

■ *Liver function.* Drugs absorbed by the small intestine are transported to the liver before being circulated to the rest of the body. The liver may metabolize much of the drug before it enters the circulatory system. This mechanism is referred to as the **first-pass effect.** Liver metabolism may inactivate the drug; if so, the first-pass effect lowers the amount of active drug released into the systemic circulation. Therefore, higher drug dosages must be administered to achieve the desired effect.

■ *Blood flow.* Increased blood flow to an absorption site improves drug absorption, whereas reduced blood flow decreases absorption. More rapid absorption leads to a quicker onset of drug action. For example, the muscle area selected for IM administration can make a difference in the drug absorption rate. Blood flows faster through the deltoid muscle (in the upper arm) than through the gluteal muscle (in the buttocks). The gluteal muscle, however, can accommodate a larger volume of drug than the deltoid muscle.

■ *Pain and stress.* Pain and stress can decrease the amount of drug absorbed. This may be due to a change in blood flow, reduced movement through the GI tract, or gastric retention triggered by the autonomic nervous system's response to pain.

■ *Stomach contents.* Solid foods and high-fat meals slow down the rate at which contents leave the stomach and enter the intestines, delaying intestinal absorption of a drug. However, some drugs, such as griseofulvin, are better absorbed if eaten with a fatty meal.

■ *Formulation.* Drug formulation (such as tablets, capsules, liquids, sustained-release formulas, inactive ingredients, and coatings) affects the drug absorption rate and the time needed to reach peak blood concentration levels.

■ *Interactions.* Combining one drug with another drug or with food can cause interactions that increase or decrease drug absorption, depending on the substances involved.

Distribution

Drug distribution is the process by which the drug is delivered to body tissues and fluids. Distribution of an absorbed drug within the body depends on several factors:

■ *Blood flow.* After a drug has reached the bloodstream, its distribution in the body depends on blood flow. The drug is quickly distributed to the organs with a large supply of blood. These organs include the heart, liver, and kidneys. Distribution to other internal organs, skin, fat, and muscle is slower.

■ *Solubility.* The ability of a drug to cross a cell membrane depends on whether the drug is water- or lipid (fat)-soluble. Lipid-soluble drugs easily cross through cell membranes, whereas water-soluble drugs can't. Lipid-soluble drugs can also enter the brain by crossing the blood-brain barrier (a membrane that protects the blood vessels in the brain from harmful substances).

■ *Protein binding.* As a drug travels through the body, it comes in contact with proteins such as the plasma protein albumin. The drug can remain free or bind to the protein. The portion of a drug that's bound to a protein is inactive and can't exert a therapeutic effect. Only the free, or unbound, portion remains active. A drug is said to be highly protein-bound if more than 80 percent of the drug is bound to protein.

Metabolism

Drug metabolism, or biotransformation, is the process by which the body changes a drug from its dosage form to a more water-soluble form that can then be excreted. Drugs can be metabolized in several ways. Most drugs are metabolized into inactive metabolites (products of metabolism), which are then excreted. Other drugs are converted to active metabolites, which are capable of exerting their own pharmacologic action. Metabolites may undergo further metabolism or may be excreted from the body unchanged. Some drugs can be administered as inactive drugs, called **prodrugs,** which don't become active until they're metabolized.

Several factors can affect biotransformation:

■ *Location.* Enzymes in the liver metabolize the majority of drugs. However, metabolism can also occur in the plasma, kidneys, and membranes of the intestines. In contrast, some drugs inhibit or compete for enzyme metabolism, which can cause the accumulation of drugs when they're given together. This accumulation increases the potential for an adverse reaction or drug toxicity.

- *Disease.* Certain diseases can reduce metabolism. These include liver diseases, such as cirrhosis, and heart failure, which reduces circulation to the liver.
- *Genetics.* Genetics allows some people to metabolize drugs rapidly and others to metabolize them more slowly.
- *Environment.* Environment can alter drug metabolism. For example, cigarette smoke and alcohol may affect the rate of metabolism of some drugs. A stressful environment, such as prolonged illness, surgery, or injury, can also change how a person metabolizes drugs.
- *Age.* Developmental changes can also affect drug metabolism. For instance, infants have immature livers that reduce the rate of metabolism, and older adult patients experience a decline in liver size, blood flow, and enzyme production that also slows metabolism.
- *Enzyme suppression or enhancement.* The way a drug is metabolized can be influenced by inhibition (the suppression of an enzyme) and induction (the enhancement of an enzyme). A big concern is the occurrence of drug interactions as a result of inhibition and induction. For instance, when a drug is vital to the health of the patient, such as an anticonvulsant drug or blood pressure medicine, it's important to understand that other drugs and substances can interfere with how quickly or slowly a drug is metabolized. Substances such as nicotine, found in cigarettes, can induce enzymes, and grapefruit juice can inhibit enzymes, so awareness of a patient's lifestyle is another factor to consider.

Excretion

Drug excretion refers to the elimination of drugs from the body. Most drugs are excreted by the kidneys and leave the body through urine. Drugs can also be excreted through the lungs, exocrine (sweat, salivary, or mammary) glands, and intestinal tract.

Clearance

The rate at which a drug is eliminated, or cleared, from the body is known as its clearance. The kidneys do most of the work of clearing a drug from the body after it has been metabolized (renal clearance). The liver also works to clear drugs from the system (hepatic clearance).

To test the rate of clearance, health care providers can perform a blood test to measure the level of creatinine (a waste product) in the blood. Or a urine test may be performed to find out whether the amount of creatinine in urine collected for 12 to 24 hours is relative to the level of creatinine in the blood (creatinine clearance).

Half-Life

The half-life of a drug is the time it takes for half of the drug to be eliminated by the body. Factors that affect a drug's half-life include the drug's rate of absorption, metabolism, and excretion. Knowing how long a drug remains in the body helps to determine how frequently it should be administered.

A drug that's given only once is eliminated from the body almost completely after four or five half-lives. But a

AT THE COUNTER

Interaction Alert

You are processing a prescription when the computer system alerts you to a drug interaction. What should you do?

You should alert the pharmacist. There are many types of interactions that a drug may have with another drug, food, or an existing disease state. Pharmacists are trained to identify which interactions require action. Only a pharmacist should override an interaction on the computer system.

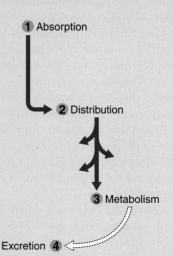

HOW IT WORKS

How the Pharmacokinetic Process Works

A drug moves through the body in four phases: absorption, distribution, metabolism, and excretion (figure 1-1).

1 Absorption

2 Distribution

3 Metabolism

Excretion **4**

FIGURE 1-1   (1) First, the drug is absorbed by the body. (2) Next, the drug is distributed to various tissues. (3) Then, the drug is metabolized, or changed into a form that can be excreted. (4) Finally, the drug is excreted, or removed from the body.

drug that's administered several times at regular intervals reaches a steady concentration (or steady state) in the body after about four or five half-lives. Steady state occurs when the rate of drug administration equals the rate of drug excretion.

Onset, Peak, and Duration

In addition to absorption, distribution, metabolism, and excretion, three other factors play important roles in a drug's pharmacokinetics:

- *Onset of action.* The onset of action refers to the time interval from when the drug is administered to when its therapeutic effect actually begins. Rate of onset varies, depending on the route of administration and other pharmacokinetic properties.
- *Peak concentration.* As the body absorbs more of the drug, blood concentration levels increase. The peak concentration level is reached when the absorption rate equals the elimination rate. However, the time of peak concentration isn't always the time of peak response.
- *Duration of action.* The duration of action is the length of time the drug produces its therapeutic effect.

PHARMACODYNAMICS

Pharmacodynamics is the study of the drug mechanisms that produce biochemical or physiologic changes in the body. Drug action is the interaction at the cellular level between a drug and cellular components, such as the complex proteins that make up the cell membrane, enzymes, or target receptors. The response resulting from this drug action is the drug effect. The following sections describe different types of drug effects.

Cell Function

A drug can modify cell function or rate of function, but it can't impart a new function to a cell or to target tissue. Therefore, the drug effect depends on what the cell is capable of accomplishing.

A drug can alter the target cell's function by:

- modifying the cell's physical or chemical involvement
- interacting with a receptor (a specialized location on a cell membrane or inside a cell)

Agonists and Antagonists

Many drugs work by stimulating or blocking drug receptors. A drug attracted to a receptor displays an affinity for that receptor. When a drug displays an affinity for a receptor and stimulates it, the drug acts as an **agonist**. If a drug has an affinity for a receptor but does not initiate a response after binding, it's called an **antagonist**. An antagonist prevents a response from occurring.

Antagonists can be competitive or noncompetitive.

- A **competitive antagonist** competes with the agonist for receptor sites. Because this type of receptor binds reversibly to the receptor site, administering larger doses of an agonist can overcome the antagonist's effects.
- A **noncompetitive antagonist** binds to receptor sites and blocks the effects of the agonist. Administering larger doses of the agonist can't reverse the antagonist's action.

T I P Competitive antagonists fight their way to receptor sites, but larger doses of an agonist can "beat" the antagonist's effects.

Nonselective Drugs

If a drug acts on a variety of receptors, it's said to be nonselective and can cause multiple and widespread effects. In addition, some receptors are classified further by their specific effects. For example, beta receptors typically produce increased heart rate and bronchial relaxation as well as other systemic effects. Beta receptors, however, can be further divided into beta$_1$ receptors, which act primarily on the heart, and beta$_2$ receptors, which act primarily on smooth muscles and gland cells.

Drug Potency

Drug potency (strength) refers to the relative amount of a drug required to produce a desired response. Drug potency is also used to compare two drugs. If drug X produces the same response as drug Y at a lower dose, then drug X is more potent than drug Y.

As its name implies, a **dose-response curve** is used to graphically represent the relationship between the dose of a drug and the response it produces. (See *How It Works: Dose-Response Curve.*) On the dose-response curve, a low dose usually corresponds to a low response. At a low dose, a dosage increase produces only a slight increase in response. With further dosage increases, the drug response rises significantly. After a certain point, however, an increase in dose yields little or no increase in response. At this point, the drug is said to have reached maximum effectiveness.

Therapeutic Index

Most drugs produce multiple effects. The relationship between a drug's desired therapeutic effects and the adverse reactions it produces is called the drug's **therapeutic index**. It's also referred to as its **margin of safety**.

The therapeutic index usually measures the difference between:

- an effective dose for 50 percent of the patients treated
- the minimal dose at which adverse reactions occur

HOW IT WORKS

Dose-Response Curve

Figure 1-2 shows the dose-response curve for two different drugs. As you can see, at low doses of each drug, a dosage increase results in only a small increase in drug response (for example, from point A to point B). At higher doses, an increase in dosage produces a much greater response (from point B to point C). As the dosage continues to climb, however, an increase in dosage produces very little increase in response (from point C to point D).

This graph also shows that drug X is more potent than drug Y because it produces the same response, but at a lower dose (compare point A to point E).

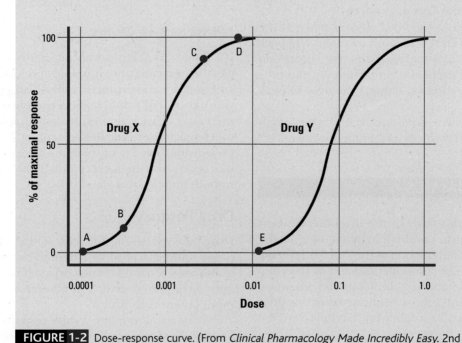

FIGURE 1-2 Dose-response curve. (From *Clinical Pharmacology Made Incredibly Easy*. 2nd Ed. Philadelphia, PA: Lippincott Williams & Wilkins; 2005.)

Drugs with a narrow, or low, therapeutic index have a narrow margin of safety. This means that there's a narrow range of safety between an effective dose and a lethal one. On the other hand, a drug with a high therapeutic index has a wide margin of safety and poses less risk of toxic (harmful) effects.

PHARMACOTHERAPEUTICS

Pharmacotherapeutics is the use of drugs to treat disease. When choosing a drug to treat a particular condition, health care providers consider not only the drug's effectiveness but also other factors, such as the type of therapy the patient will receive.

Habits and Lifestyle

A patient's overall health and other individual factors can alter that patient's response to a drug. Also, because no two people are identical physiologically or psychologically, patients' responses to a drug can vary greatly, depending upon such factors as:

- age
- cardiovascular function
- diet
- general health
- drug interactions
- GI function
- liver function
- infection

- kidney function
- gender

Coinciding medical conditions and personal lifestyle characteristics must be considered when selecting drug therapy.

Tolerance and Dependence

It's important to remember that certain drugs have a tendency to create drug tolerance and drug dependence in patients. **Drug tolerance** occurs when a patient develops a decreased response to a drug over time. The patient then requires larger doses to produce the same response.

Drug tolerance differs from **drug dependence**, in which a patient displays a physical or psychological need for the drug. Physical dependence produces withdrawal symptoms when the drug is stopped, whereas psychological dependence is based on a desire to continue taking the drug to relieve tension and avoid discomfort.

***

T I P Be careful to note a patient's history with drugs that can lead to dependence. The frequency, dosage, and condition being treated may require a call to the physician.

DRUG INTERACTIONS

Drug interactions can occur between drugs or between drugs and foods. They can interfere with the results of a laboratory test or produce physical or chemical incompatibilities. The more drugs a patient receives, the greater the chances that a drug interaction will occur. For example, toxic drug levels can occur when a drug's metabolism and excretion are inhibited by another drug, while some drug interactions affect excretion only.

Other potential drug interactions include:

- additive effects
- potentiation
- antagonistic effects
- decreased or increased absorption
- protein-binding competition
- food interactions

Drug interactions can also alter laboratory tests and can produce changes seen on a patient's electrocardiogram.

Additive Effects

Additive effects can occur when two drugs with similar actions are administered to a patient. The effects are equivalent to the sum of either drug's effects if administered alone in higher doses.

Giving two drugs together, such as two analgesics (pain relievers), has several potential advantages: lower doses of each drug, decreased probability of adverse reactions, and greater pain control than from one drug given alone (most likely because of different mechanisms of action). There's a decreased risk of adverse effects when giving two drugs for the same condition because the patient is given lower doses of each drug—the higher the dose, the greater the risk of adverse effects.

Potentiation and Antagonistic Effects

A synergistic effect, also called **potentiation**, occurs when two drugs that produce the same effect are given together and one drug enhances the effect of (potentiates) the other drug. This produces greater effects than when each drug is taken alone.

An **antagonistic effect** occurs when the combined response of two drugs is less than the response produced by either drug alone.

Absorption Effects

Two drugs given together can change the absorption of one or both of the drugs. Drugs that change the acidity of the stomach can affect the ability of another drug to dissolve in the stomach. Also, some drugs can interact and form an insoluble compound that can't be absorbed. Sometimes, an absorption-related drug interaction can be avoided by administering the drugs at least two hours apart.

Protein-binding Competition

After a drug is absorbed, the blood distributes it throughout the body as a free drug or as a drug that's bound to plasma protein. When two drugs are given together, they can compete for protein-binding sites, leading to an increase in the effects of one drug as that drug is displaced from the protein and becomes a free, unbound drug.

Food Interactions

Interactions between drugs and food can alter the therapeutic effects of the drug. Food can also alter the rate and amount of drug absorbed from the GI tract, affecting bioavailability—the amount of a drug dose that's made available to the systemic circulation. Drugs can also impair vitamin and mineral absorption.

Some drugs stimulate enzyme production, increasing metabolic rates and the demand for vitamins that are enzyme cofactors (which must unite with the enzyme for the enzyme to function). Dangerous interactions can also occur. For instance, when food that contains tyramine (such as aged cheddar cheese) is eaten by a person taking a monoamine oxidase inhibitor, hypertensive crisis can occur. Grapefruit can inhibit the metabolism of certain medications, such as fexofenadine, cyclosporine, and nifedipine, resulting in toxic blood levels. Because of all the interactions food can have with drug metabolism, being aware of drug interactions is essential.

ADVERSE DRUG REACTIONS

A drug's desired effect is called the **expected therapeutic response**. An **adverse reaction** (also called a **side effect** or **adverse effect**), on the other hand, is a harmful, undesirable response to a drug. Adverse drug reactions can range from mild effects that disappear when the drug is discontinued to debilitating diseases that become chronic. Adverse reactions can appear shortly after starting a new medication, but may become less severe over time.

Adverse drug reactions can be classified as dose-related or patient sensitivity-related.

Dose-Related Reactions

Most adverse drug reactions result from the known pharmacologic effects of a drug and are typically dose related. These types of reactions can be predicted in most cases. The four major types of dose-related reactions are discussed below.

Secondary Effects

A drug typically produces not only a major therapeutic effect but also secondary effects that can be harmful or beneficial. For example, morphine used for pain control can lead to two undesirable secondary effects: constipation and respiratory depression. Diphenhydramine used as an antihistamine produces sedation as a secondary effect and is sometimes used as a sleep aid.

Hypersusceptibility

A patient can be hypersusceptible to the pharmacologic actions of a drug. Such a patient experiences an excessive therapeutic response or secondary effects even when given the usual therapeutic dose. Hypersusceptibility typically results from altered pharmacokinetics (absorption, metabolism, and excretion), which leads to higher-than-expected blood concentration levels. Increased receptor sensitivity

also can increase the patient's response to therapeutic or adverse effects.

Overdose

A toxic drug reaction can occur when an excessive dose is taken, either intentionally or by accident. The result is an exaggerated response to the drug that can lead to brief changes or more serious reactions, such as respiratory depression, cardiovascular collapse, and even death. To avoid toxic reactions, chronically ill or older adult patients often receive lower drug doses.

Iatrogenic Effects

Iatrogenic effects are adverse drug reactions that can mimic pathologic disorders. For example, drugs such as antineoplastics, aspirin, corticosteroids, and indomethacin commonly cause GI irritation and bleeding. Other examples of iatrogenic effects include induced asthma with propranolol, induced nephritis (kidney inflammation) with methicillin, and induced deafness with gentamicin.

Sensitivity-Related Interactions

Patient sensitivity-related adverse reactions aren't as common as dose-related reactions. Sensitivity-related reactions result from a patient's unusual and extreme sensitivity to a drug. These adverse reactions arise from a unique tissue response rather than from an exaggerated pharmacologic action. Extreme patient sensitivity can occur as a drug allergy or an idiosyncratic response.

A drug allergy occurs when a patient's immune system identifies a drug, a drug metabolite, or a drug contaminant as a dangerous foreign substance that must be neutralized or destroyed. Previous exposure to the drug or to one with similar chemical characteristics sensitizes the patient's immune system, and subsequent exposure causes an allergic reaction (hypersensitivity). An allergic reaction not only directly injures cells and tissues, but also produces broader systemic damage by initiating cellular release of vasoactive and inflammatory substances. This type of severe allergic reaction is also called an **anaphylactic reaction**.

The allergic reaction can vary in intensity from a mild reaction with a rash and itching to an immediate, life-threatening reaction with circulatory collapse and swelling of the larynx and bronchioles.

Some sensitivity-related adverse reactions don't result from pharmacologic properties of a drug or from an allergy but are specific to the individual patient. These are called **idiosyncratic responses**. Some idiosyncratic responses have a genetic cause.

QUICK QUIZ

Answer the following multiple-choice questions.

1. What is the clearest, most precise way to refer to a drug?
   a. by the generic name
   b. by the chemical name
   c. by the brand name
   d. by the trade name
2. Which of the following is *not* a route of drug administration?
   a. intramuscular
   b. buccal
   c. extradermal
   d. sublingual
3. Drugs can be derived from:
   a. plants.
   b. animals.
   c. minerals.
   d. all of the above
4. Which organ primarily metabolizes *most* drugs?
   a. the lungs
   b. the kidneys
   c. the liver
   d. the small intestine
5. When the absorption rate of a drug equals the elimination rate, the drug has reached its:
   a. peak concentration level.
   b. half-life.
   c. onset of action.
   d. potentiation.

Please answer each of the following questions in one to three sentences.

1. Explain the difference between drug tolerance and drug dependence.

2. Name four types of drug interactions.

3. What are the steps of pharmacokinetics?

4. Briefly explain the difference between competitive and noncompetitive antagonists.

5. What's the difference between an allergic reaction and an adverse reaction?

Answer the following questions as either true or false.

1. ___ The U.S. Food and Drug Administration sets the guidelines for drug naming.
2. ___ Tablets can be given orally, vaginally, or rectally.
3. ___ Passive transport requires the cell to produce energy to equalize the concentration of drug on both sides of a membrane.
4. ___ Drugs are immediately excreted after they've been absorbed into the body.
5. ___ Drug potency refers to the relative amount of a drug required to produce a desired response.

Match the description in the left column with the correct route of administration from the right column.

1. injected directly into the muscle   a. subcutaneous
2. injected just beneath the skin   b. intravenous
3. injected into a vein   c. intramuscular
4. inhaled into the lungs   d. sublingual
5. placed under the tongue   e. respiratory

CHAPTER 2

Autonomic Nervous System Drugs

CHAPTER OBJECTIVES

- Match trade and generic names of commonly used autonomic nervous system drugs
- Identify uses of commonly used autonomic nervous system drugs
- Match autonomic nervous system drugs to the appropriate classification
- Identify common adverse reactions of commonly used autonomic nervous system drugs
- Describe the mechanism of action of cholinergic agonists
- Compare the mechanisms of action of direct-acting, indirect-acting, and dual-acting adrenergic drugs
- Identify the effects that alpha-adrenergic blockers have on the body
- Identify the effects on the body of beta-adrenergic blockers, including beta$_1$, beta$_2$, and nonselectives

KEY TERMS

acetylcholine—a neurotransmitter in the parasympathetic nervous system required for memory and thinking

adrenergic drugs—drugs that imitate the effects produced by the sympathetic nervous system, which activates the body's "fight-or-flight" response; also known as *sympathomimetic drugs*

adrenergic blocking drugs—drugs that block the transmission of impulses at adrenergic receptor sites; used to disrupt sympathetic nervous system function; also referred to as *sympatholytic drugs*

alpha-adrenergic blockers (or *alpha blockers*)—drugs that operate by interrupting the actions of the catecholamines epinephrine and norepinephrine at alpha$_1$ and alpha$_2$ receptors

anticholinergic drugs—see *cholinergic blocking drugs*

anticholinesterase drugs—drugs that work by slowing down or blocking the destruction of acetylcholine at the cholinergic receptor sites

asthenia—weakness; loss of strength

beta-adrenergic blockers (or *beta blockers*)—the most widely used adrenergic blocking drugs; prevent stimulation of the sympathetic nervous system by inhibiting the action of catecholamines at beta-adrenergic receptors

bradycardia—slow heart rate, usually at a rate less than 60 beats per minute

bronchospasm—spasm or constriction of the bronchi resulting in difficulty breathing

cardioselective beta-adrenergic blockers—selective beta-adrenergic blocking drugs that primarily affect beta$_1$-receptor sites and reduce stimulation of the heart

cholinergic agonists—drugs that imitate the action of the neurotransmitter acetylcholine

cholinergic drugs—drugs that promote the action of the neurotransmitter acetylcholine; also called *parasympathomimetic drugs* because they produce effects that imitate parasympathetic nerve stimulation

cholinergic blocking drugs—drugs that interrupt parasympathetic nerve responses in both the central and autonomic nervous systems; also referred to as *anticholinergic drugs* because they stop acetylcholine from activating cholinergic receptors

dyspnea—labored or difficult breathing; shortness of breath

edema—accumulation of excess water in the body; swelling

glaucoma—a group of diseases of the eye characterized by increased intraocular pressure; results in changes within the eye, visual field defects, and eventually blindness (if left untreated)

hyperglycemia—high blood glucose (sugar) level

hypertension—high blood pressure; usually defined as a systolic pressure above 140 mm Hg or a diastolic pressure above 90 mm Hg

hypotension—abnormally low blood pressure

myocardial infarction—heart attack

noncatecholamine adrenergic drugs—direct-acting, indirect-acting, or dual-acting drugs that stimulate the sympathetic nervous system

orthostatic hypotension—a drop in blood pressure that can occur when a patient moves from a lying or sitting position to standing up straight

parasympathomimetic drugs—drugs that produce effects that imitate parasympathetic nerve stimulation
sympatholytic drugs—see *adrenergic blocking drugs*
sympathomimetic drugs—see *adrenergic drugs*
tachycardia—rapid heart rate (above 100 beats per minute)

target organ—the organ intended to receive the therapeutic dose of a medication
vertigo—an abnormal feeling of spinning or rotation motion that may occur with motion sickness and other disorders

The nervous system includes the brain, spinal cord, and nerves. The involuntary division of the nervous system is called the autonomic nervous system, making reference to its automatic activity. It regulates the action of the glands, the smooth muscles of hollow organs and vessels, and the heart muscle.

The autonomic nervous system is further subdivided into a sympathetic nervous system and a parasympathetic nervous system based on how each system affects different organs. You'll learn more about these two systems and the drugs that mimic their actions later in this chapter.

Autonomic nervous system drugs are used to treat a wide variety of conditions. Because these drugs affect the nervous system, they can produce effects in many areas throughout the body. In this chapter, you'll learn about the autonomic nervous system drugs that are used to treat conditions such as:

- dementia caused by Alzheimer disease
- muscle fatigue and muscle weakness
- asthma and other breathing difficulties
- abnormally high or low blood pressure
- heart conditions

CHOLINERGIC DRUGS

Cholinergic drugs support the action of the neurotransmitter **acetylcholine**. They are also called **parasympathomimetic drugs** because they produce effects that mimic parasympathetic nerve stimulation. The parasympathetic nervous system is the part of the nervous system that helps the body save energy. It produces certain responses in the body that are designed to use less energy. They include (but are not limited to) the following:

- decreasing blood pressure
- decreasing heart rate
- increasing saliva production
- causing slower/more shallow breathing
- constricting eye pupils

There are two main classes, or groups, of cholinergic drugs.

- **Cholinergic agonists** imitate the action of the neurotransmitter acetylcholine.
- **Anticholinesterase drugs** work by stopping the destruction of acetylcholine at cholinergic receptor sites. (See *How Cholinergic Drugs Work.*)

HOW IT WORKS

How Cholinergic Drugs Work

Cholinergic drugs fall into one of two major classes: cholinergic agonists and anticholinesterase drugs. Here's how these drugs achieve their effects.
Cholinergic agonists (figure 2-1A):

1. When a neuron in the parasympathetic nervous system is stimulated, the neurotransmitter acetylcholine is released.
2. Acetylcholine crosses the synapse (the space between adjacent neurons) and interacts with receptors in or on an adjacent neuron. Cholinergic agonists stimulate cholinergic receptors, mimicking the action of acetylcholine.

Anticholinesterase drugs (figure 2-1B):

1. After acetylcholine stimulates the cholinergic receptor, it's destroyed by the enzyme acetylcholinesterase.
2. Anticholinesterase drugs inhibit acetylcholinesterase. As a result, acetylcholine isn't broken down and begins to accumulate, leading to prolonged acetylcholine effects.

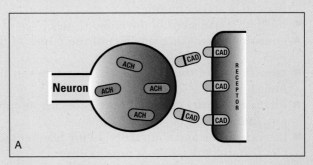

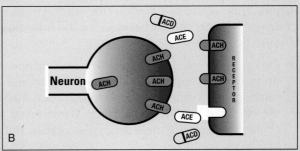

FIGURE 2-1 Cholinergic agonists (A) and anticholinesterase drugs (B). In both parts of the figure, ACH is acetylcholine, CAD is cholinergic agonist drug, ACE is acetylcholinesterase, and ACD is anticholinesterase drug. (From *Clinical Pharmacology Made Incredibly Easy.* 2nd Ed. Philadelphia, PA: Lippincott Williams & Wilkins; 2005.)

Cholinergic Agonists

These drugs directly arouse cholinergic receptors by imitating the action of the neurotransmitter acetylcholine. The ways in which the body processes these drugs can vary widely. It also depends on how each cholinergic agonist interacts with or attaches to the nervous system (receptors).

Cholinergic agonists are rarely given through an intramuscular (IM) or intravenous (IV) injection. This is because they're almost immediately broken down by cholinesterases (enzymes) in the spaces between tissues and inside the blood vessels, so they never get to do their job. In addition to that, they work very quickly and can cause a *cholinergic crisis* (a drug overdose that can produce muscle weakness and paralysis in the muscles used in breathing).

T I P When filling a prescription for cholinergic agonists, remember that these drugs are rarely given by IM or IV injection. Instead, they're usually administered topically, as eye drops, or orally.

Cholinergic agonists work by acting like acetylcholine on the neurons in certain organs of the body. These organs are referred to as **target organs**. When cholinergic agonists combine with receptors (the part of the cell that receives the signal from the drug) on the cell membranes of target organs, they stimulate the muscle and produce:

- salivation
- **bradycardia** (a slow heart rate, usually at a rate of less than 60 beats per minute)
- dilation (expansion) of the blood vessels
- constriction (making smaller) of the pupils of the eyes
- constriction of the bronchioles (tiny tubes in the lungs)
- increased activity of the GI tract (stomach, esophagus, intestines)
- increased tone and contraction of the bladder muscles (causing the frequent urge to urinate)

Cholinergic agonists have specific interactions with other drugs. Patients should be aware of the following interactions:

- Other cholinergic drugs, particularly anticholinesterase drugs (such as ambenonium, edrophonium, neostigmine, physostigmine, and pyridostigmine), increase the effects of cholinergic agonists. When taken with cholinergic agonists, these drugs also increase the risk of toxicity (overdose).
- Cholinergic blocking drugs (such as atropine, belladonna, homatropine, methantheline, methscopolamine, propantheline, and scopolamine) reduce the effects of cholinergic drugs.
- Quinidine, a medication used to treat heart arrhythmia, also reduces the effectiveness of cholinergic agonists.

The following sections include brief description of several cholinergic agonists.

Acetylcholine

Acetylcholine (Miochol-E) is administered by ophthalmic injection to reduce eye pressure in patients during eye surgery. This drug doesn't go through the nervous system very well, and most of its effects on the nervous system are minor, causing parasympathetic action. Acetylcholine is destroyed in the body very quickly.

Bethanechol and Carbachol

Bethanechol (Urecholine) is used to treat weak bladder conditions and postoperative and postpartum (after birth) urine retention. It comes in tablet form and is administered by mouth.

In the form of an ophthalmic solution, carbachol (Isopto Carbachol) may be administered topically, with eye drops. This form of the drug is used to reduce eye pressure in patients who have **glaucoma** (a group of diseases of the eye characterized by increased pressure within the eyeball).

Cevimeline and Pilocarpine

Cevimeline (Evoxac) is used to treat dry mouth in patients with Sjögren syndrome (a disorder in which the body's immune system attacks its own moisture-producing glands). This drug is given by mouth in capsule form.

Pilocarpine (Isopto Carpine, Pilopine HS) comes in the form of an ophthalmic gel or solution and is administered topically, with gel or eye drops. This drug is used to reduce eye pressure in patients with glaucoma. Pilocarpine hydrochloride (Salagen) is also given by mouth in the form

 PROCEED WITH CAUTION

Adverse Reactions to Cholinergic Agonists

The adverse reactions for cholinergic agonists vary from drug to drug. Most adverse reactions are related to the muscle stimulated.

Adverse reactions may include:

- abdominal cramps
- diarrhea
- nausea
- rhinitis, sinusitis, upper respiratory tract infections
- headache
- increased sweating

Drugs used in the eye have direct effects on the eye and may cause:

- brief stinging and burning upon application
- nearsightedness
- blurred vision
- eyebrow pain

of tablets. In this form, it's used to treat dry mouth caused by radiation therapy or Sjögren syndrome.

Anticholinesterase Drugs

Anticholinesterase drugs block the action of the enzyme acetylcholinesterase (which breaks down the neurotransmitter acetylcholine) at cholinergic receptor sites. These drugs prevent the breakdown of acetylcholine. As acetylcholine builds up, it continues to stimulate the cholinergic receptors. Anticholinesterase drugs are divided into two categories:

- *Irreversible anticholinesterase drugs.* These drugs have long-lasting effects and are used mainly as insecticides or as nerve gas in chemical warfare. Most irreversible anticholinesterase drugs don't have therapeutic usefulness and will not be prescribed by a physician.
- *Reversible anticholinesterase drugs.* These drugs have a short duration of action, and many are used therapeutically.

Anticholinesterase drugs affect how acetylcholine acts at receptor sites. They can cause a stimulant or depressant effect on cholinergic receptors, depending on the site, the dose of the drug, and the duration of action. For example, reversible anticholinesterase drugs block the breakdown of acetylcholine for minutes to hours. However, irreversible anticholinesterase drugs can do that for days to weeks.

The following drug interactions can occur with anticholinesterase drugs.

- If taken with other cholinergic drugs, especially cholinergic agonists (such as carbachol, bethanechol, and pilocarpine), the risk of toxic reaction is increased.
- Certain drugs can reduce the effects of anticholinesterase drugs and possibly hide early signs of a cholinergic crisis. These drugs include aminoglycoside antibiotics, anesthetics, cholinergic blocking drugs (such as atropine, propantheline, belladonna, and scopolamine), magnesium, corticosteroids, and antiarrhythmic drugs.
- Other drugs with cholinergic-blocking properties can cancel out the effects of anticholinesterase drugs. These drugs include bladder relaxants, tricyclic antidepressants, and antipsychotics.

The following sections include brief descriptions of anticholinesterase drugs

Ambenonium

Ambenonium (Mytelase) is used to increase muscle contraction in patients with myasthenia gravis (a disease that causes skeletal muscle fatigue). It is administered by mouth in the form of tablets.

Donepezil

Donepezil (Aricept) is used to treat mild to moderate dementia in patients with Alzheimer disease. It's used to help their thinking and remembering. It is administered by mouth in tablet or oral solution form. Aricept ODT is an orally disintegrating tablet, which dissolves on the tongue and does not require swallowing. The orally disintegrating tablet is a dosage form that is useful for patients who have trouble swallowing.

There are several drug interactions that can occur with donepezil.

- Donepezil's rate of elimination can be increased if it's taken with carbamazepine, rifampin, phenytoin, dexamethasone, or phenobarbital.
- Donepezil may have increased effects when it's taken with drugs such as cimetidine or erythromycin, which inhibit cytochrome P-450 enzymes. These enzymes, which are produced in the liver, help remove drugs from the bloodstream. When these enzymes are inhibited, the clearance of certain drugs from the blood is decreased.

Galantamine

The drug galantamine (Razadyne, Razadyne ER) is used to treat mild to moderate dementia in patients with Alzheimer disease. Razadyne is administered by mouth in oral solution or tablet form. Razadyne ER is administered in extended-release capsule form, which allows for once daily dosing instead of twice daily dosing with the tablet or oral solution. Like donepezil, galantamine may have increased effects when taken with cimetidine or erythromycin (drugs that inhibit cytochrome P-450 enzymes).

T I P Older adult patients often take several different drugs for a variety of conditions, increasing the risk of drug interactions. It's especially important that these patients be aware of the drug interactions that may occur with the medications they're taking.

Edrophonium and Neostigmine

Edrophonium (Enlon, Reversol) is administered intravenously to diagnose myasthenia gravis.

Neostigmine is used to increase bladder tone or to increase muscle contraction in patients with myasthenia gravis. It comes in two forms:

- Neostigmine bromide (Prostigmin) is administered by mouth in tablet form.
- Neostigmine methylsulfate is administered by IV, IM, or SubQ injection.

Neostigmine is not absorbed very well in the GI tract. The patient will need to take a higher dose (but less frequently) if taking it orally, as the oral dose acts longer in the body. If a quicker effect is needed, however, neostigmine can be given by IM or IV injection.

Physostigmine

This drug is used to counteract the effects of the following types of drugs:

- anticholinergic drugs (cholinergic blocking drugs)
- tricyclic antidepressants
- belladonna alkaloids
- narcotics

Physostigmine can cross the blood-brain barrier (a membrane that protects the blood vessels in the brain by preventing certain substances from entering the brain). It is administered by IV or IM injection.

Pyridostigmine

Pyridostigmine (Mestinon, Mestinon Timespan, Regonol) is used to increase muscle contraction in patients with myasthenia gravis. It also increases the effects of the antidotes used to counteract harmful nerve agents. It can be taken by mouth in syrup, tablet, or extended-release tablet form. It can also be administered by IV or IM injection.

Rivastigmine

This medication is used to treat mild to moderate dementia in patients who suffer from Alzheimer disease. It has been found to help these patients' thinking and remembering. Rivastigmine (Exelon) is administered by mouth in capsule and oral solution form. It is also available in the form of a transdermal patch.

> **! PROCEED WITH CAUTION**
>
> ### Adverse Reactions to Anticholinesterase Drugs
>
> Most of the harmful reactions that result from the use of these drugs are due to increased action of acetylcholine at receptor sites. Adverse reactions may include:
>
> - nausea, vomiting
> - diarrhea
> - irregular heartbeat (cardiac arrhythmia)
> - headache
> - anorexia (loss of appetite and weight loss)
> - pruritus (itching of the skin)
> - insomnia (poor sleep or lack of sleep)
> - difficulty breathing, wheezing (labored breathing), increased bronchial secretions and chest tightness
> - seizures
> - increased urination (called *nocturnia* when it disrupts sleep at night)
> - muscle weakness or cramps
> - abdominal cramps or pain
> - restlessness, excitability (especially in older adults)
> - increased salivation
> - dizziness

TIP The pharmacist will inform patients about possible drug interactions. For example, cigarette use has been shown to cause the drug rivastigmine to be eliminated from the body faster.

Tacrine

Like donepezil, galantamine, and rivastigmine, tacrine (Cognex) is used to treat mild to moderate dementia in patients with Alzheimer disease. Tacrine is administered by mouth in capsule form.

The main drug interaction associated with tacrine is that it may have increased effects when taken with drugs that are known to inhibit cytochrome P-450 enzymes (for example, cimetidine or erythromycin).

Liver toxicity, which can be life threatening, is a common adverse effect of tacrine.

CHOLINERGIC BLOCKING DRUGS

Cholinergic blocking drugs interrupt parasympathetic nerve responses in both the central and autonomic nervous systems. They are also referred to as **anticholinergic drugs** because they stop acetylcholine from activating cholinergic receptors.

Cholinergic blockers are divided into three groups of drugs:

- belladonna alkaloids
- quaternary ammonium drugs (synthetic derivatives of belladonna alkaloids)
- tertiary amines

Cholinergic blockers can have paradoxical (opposite from intended) effects on the body. These effects are dependent on the dosage and the condition being treated. Cholinergic blockers can create either a stimulating or depressing effect on the target organ. In the brain, however, they do both. Low levels of medication stimulate activity in the brain, whereas higher levels depress brain activity. The effects of the drug are also determined by the disorder the patient has. For example, Parkinson disease is distinguished by low dopamine levels. This intensifies the stimulating effects of acetylcholine. Cholinergic blockers lessen this effect; however, in other disorders, cholinergic blockers stimulate the central nervous system.

TIP Check and double-check! When filling a prescription for cholinergic blocking drugs, make sure the dosage matches the diagnosis.

Cholinergic blockers are frequently used to treat disorders of the GI tract and related complications. For example, cholinergic blocking drugs are given by injection before some diagnostic procedures (such as endoscopy and sigmoidoscopy) to relax the GI smooth muscle.

Cholinergic blockers are also used as cycloplegics, which means they:

- change the shape of the eye lens
- paralyze the ciliary muscles (the muscles in the eye used for fine focusing)

Additionally, these drugs act as mydriatics (pupil dilators). This makes it easier for physicians to detect nearsightedness or farsightedness during an eye exam or to do surgery on the eye.

Cholinergic blockers slow down the process of food and medications passing through the stomach. Therefore, these drugs remain in contact with the mucous membranes of the GI tract for an extended period of time. The amount of the drug that is absorbed increases, which increases the risk of adverse effects.

Drugs that increase the effects of cholinergic blockers include:

- disopyramide
- tricyclic and tetracyclic antidepressants
- cyclobenzaprine (a muscle relaxant)
- antidyskinetics such as amantadine, which is used to treat Parkinson disease
- antipsychotic drugs, such as haloperidol, thioxanthenes, and phenothiazines
- orphenadrine, which is used to treat pain from muscle injury
- antiemetics (used to relieve nausea and vomiting) and antivertigo drugs such as cyclizine, diphenhydramine, buclizine, and meclizine

Drugs that decrease the effects of cholinergic blockers include:

- anticholinesterase drugs, such as pyridostigmine and neostigmine
- cholinergic agonists such as bethanechol

There can be other drug interactions with cholinergic blockers:

- When taken with a cholinergic blocker, morphine and other opiate-like analgesics (painkillers) can further slow the movement of food and drugs through the GI system.
- When digoxin (a cardiac medication) is taken with a cholinergic blocker, the risk for digoxin toxicity increases.
- Nitroglycerin tablets taken under the tongue have a reduced absorption in the body when taken with cholinergic blockers.

Belladonna Alkaloids

The major cholinergic blocking drugs are the belladonna alkaloids. These drugs are absorbed from the:

- GI tract
- eyes
- skin
- mucous membranes

 PROCEED WITH CAUTION

Adverse Reactions to Cholinergic Blockers

Adverse effects of these drugs may include:

- **tachycardia** (increased heart rate), palpitations
- dry mouth
- decreased sweating
- reduced bronchial secretions
- headache
- restlessness
- insomnia
- dizziness
- blurred vision
- mydriasis (abnormally dilated pupils)
- constipation
- confusion or excitement in older adult patients
- urinary hesitancy or retention

Many of these reactions, such as dry mouth and urinary retention, occur because anticholinergic drugs draw water out of cells. Patients who are taking these medications should be advised to drink plenty of water or suck on sugar-free hard candy. For severe cases of dry mouth, the physician may prescribe an artificial saliva product.

For ophthalmic preparations, a common adverse reaction is blurred vision.

Adverse reactions to transdermal forms of cholinergic blockers include:

- severe itching of the skin
- local irritation

Drug dosage plays an important role when it comes to cholinergic blockers and adverse reactions. The difference between a toxic dose and a therapeutic dose can be small.

The belladonna alkaloids are the only cholinergic blockers that easily cross into the blood system of the brain (the blood-brain barrier).

The belladonna alkaloids are used with morphine to treat pain caused by stones in the bile duct (biliary colic). These drugs, particularly atropine and hyoscyamine, are also good antidotes to cholinergic and anticholinesterase drugs.

Atropine

Atropine has many uses and many trade names. Under the trade names Sal-Tropine and Atreza, it can be administered by mouth in tablet form. The brand name Isopto Atropine is administered ophthalmically. Atropine may also be administered by IV, IM, or SubQ injection. In these forms, atropine is often used:

- to treat arrhythmia (irregular heartbeat) caused by anesthetics, succinylcholine (used to cause brief but complete muscle relaxation), or choline esters (nerve ending enzymes)

HOW IT WORKS

How Atropine Speeds the Heart Rate

To understand how atropine affects the heart, first consider how the heart's electrical conduction system functions (figure 2-2).

Without the Drug

When the neurotransmitter acetylcholine is released, the vagus nerve stimulates the sinoatrial (SA) node (the heart's pacemaker) and the atrioventricular (AV) node, which controls conduction between the atria and the ventricles of the heart. This inhibits electrical conduction and causes the heart rate to slow down.

With the Drug

Atropine, a cholinergic blocking drug, competes with acetylcholine for cholinergic receptor sites on the SA and AV nodes. By blocking acetylcholine, atropine speeds up the heart rate.

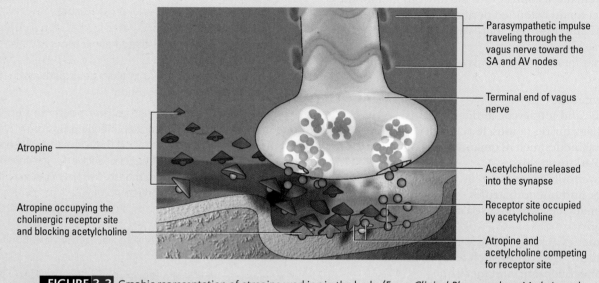

FIGURE 2-2 Graphic representation of atropine working in the body. (From *Clinical Pharmacology Made Incredibly Easy.* 2nd Ed. Philadelphia, PA: Lippincott Williams & Wilkins; 2005.)

- to treat symptomatic sinus bradycardia (when the heart beats too slowly, causing low blood pressure or dizziness)
- as an antidote for nerve agents
- to treat organophosphate pesticide poisoning
- before surgery to decrease gastric, oral, and respiratory secretions

In addition, atropine can be applied topically in the form of an ophthalmic ointment or ophthalmic solution. In these forms, it can be used as a cycloplegic.

Belladonna

Belladonna is commonly seen today in combination form with other drugs, which are administered in the following ways:

- by mouth in tablet form (Spastrin)
- rectally in the form of suppositories (B&O Supprettes)

Belladonna is used, in addition to other drugs, to treat peptic ulcer disease. It has also been used to treat irritable bowel syndrome (but only if other treatment options, such as changes in diet, have not been effective). Additionally, rectal suppositories that contain belladonna have been prescribed for patients who have recently undergone genital or urinary surgery. These suppositories are classified as Schedule II drugs. In these cases, belladonna is used as a pain reliever when non-opiate pain relievers have been ineffective.

Hyoscyamine

Hyoscyamine is available under a variety of trade names, including Anaspaz, Colidrops, Colytrol Pediatric, Cystospaz, Cystospaz-M, HyoMax, Hyosyne, Levbid, Levsin, Levsin SL, Medispaz, Spasdel, Symax, Symax Duotab, and Symax SR. The drug is generally administered by mouth in the form of tablets (including dissolving, sublingual, biphasic-release, and extended-release tablets), extended-release capsules, oral drops, and oral liquid. Levsin can also be administered by injection.

Like atropine, hyoscyamine is used to counteract the effects of neuromuscular blocking drugs by competing for the same receptor sites. This drug has several other uses. It is:

- used to treat disorders of the GI tract caused by spasm
- given before surgery to reduce secretions
- used as therapy for peptic ulcers and inflammation of the urinary bladder

A common adverse effect of hyoscyamine, which is not seen with other cholinergic blockers, is paralytic ileus (bowel obstruction caused by paralysis of the bowel wall).

Methscopolamine

The drug methscopolamine (Pamine) is used as therapy for patients who have peptic ulcers. It is administered by mouth in tablet form 30 minutes before meals and at night before sleep. While other cholinergic blockers may cause insomnia, methscopolamine may cause drowsiness; therefore, the dose at bedtime can be given without causing insomnia.

T I P For methscopolamine to be effective, this drug must be taken exactly as directed. Patients are usually instructed to take methscopolamine 30 minutes before meals and at night before sleep.

Scopolamine

Scopolamine comes in a variety of dosage forms and has several different therapeutic uses.

- Scopolamine is administered by mouth, in tablet form (Scopace, Maldemar), or by transdermal patch (Transderm-Scōp) to prevent nausea and vomiting from motion sickness.
- Like other belladonna alkaloids, scopolamine can affect the brain. For example, when combined with the pain reliever morphine, scopolamine hydrobromide can be administered by injection to bring about drowsiness and amnesia in a patient who is having surgery.
- Scopolamine (Isopto Hyoscine) is administered topically, as eye drops. This form of the drug is used to dilate the pupils prior to an eye exam or eye surgery. It's also used to treat other eye conditions.

AT THE COUNTER

Scopolamine Transdermal Patches

Mr. Smith comes into the pharmacy to pick up his prescription for scopolamine transdermal patches. He is excited about the seven-day Caribbean cruise he is leaving for in a couple of days and tells you all about it. The pharmacist counsels him on the proper use of the patch and tells him about possible adverse reactions.

A few hours later, Mr. Smith calls the pharmacy to ask why he was given only three patches when he is going to be gone for seven days. What should you tell him?

The patch helps prevent nausea and vomiting for motion sickness for up to three days, so he needs only three patches for his seven-day cruise.

Common adverse effects of scopolamine, which are not common with other cholinergic blockers, include the following:

- nausea
- vomiting
- epigastric distress (discomfort in the abdomen)

Synthetic Derivatives (Quaternary Ammonium Drugs)

All cholinergic blockers can be used to treat spastic or hyperactive conditions of the GI tract and urinary tract (because they ease muscles and lower the secretions of the GI tract). They can also be used to treat urinary incontinence, as they relax the bladder. Because they tend to have fewer negative reactions than the belladonna alkaloids, the quaternary ammonium compounds are the preferred medications for these conditions.

Glycopyrrolate

Glycopyrrolate (Robinul, Robinul Forte) is used in therapy for peptic ulcers and other GI disorders. It is also given before surgery to reduce secretions and prevent a drop in heart rate during anesthesia. This drug may be administered by IV, IM, or SubQ injection. It can also be administered by mouth in tablet form.

Propantheline

The drug propantheline is used as therapy for patients who have peptic ulcers. It's administered by mouth in tablet form 30 minutes before meals and at night before sleep.

Tertiary Amines

The tertiary amines are used chiefly to treat functional GI disorders and overactive bladder conditions.

Dicyclomine

The drug dicyclomine (Bentyl) is used to treat irritable bowel syndrome and other functional GI disorders. It can be administered by mouth in capsule, syrup, solution, or tablet form. Dicyclomine can also be administered by IM injection.

Oxybutynin

Oxybutynin (Ditropan XL, Oxytrol) is used to treat patients who have overactive bladder conditions. It can be administered by mouth in solution, tablet, and extended-release tablet form. It's also administered by transdermal patch patch and topical gel.

T I P If you notice the letters *LA, CR, ER,* or *XL* after a drug's trade name, then it's probably an extended-release form of the drug. Extended-release formulations are very popular because they allow the patient to take fewer doses per day yet have the effects of the medication continue.

Tolterodine

The drug tolterodine (Detrol, Detrol LA) is used to treat overactive bladder in patients with symptoms of urinary frequency, urgency, or urge incontinence. It can be administered by mouth in the form of tablets or extended-release capsules.

ADRENERGIC DRUGS

Adrenergic drugs are also referred to as **sympathomimetic drugs**. They bring about effects similar to those produced by the sympathetic nervous system, which activates the body's "fight-or-flight" response. This response helps the body avoid or prepare to confront a crisis situation. For example, when you're faced with a crisis, your body might respond with an increased heart rate, muscle tension, increased blood pressure, and deeper and heavier breathing.

Adrenergic drugs are put into two groups, based on chemical structure: catecholamines (both synthetic and naturally occurring) and noncatecholamines.

These drugs are also classified by how they act in the body:

- *Indirect-acting.* These drugs generate the release of a neurotransmitter (usually norepinephrine).
- *Direct-acting.* Drugs that are direct-acting act directly on the organ or tissue in which the nerve is stimulated by the sympathetic nervous system.
- *Dual-acting.* These drugs have both indirect and direct actions.

The therapeutic uses of adrenergics depend on which receptors they stimulate and to what degree. These drugs can affect:

- beta-adrenergic receptors
- alpha-adrenergic receptors
- dopamine receptors

Most adrenergic drugs work by stimulating alpha and beta receptors, thus imitating the action of epinephrine and norepinephrine. Dopaminergic drugs, however, act mainly on receptors in the sympathetic nervous system stimulated by dopamine.

Catecholamines

All catecholamines have the same basic chemical structure. Therefore, they all share certain properties:

- stimulating the nervous system
- raising the heart rate
- tightening the peripheral blood vessels
- dilating (opening) the bronchi

Catecholamines are destroyed by digestive enzymes and therefore can't be taken by mouth. Instead, they are

HOW IT WORKS

Understanding Adrenergics

Adrenergic drugs are distinguished by how they achieve their effect. Figure 2-3 shows the action of direct-, indirect-, and dual-acting adrenergics.

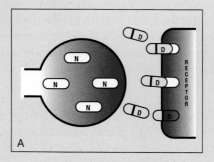

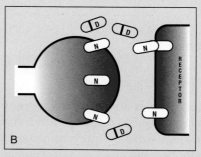

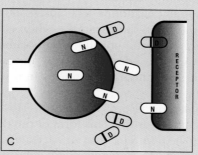

FIGURE 2-3 Direct-acting adrenergics directly stimulate adrenergic receptors (A). Indirect-acting adrenergics stimulate the release of norepinephrine from nerve endings into the synapse (B). Dual-acting adrenergics stimulate both adrenergic receptor sites and the release of norepinephrine from nerve endings (C). In all three parts of the figure, N is norepinephrine and D is adrenergic drug. (From *Clinical Pharmacology Made Incredibly Easy.* 2nd Ed. Philadelphia, PA: Lippincott Williams & Wilkins; 2005.)

given either sublingually (under the tongue) or by SubQ or IM injection. Sublingually, catecholamines are absorbed quickly through the mucous membranes, and any remainder is broken down (metabolized) by swallowed saliva if they are not completely absorbed under the tongue. In contrast, when a drug is injected under the skin, absorption gets slowed down because the drug causes constriction in the blood vessels around the area where the needle enters. However, IM injections don't have the same problem, as there is not as much constriction of the blood vessels near the injection site, so the drug can be absorbed more quickly.

Primarily, catecholamines are direct-acting. They either cause an inhibitory (slowing) or excitatory (escalating) effect, depending on the receptors with which they combine. If they combine with beta receptors, the typical response is inhibitory. If they combine with alpha receptors, the typical response is excitatory (except in the intestines, where these drugs have a relaxing effect).

TIP A good trick to remember how catecholamines affect alpha and beta receptors: *A* stands for *alpha* (receptors) and also for *activate* (excitatory response). *B* stands for *beta* (receptors) and also for *block* (inhibitory response).

Catecholamines can have different clinical effects on the body depending on the dosage and route of administration. They are called *potent inotropes*, which means they cause the heart to contract more forcefully. As a result, the ventricles of the heart empty more completely with each heartbeat, which increases the work the heart has to do, as well as the amount of oxygen that's required for the heart to work.

Catecholamines can also cause the heart to have abnormal rhythms. This happens when they cause the Purkinje fibers (a complex web of fibers that carry electrical impulses into the ventricles) to fire on their own.

The effects of natural catecholamines (those produced by the body) can differ from the effects of manufactured catecholamines. Manufactured catecholamines have a short duration of action, which limits how useful they are therapeutically.

Drug interactions involving catecholamines can be serious.

- Alpha-adrenergic blockers, such as phentolamine, can produce **hypotension** (abnormally low blood pressure).
- Beta-adrenergic blockers, such as propranolol, can lead to bronchial constriction and breathing difficulties.
- Other adrenergics can enhance adverse effects. These drugs can also produce additive (synergistic) effects, such as arrhythmias and **hypertension** (abnormally high blood pressure). An increased risk of hypertension may also occur when adrenergic drugs are given with other drugs that can cause hypertension.
- When they interact with catecholamines, tricyclic antidepressants can lead to hypertension.

Dobutamine

The drug dobutamine stimulates the heart's beta$_1$ receptors, so it's used to treat low cardiac output caused by heart disease or cardiac surgery. It's administered by IV injection, and common adverse effects include high blood pressure and increased heart rate.

Dopamine

This drug is administered by IV injection and is used:

- to treat acute allergic reactions to drugs
- to increase cardiac output
- to correct low blood pressure

Because dopamine primarily stimulates the dopamine receptors, it's also used in low doses to improve blood flow to the kidneys by dilating the renal blood vessels.

Epinephrine

The drug epinephrine is administered by inhalation through an aerosol or a nebulizer inhaler. It can also be administered by IV, IM, or SubQ injection. As a result, epinephrine has several different trade names and dosage forms, which are sold either over the counter or as a prescription drug.

For inhalation either nasally or orally:

- Adrenalin
- Primatene Mist

For injection:

- Adrenalin
- EpiPen
- EpiPen Jr.
- Twinject

⚠ PROCEED WITH CAUTION

Adverse Reactions to Catecholamines

Adverse reactions to catecholamines can include:

- dizziness
- restlessness
- drowsiness
- headache
- nausea
- vomiting
- palpitations, tachycardia
- anxiety or nervousness
- tremors
- angina (chest pain)
- stroke
- hypotension (low blood pressure)
- hypertension or a hypertensive crisis
- cardiac arrhythmias
- increased blood glucose levels (caution in diabetic patients)
- tissue necrosis and sloughing (if the drug is given by IV and leaks into the surrounding tissue)

Some dental preparations also contain epinephrine, although these are usually found only in dentists' offices and not in pharmacies.

Because epinephrine stimulates both alpha and beta receptors, it has several uses. For example, it's used to treat:

- acute allergic reactions to drugs, including anaphylactic shock
- acute asthma attacks
- cardiac arrest

Epinephrine may cause **hyperglycemia** (high blood sugar) in diabetic patients. For this reason, these patients may require an increased dose of insulin or oral antidiabetic agents.

Norepinephrine

As you read earlier in this chapter, when catecholamines combine with beta receptors, they usually produce an inhibitory response. However, in heart cells, norepinephrine (Levophed) causes excitatory effects. Norepinephrine also stimulates alpha receptors. For this reason, it's administered by IV injection to treat the following conditions:

- low blood pressure caused by relaxation of the blood vessels
- low blood pressure as a result of blood loss (such as from hemorrhage)
- severely low blood pressure during cardiac arrest

Isoproterenol

Like dobutamine, isoproterenol (Isuprel) stimulates only beta receptors. It's used to treat:

- heart block (a delay or interruption in the conduction of electrical impulses between the heart's atria and ventricles)
- bradycardia in patients who have recently undergone cardiac surgery
- acute allergic reactions to drugs

This drug is administered by IV injection. A rapid rise and fall in blood pressure is often seen with isoproterenol.

Noncatecholamines

Noncatecholamine adrenergic drugs have a wide range of therapeutic uses because of the variety of effects they can have on the body.

Although these drugs are all excreted in urine, they're absorbed in different ways. Absorption of noncatecholamines depends on the administration route.

Noncatecholamines can be:

- direct-acting
- indirect-acting
- dual-acting (unlike catecholamines, which are primarily direct-acting)

PROCEED WITH CAUTION

Adverse Reactions to Noncatecholamines

Adverse reactions to noncatecholamine drugs can include:

- irritability
- seizures
- restlessness, nervousness
- anxiety or overexcitement, hyperactivity
- headache
- shaking, tremor
- drowsiness or insomnia
- light-headedness, dizziness
- **vertigo** (an abnormal feeling of spinning or rotation motion)
- hypotension or hypertension
- palpitations
- incoherence
- angina
- pallor (pale skin) or flushing
- irregular heart rhythm
- bradycardia or tachycardia
- cerebral hemorrhage
- tingling or coldness in the arms or legs
- cardiac arrest
- nausea
- vomiting

With oral and nasal inhalers, adverse reactions may also include:

- local irritation of the nose (nasal)
- local irritation of the throat (oral)
- rhinitis (nasal)
- cough (oral)

Additionally, the eye drop formulations may cause local stinging or burning.

These drugs stimulate the sympathetic nervous system, producing a variety of effects in the body.

The following are a few examples of drugs that interact with noncatecholamines.

- Anesthetics (general), cyclopropane, and halogenated hydrocarbons can cause arrhythmias.
- Monoamine oxidase inhibitors can cause severe hypertension and even death.
- When taken with some noncatecholamines, oxytocic drugs (which stimulate the uterus to contract) can cause hypertensive crisis or stroke.
- Tricyclic antidepressants can cause hypertension and arrhythmias.
- Urine alkalizers, such as acetazolamide and sodium bicarbonate, slow the body's excretion of noncatecholamines, prolonging their duration of action.

Phenylephrine

Phenylephrine is a direct-acting noncatecholamine that stimulates alpha receptors. It is also often used in topical hemorrhoid preparations, often in combination with other ingredients, to help shrink the inflamed blood vessels of the rectum. It comes in several different forms:

- *Ophthalmic solution.* As an ophthalmic solution, phenylephrine (AK-Dilate, Mydfrin, Neofrin) is used to treat abnormal dilation of the pupils and minor eye irritations. In this form, the drug is administered topically to the eye as a drop.
- *Nasal solution.* In nasal solution form, phenylephrine (Neo-Synephrine, Sinex, 4-Way) is used to treat nasal congestion. It is administered by nasal drops or nasal spray. These dosage forms are available over the counter.
- *Injection.* When administered by injection, phenylephrine causes the constriction of blood vessels. This form of the drug is used to maintain blood pressure during spinal or inhaled anesthesia. It's also used to treat mild to severe hypotension and shock. Routes of administration include IV, IM, or SubQ injection.
- *Oral tablets (regular, dissolving, and chewable forms), oral liquid, and oral dissolving film.* This drug also comes in oral form. It's now included as a replacement for pseudoephedrine in many over-the-counter products, such as Lusonal, Nasop, Nasop 12, Sudafed PE, and PediaCare. These medications are used to treat nasal congestion.

Albuterol

Albuterol (AccuNeb, Proventil, Proventil HFA, Ventolin HFA, Proair HFA, VoSpire ER) selectively stimulates $beta_2$ receptors. It's used to dilate the bronchioles and to treat or prevent breathing difficulties.

This drug is administered by mouth in the form of syrup, tablets, or extended-release tablets. It may also be inhaled as a nebulizer solution or an inhalation suspension. When albuterol is inhaled, it is absorbed gradually from the bronchi, which results in lower drug levels in the body. In this form, the drug is excreted within 24 hours. Oral albuterol, however, is usually excreted within three days.

Ephedrine

Ephedrine is a dual-acting noncatecholamine. This drug is used to dilate the bronchioles and to treat nasal decongestion. It's also used to treat low blood pressure. Ephedrine comes in an injection for administration:

- by IV, IM, or SubQ injection

Ephedrine is often found in combination with other ingredients.

Formoterol

Formoterol (Foradil Aerolizer, Perforomist) is used to dilate the bronchioles and to treat and prevent breathing difficulties. It is administered by inhalation of a powder packaged in capsules and as a nebulizer solution. Adverse effects with formoterol are uncommon.

Levalbuterol

Similar to albuterol and formoterol, levalbuterol (Xopenex, Xopenex HFA) is used to dilate the bronchioles and to prevent or treat breathing difficulties. It comes in the form of a nebulizer solution or a pressurized suspension and must be administered by inhalation. Common adverse effects of this drug are rhinitis and viral infection.

Metaproterenol

Like albuterol, metaproterenol selectively stimulates $beta_2$ receptors. It's used to dilate the bronchioles to treat asthma and breathing difficulties. This drug is administered by inhalation in the form of a nebulizer solution. In addition, metaproterenol can be administered by mouth in tablet or oral solution form.

Pirbuterol

The drug pirbuterol (Maxair Autohaler) is used to dilate the bronchioles, to prevent and reverse breathing difficulties, and to treat asthma. It is administered by inhalation in the form of an inhaler. Adverse effects with pirbuterol are uncommon.

T I P Patients should be made aware of all adverse effects, even if they are uncommon.

Salmeterol

Salmeterol (Serevent, Diskus) is used to dilate the bronchioles to treat asthma and breathing difficulties. It is administered by inhalation in the form of an inhalation powder. In addition to the adverse effects seen with other noncatecholamines, salmeterol can also cause:

- heartburn
- GI distress
- diarrhea

Terbutaline

Like albuterol and metaproterenol, terbutaline selectively stimulates $beta_2$ receptors. This drug is administered by mouth in tablet form or by SubQ injection. It's used:

- to dilate the bronchioles and to relax bronchial smooth muscle
- to treat breathing difficulties
- to stop preterm labor

Patients who are taking terbutaline should be aware of possible drug interactions. For example, low blood pressure can occur if terbutaline is taken with general anesthetics, cyclopropane, or halogenated hydrocarbons. Terbutaline can also inhibit the effects of oxytocic drugs (drugs that stimulate the uterus to contract).

ADRENERGIC BLOCKING DRUGS

Adrenergic blocking drugs are used to disrupt sympathetic nervous system function. They are also referred to as **sympatholytic drugs**. These drugs block the transmission of impulses at adrenergic neurons or adrenergic receptor sites. At these sites, adrenergic blocking drugs can:

- reduce available norepinephrine
- disrupt the action of adrenergic drugs
- prevent the action of cholinergic drugs

Alpha-Adrenergic Blockers

Alpha-adrenergic blockers (or **alpha blockers**) operate by interrupting the actions of the catecholamines epinephrine and norepinephrine at alpha$_1$ and alpha$_2$ receptors. The outcome of this process is:

- relaxation of the smooth muscle in blood vessels
- increased dilation of blood vessels
- decreased blood pressure

Alpha-adrenergic blockers work in one of two ways:

- They interfere with the synthesis, storage, release, and reuptake of norepinephrine by neurons.
- They antagonize epinephrine, norepinephrine, or adrenergic drugs at alpha receptor sites.

These drugs occupy alpha receptor sites on the smooth muscle of the blood vessels. (See *How Alpha-Adrenergic Blockers Affect Peripheral Blood Vessels.*) This prevents catecholamines from occupying and stimulating these same receptor sites. As a result, blood vessels dilate, and local blood flow to the skin and other organs is increased. The dilation of blood vessels also helps to decrease blood pressure.

The therapeutic effect of an alpha-adrenergic blocker depends on the extent of blood vessel constriction in the body before the medication is taken. For example, if a patient takes the drug while he is lying down, he will experience only a small change in blood pressure. In this position, the patient's veins are not constricted, so the alpha-adrenergic blocker will cause little change. When a patient stands up, though, norepinephrine is released to constrict the blood vessels and direct blood back up to the heart. Alpha-adrenergic drugs keep the veins from constricting, and, instead, blood pools in the legs. This causes a drop in blood pressure called **orthostatic hypotension**.

Phentolamine

The drug phentolamine is administered by IV or IM injection to control or prevent hypertension. It's also used to treat necrosis (death) of the skin at the site where norepinephrine or dopamine was administered by IV injection.

HOW IT WORKS

How Alpha-Adrenergic Blockers Affect Peripheral Blood Vessels

By occupying alpha receptor sites, alpha-adrenergic blocking drugs cause the blood vessel walls to relax (figure 2-4). This leads to dilation of the blood vessels and reduced peripheral vascular resistance (the pressure that blood must overcome as it flows in a vessel).

These effects can cause orthostatic hypotension, a drop in blood pressure that occurs when changing position from lying down to standing. Redistribution of blood to the dilated blood vessels of the legs causes hypotension.

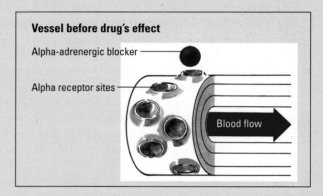

Vessel before drug's effect

Alpha-adrenergic blocker

Alpha receptor sites

Blood flow

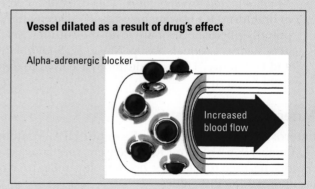

Vessel dilated as a result of drug's effect

Alpha-adrenergic blocker

Increased blood flow

FIGURE 2-4 Graphic representation of alpha-adrenergic blockers work on peripheral blood vessels. (From *Clinical Pharmacology Made Incredibly Easy.* 2nd Ed. Philadelphia, PA: Lippincott Williams & Wilkins; 2005.)

Common adverse effects of phentolamine, in addition to those seen with most alpha-adrenergic blockers, include:

- diarrhea
- nausea
- vomiting

Prazosin

Prazosin (Minipress) is used to treat hypertension and benign enlargement of the prostate gland. It is administered by mouth in capsule form.

PROCEED WITH CAUTION

Adverse Reactions to Alpha-Adrenergic Blockers

Most adverse reactions associated with this class of drugs are caused by dilation (widening) of the blood vessels. These reactions include:

- **edema** (accumulation of excess water in the body; swelling)
- difficulty breathing
- bradycardia or tachycardia
- angina
- heart attack
- light-headedness, dizziness
- headache
- nasal congestion
- **asthenia** (weakness; loss of strength)
- spasm of blood vessels in the brain
- a shocklike state
- orthostatic hypotension or severe hypertension
- flushing
- arrhythmias

An interesting adverse effect of prazosin is called *first-dose syncope*, which occurs especially with the first dose taken. First-dose syncope is a result of a decrease in blood pressure and causes the patient to faint. As a result, the first dose should always be taken when the patient is going to bed. Since the first dose is taken at bedtime, most patients will continue to take the medication daily at bedtime.

Doxazosin

Like prazosin, doxazosin (Cardura, Cardura XL) is used to treat hypertension and benign enlargement of the prostate gland. It's administered by mouth in immediate- or extended-release tablet form.

AT THE COUNTER

Terazosin and Dizziness

Ms. Jones calls the pharmacy to ask a question about her blood pressure medication. She remembers that the "little red pill" is her terazosin. She wants to stop taking it because she says that it makes her feel dizzy and light-headed, especially when she has been sitting or lying down. What is this phenomenon called, and what should you tell her?

Ms. Jones has been experiencing orthostatic hypotension. Alpha-adrenergic drugs (such as terazosin) cause a small change in blood pressure when lying down, so when she stands up too quickly it makes her feel light-headed. Orthostatic hypotension is a common side effect, and she should not stop taking the drug. Instead, suggest that she speak with the pharmacist about ways to manage the adverse effect.

TIP Whenever you come across a generic name that ends in *-zosin*, it is most likely an alpha-adrenergic blocker. This naming pattern makes these drugs easy to classify correctly.

Terazosin

Terazosin (Hytrin) is another medication used to treat hypertension and benign enlargement of the prostate gland. This drug is taken by mouth in tablet or capsule form.

Beta-Adrenergic Blockers

Beta-adrenergic blockers (or **beta blockers**) are the most widely used adrenergic blocking drugs. These drugs prevent stimulation of the sympathetic nervous system by inhibiting the action of catecholamines at beta-adrenergic receptors. Beta-adrenergic blockers are classified as *selective* or *nonselective*.

These drugs are distributed widely in bodily tissues. However, the highest concentrations appear in the:

- liver
- heart
- lungs
- saliva

Beta-adrenergic blockers have widespread effects in the body and are therefore used to treat a variety of conditions. Their therapeutic usefulness is based largely on how they affect the heart. (See *How Beta-Adrenergic Blockers Work*.) For example, these drugs can be prescribed after a heart attack to prevent another heart attack from occurring or to treat:

- hypertension
- angina
- supraventricular arrhythmias (irregular heartbeats that originate in the atria, SA node, or atrioventricular node of the heart)
- hypertrophic cardiomyopathy (a disease of the heart muscle)
- cardiovascular symptoms associated with overproduction of thyroid hormones (a condition known as thyrotoxicosis)

However, their usefulness is not limited to heart conditions. Beta-adrenergic blockers can also be used to treat:

- anxiety
- essential tremor
- migraine headaches
- open-angle glaucoma
- tumor of the adrenal gland (pheochromocytoma)

Many drugs can interact with beta-adrenergic blockers to cause potentially dangerous effects. Some of the most serious drug interactions can cause cardiac or respiratory depression, arrhythmias, severe breathing difficulties, and severe hypotension. The following drug interactions may occur:

PROCEED WITH CAUTION

Adverse Reactions to Beta-Adrenergic Blockers

There are generally few adverse reactions to beta-adrenergic blockers. When these reactions occur, however, they are drug- or dose- dependent and can include:

- bradycardia
- heart failure
- hypotension
- dizziness, light-headedness
- nervousness
- peripheral vascular insufficiency
- fatigue, lethargy
- asthenia
- diarrhea or constipation
- nausea and vomiting
- abdominal discomfort
- flatulence
- anorexia
- atrioventricular block
- bronchospasm
- anorexia
- rash
- fever and sore throat
- spasm of the larynx
- respiratory distress (allergic response)

Common adverse reactions for the ophthalmic dosage forms may include:
- syncope
- transient eye stinging and burning
- hypotension

- When drugs such as cimetidine, digoxin, or verapamil are taken with beta-adrenergic blockers, increased effects or toxicity can occur.
- Decreased effects can occur when rifampin, antacids, calcium salts, barbiturates, or anti-inflammatory drugs are taken with beta-adrenergic blockers.
- Lidocaine toxicity may occur when lidocaine is taken with beta-adrenergic blocking drugs.
- For diabetic patients, altered dosage of insulin and oral antidiabetic drugs may be necessary when these drugs are taken with beta-adrenergic blockers.

Nonselective Beta-Adrenergic Blockers

These drugs affect:

- $beta_1$ receptors (found mainly in the heart)
- $beta_2$ receptors (found in the bronchi, uterus, and blood vessels)

Nonselective beta-adrenergic blockers reduce stimulation of the heart and also produce constriction in the bronchioles of the lungs. For example, nonselective beta-adrenergic blockers can cause bronchospasm in patients who suffer from chronic obstructive lung disease. (**Bronchospasm** is a spasm or constriction of the bronchi resulting in difficulty breathing.) However, this particular adverse effect isn't seen when these drugs are given at lower doses.

Several serious drug interactions can occur with nonselective beta-adrenergic blockers:

- These drugs impair the ability of theophylline to induce bronchodilation.
- Clonidine, when taken with a nonselective beta-adrenergic blocker, can cause life-threatening hypertension during clonidine withdrawal.
- When taken with nonselective beta-adrenergic blocking drugs, adrenergics can cause hypertension and bradycardia.

Carvedilol

The drug carvedilol (Coreg, Coreg CR) is used to treat hypertension, angina, and cardiomyopathy (a disease of the heart muscle). It is administered by mouth in tablet and extended-release capsule forms. In addition to the common adverse reactions seen with most beta-adrenergic blockers, carvedilol may also cause:

- postural hypertension
- hyperglycemia
- weight gain
- upper respiratory tract infection
- hypersensitivity reactions

TIP Whenever you come across a generic name that ends in *-lol*, it's probably a beta-adrenergic blocking drug.

Labetalol and Levobunolol

Labetalol (Trandate) is used to treat hypertension. It may be taken by mouth in tablet form or administered by IV injection. A common adverse effect of this medication is orthostatic hypotension.

The drug levobunolol (Betagan) is used to treat open-angle glaucoma. It's administered by eye drops in the form of an ophthalmic solution.

Penbutolol and Pindolol

Like labetalol, penbutolol (Levatol) is used to treat hypertension. This drug is administered by mouth in tablet form. Pindolol is another drug that is used to treat hypertension. It is administered by mouth in tablet form.

Sotalol

The drug sotalol (Betapace, Betapace AF) is used to treat life-threatening ventricular arrhythmias. It is administered by mouth in tablet form. Common adverse effects of this drug, in addition to those seen with other beta-adrenergic blockers, may include:

- headache
- palpitations
- chest pain

HOW IT WORKS

How Beta-Adrenergic Blockers Work

By occupying beta receptor sites, beta-adrenergic blockers prevent catecholamines (norepinephrine and epinephrine) from occupying these sites and exerting their stimulating effects. Figure 2-5 shows the effects of beta-adrenergic blockers on the heart, lungs, and blood vessels.

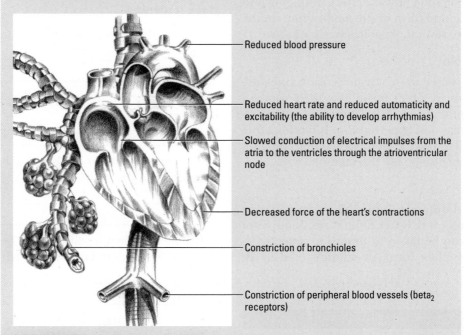

Reduced blood pressure

Reduced heart rate and reduced automaticity and excitability (the ability to develop arrhythmias)

Slowed conduction of electrical impulses from the atria to the ventricles through the atrioventricular node

Decreased force of the heart's contractions

Constriction of bronchioles

Constriction of peripheral blood vessels (beta$_2$ receptors)

FIGURE 2-5 Beta-adrenergic blockers work on the heart, lungs, and blood vessels. (From *Clinical Pharmacology Made Incredibly Easy*. 2nd Ed. Philadelphia, PA: Lippincott Williams & Wilkins; 2005.)

- nausea
- vomiting
- **dyspnea** (labored or difficult breathing; shortness of breath)

Nadolol

This medication is used to treat angina and hypertension. It is administered by mouth in tablet form. Common adverse effects of nadolol (Corgard) may also include:

- increased airway resistance
- bradycardia, which is life threatening
- heart failure, which is life threatening

Propranolol

The drug propranolol (Inderal, Inderal LA) has a number of therapeutic uses. It is prescribed to treat:

- cardiac arrhythmias
- **myocardial infarction** (heart attack)
- angina
- hypertension
- migraine headaches

This drug can be taken by mouth in the form of tablets, solution, or extended-release capsules, or administered by IV injection.

Timolol

As an extended-release ophthalmic gel or solution, timolol (Betimol, Istalol, Timoptic, Timoptic-XE) is used to treat open-angle glaucoma. The oral form of timolol, administered in tablet form, is used to treat hypertension, myocardial infarction, and migraine headaches. When taken orally, timolol may cause pulmonary edema.

Selective Beta-Adrenergic Blockers

Selective beta-adrenergic blocking drugs primarily affect beta$_1$-receptor sites and reduce stimulation of the heart. Because of this, they are frequently called **cardioselective beta-adrenergic blockers**.

Acebutolol and Atenolol

Acebutolol (Sectral) is administered by mouth in the form of capsules to treat hypertension and ventricular arrhythmias. The drug atenolol (Tenormin) is used to treat hypertension and angina. It is taken by mouth in tablet form.

Betaxolol

Betaxolol (Betoptic S) can be administered topically, by eye drops (as an ophthalmic solution or suspension) to treat open-angle glaucoma. Additionally, betaxolol (Kerlone) can be taken orally in tablet form to treat hypertension.

When the ophthalmic solution or suspension is instilled in the eye, a common adverse effect is stinging and brief discomfort. The oral form of the medication, on the other hand, can cause several possible adverse effects.

Bisoprolol and Esmolol

Bisoprolol (Zebeta) is used to treat hypertension and is administered by mouth in tablet form. The drug esmolol (Brevibloc) is administered by IV injection to treat supraventricular arrhythmias and hypertension. It has few common adverse effects. However, hypotension is one common adverse effect that can also be life threatening.

Metoprolol Tartrate

Metoprolol tartrate (Lopressor, Toprol XL) is used to treat hypertension, angina, and heart failure resulting from cardiomyopathy. It can be taken by mouth in immediate- or extended-release tablet form, or administered by IV injection.

QUICK QUIZ

Answer the following multiple-choice questions.

1. Which of the following is *not* a possible adverse reaction to cholinergic blocking drugs?
   a. dry mouth
   b. orthostatic hypotension
   c. decreased sweating
   d. increased heart rate
2. Cholinergic agonists are used:
   a. to reduce eye pressure in patients who have glaucoma.
   b. to treat weak bladder conditions.
   c. to treat dry mouth caused by Sjögren syndrome.
   d. all of the above
3. By which route of administration are the cholinergic drugs carbachol and pilocarpine commonly given?
   a. oral (in capsule form)
   b. sublingual
   c. topical (eye drops)
   d. SubQ injection
4. Which response does the sympathetic nervous system activate in the body?
   a. "shut down"
   b. "fight or flight"
   c. "overstimulation"
   d. "relaxation"

5. Which of the following is *not* a possible drug interaction with cholinergic blockers?
   a. Morphine further slows the movement of food and drugs through the GI system.
   b. The risk for digoxin toxicity is increased.
   c. Clonidine can cause life-threatening hypertension.
   d. The body's absorption of nitroglycerin (administered sublingually) is reduced.

Please answer each of the following questions in one to three sentences.

1. Identify three common uses of anticholinesterase drugs.

   _____

   _____

2. Name four cholinergic agonists.

   _____

   _____

3. What are at least three effects that beta-adrenergic blockers have on the body?

   _____

   _____

4. Briefly explain the differences between direct-acting, indirect-acting, and dual-acting adrenergics.

   _____

   _____

5. How do cholinergic agonists work in the body? What is their mechanism of action?

   _____

   _____

Answer the following questions as either true or false.

1. ___ Alpha-adrenergic blockers cause increased dilation of the blood vessels.
2. ___ Cholinergic agonists are most often given by IV injection.
3. ___ Catecholamine drugs all have different chemical structures. Therefore, these drugs have a wide variety of therapeutic uses.
4. ___ Target organs are the organs in the body that are intended to be affected by a particular drug.
5. ___ Adverse reactions to anticholinesterase drugs may include vomiting, headache, and seizures.

Match the generic name of each drug in the left column with the correct trade name from the right column.

1. cevimeline	a. Inderal
2. neostigmine	b. Brevibloc
3. oxybutynin	c. Evoxac
4. esmolol	d. Prostigmin
5. propranolol	e. Ditropan

DRUG CLASSIFICATION TABLE

Classification	Generic Name	Trade Name(s)
Cholinergic drugs	acetylcholine *a-se-teel-co'-leen*	*intraocular injection:* Miochol-E
	bethanechol *be-than'-e-kole*	*tablets:* Urecholine
	carbachol *kar'-ba-kole*	*ophthalmic solution:* Isopto Carbachol
	cevimeline *seh-vih'-meh-leen*	*capsules:* Evoxac
	pilocarpine *pye-loe-kar'-peen*	*ophthalmic solution:* Isopto Carpine *ophthalmic gel:* Pilopine HS *tablets:* Salagen
	ambenonium *am-be-noe'-nee-um*	*tablets:* Mytelase
	donepezil *doe-nep'-ah-zill*	*tablets:* Aricept *oral dissolving tablets:* Aricept ODT
	edrophonium *ed-roe-fone'-ee-yum*	*injection:* Enlon, Reversol
	galantamine *ga-lan'-ta-meen*	*tablets:* Razadyne *oral solution:* Razadyne *extended-release capsules:* Razadyne ER
	neostigmine *nee-oh-stig'-meen*	*tablets:* Prostigmin *injection:* (no longer marketed under trade name)
	physostigmine salicylate *fye-sew-stig'-meen*	*injection:* (no longer marketed under trade name)
	pyridostigmine *peer-id-oh-stig'-meen*	*tablets:* Mestinon *syrup:* Mestinon *extended-release tablets:* Mestinon Timespan *injection:* Regonol
	rivastigmine *riv-ah-stig'-meen*	*transdermal patch:* Exelon *capsules:* Exelon *oral solution:* Exelon
	tacrine *tay'-krin*	*capsules:* Cognex
Cholinergic blocking drugs	atropine *a'-troe-peen*	*tablets:* Sal-Tropine, Atreza *injection:* (no longer marketed under trade name) *ophthalmic ointment:* (no longer marketed under trade name) *ophthalmic solution:* Isopto Atropine
	belladonna *bel'-ah-dohn-a*	(no longer used as a single-ingredient product)
	belladonna alkaloids, ergotamine tartrate, and phenobarbital *bel'-ah-dohn-a er-got'-a-meen fee-noe-bar'-bi-tal*	*tablets:* Spastrin
	belladonna alkaloids and opium *bel'-ah-dohn-a oh'-pee-um*	*rectal suppositories:* B&O Supprettes

continued

DRUG CLASSIFICATION TABLE (continued)

Classification	Generic Name	Trade Name(s)
Cholinergic blocking drugs *(continued)*	hyoscyamine *high-oh-sigh'-ah-meen*	*injection:* Levsin *oral drops (solution):* Colytrol Pediatric, Spasdel *oral dissolving tablets:* Symax, HyoMax-FT *tablets:* Anaspaz, Cytospaz, Levsin, Medispaz, Spasdel *sublingual tablets:* Levsin SL, Symax, HyoMax-SL *oral solution:* Colidrops, Hyosyne, Spacol *elixir:* Spasdel *extended-release capsules:* Cytospaz-M *biphasic-release tablets:* Symax Duotab, HyoMax-DT *extended-release tablets:* Levbid, Symax SR, HyoMax-SR
	methscopolamine *meth-scoe-pol'-a-meen*	*tablets:* Pamine
	scopolamine *scoe-pol'-a-meen*	*transdermal patch:* Transderm-Scōp *tablets:* Scopace, Maldemar *ophthalmic solution:* Isopto Hyoscine *injection:* (no longer marketed under trade name)
	glycopyrrolate *glye-koe-pye'-roe-late*	*tablets:* Robinul, Robinul Forte *injection:* Robinul
	propantheline *proe-pan'-the-leen*	*tablets:* (no longer marketed under trade name)
	dicyclomine *dye-sye'-kloe-meen*	*capsules:* Bentyl *injection:* Bentyl *oral solution:* (no longer marketed under trade name) *oral syrup:* Bentyl *tablets:* Bentyl
	oxybutynin *ox-i-byoo'-ti-nin*	*tablets:* (no longer marketed under trade name) *extended-release tablets:* Ditropan XL *transdermal patch:* Oxytrol *oral solution:* (no longer marketed under trade name) *topical gel:* Gelnique
	tolterodine *toll-tear'-oh-dyne*	*tablets:* Detrol *extended-release capsules:* Detrol LA
Adrenergic drugs	dobutamine *doe'-byoo-ta-meen*	*injection:* (no longer marketed under trade name)
	dopamine *doe'-pa-meen*	*injection:* (no longer marketed under trade name)
	epinephrine *ep-i-nef'-rin*	*injection:* Adrenalin, EpiPen, EpiPen Jr., Twinject *inhalation:* Adrenalin, Primatene Mist
	norepinephrine (levarterenol) *nor-ep-i-nef'-rin*	*injection:* Levophed

continued

DRUG CLASSIFICATION TABLE *(continued)*

Classification	Generic Name	Trade Name(s)
Adrenergic drugs *(continued)*	isoproterenol *eye-sew-proe-tear'-e-nall*	*injection:* Isuprel
	phenylephrine *fen-ill-ef'-rin*	*ophthalmic solution:* AK-Dilate, Mydfrin, Neofrin *nasal solution:* Neo-Synephrine, Sinex, 4-Way *oral dissolving film:* Sudafed PE *oral dissolving tablets:* Nasop *tablets:* Sudafed PE *injection:* Neo-Synephrine *oral liquid:* PediaCare, Lusonal, Nasop *chewable tablets:* Nasop 12
	albuterol *al-byoo'-ter-ole*	*inhalation (suspension):* Proventil, Proair HFA, Proventil HFA, Ventolin HFA *nebulizer:* AccuNeb *tablets:* (no longer marketed under trade name) *syrup:* (no longer marketed under trade name) *extended-release tablets:* VoSpire ER
	ephedrine *e-fed'-rin*	*injection:* (no longer marketed under trade name) *capsules:* (no longer marketed under trade name)
	formoterol *for-moh'-te-rol*	*inhalation powder:* Foradil Aerolizer *nebulizer solution:* Perforomist
	levalbuterol *lev-al-byoo'-ter-ole*	*nebulizer solution:* Xopenex *pressurized inhaler (suspension):* Xopenex HFA
	metaproterenol *met-a-proe-ter'-e-nole*	*nebulizer solution:* (no longer marketed under trade name) *tablets:* (no longer marketed under trade name) *oral solution:* (no longer marketed under trade name)
	pirbuterol *peer-byoo'-ter-ole*	*inhaler:* Maxair Autohaler
	salmeterol *sal-mee'-ter-ol*	*inhalation powder:* Serevent, Diskus
	terbutaline *ter-byoo'-ta-leen*	*injection:* (no longer marketed under trade name) *tablets:* (no longer marketed under trade name)
Adrenergic blocking drugs	phentolamine *fen-tole'-a-meen*	*injection:* (no longer marketed under trade name)
	prazosin *pray-zoe'-sin* doxazosin *dox-aye'-zoe-sin*	*capsules:* Minipress *tablets:* Cardura *extended-release tablets:* Cardura XL
	terazosin *tear-aye'-zoe-sin*	*capsules:* Hytrin
	carvedilol *car-veh'-dih-lol*	*tablets:* Coreg *extended-release capsules:* Coreg CR

continued

DRUG CLASSIFICATION TABLE *(continued)*

Classification	Generic Name	Trade Name(s)
Adrenergic blocking drugs (*Continued*)	labetalol *lah-bet'-ah-lol*	*tablets:* Trandate *injection:* (no longer marketed under trade name)
	levobunolol *lee-voe-byoo'-noe-lol*	*ophthalmic solution:* Betagan
	penbutolol *pen-byoo'-toe-lol*	*tablets:* Levatol
	pindolol *pen'-doe-lol*	*tablets:* (no longer marketed under trade name)
	sotalol *soh'-tal-lole*	*tablets:* Betapace, Betapace AF
	nadolol *nay-doe'-lol*	*tablets:* Corgard
	propranolol *pro-pran'-oh-lol*	*injection:* Inderal *extended-release capsules:* Inderal LA *oral solution:* (no longer marketed under trade name) *tablets:* (no longer marketed under trade name)
	timolol *tye-moe'-lole*	*tablets:* (no longer marketed under trade name) *ophthalmic solution:* Betimol, Istalol, Timoptic *extended-release ophthalmic gel forming solution:* Timoptic-XE *ophthalmic gel forming solution:* (no longer marketed under trade name)
	acebutolol *a-se-byoo'-toe-lol*	*capsules:* Sectral
	atenolol *a-ten'-oh-lol*	*tablets:* Tenormin
	betaxolol *beh-tax'-oh-lol*	*ophthalmic suspension:* Betoptic S *ophthalmic solution:* (no longer marketed under trade name) *tablets:* Kerlone
	bisoprolol *bye-sew'-proe-lol*	*tablets:* Zebeta
	esmolol *ess'-moe-lol*	*injection:* Brevibloc
	metoprolol tartrate *me-toe'-proe-lol*	*tablets:* Lopressor *extended-release tablets:* Toprol XL *injection:* Lopressor

Neurologic and Neuromuscular Drugs

- Match brand and generic names of commonly used skeletal muscle relaxants
- Match commonly used skeletal muscle relaxants to the appropriate classification
- Identify common adverse reactions of commonly used skeletal muscle relaxants
- List major clinical indications of neuromuscular-blocking drugs
- Compare and contrast the mechanism of action of nondepolarizing and depolarizing blocking drugs
- Identify commonly used antiparkinsonian drugs by brand and generic names
- Describe the mechanism of action and use of commonly used antiparkinsonian drugs
- Match the brand and generic names with the appropriate classification of commonly used anticonvulsants
- Match the brand and generic names of commonly used antimigraine drugs
- Compare and contrast the routes of administration used when administering antimigraine drugs

KEY TERMS

absence seizures—seizures characterized by a brief loss of consciousness during which physical activity ceases; formerly called petit mal seizures

autonomic nervous system—the part of the peripheral nervous system concerned with functions essential to the life of the organism and not consciously controlled (for example, blood pressure, heart rate)

anticonvulsant drugs—drugs used for the management of convulsive disorders

benzodiazepine drugs—a class of drugs used to treat anxiety and seizures

centrally acting skeletal muscle relaxants—drugs that treat acute muscle spasms by acting on the central nervous system

competitive or stabilizing drugs—see *nondepolarizing blocking drugs*

diplopia—double vision

direct-acting skeletal muscle relaxants—drugs that treat spasm by acting on the muscles themselves rather than on the central nervous system

dopaminergic drugs—drugs that affect the dopamine content of the brain

hydantoins—anticonvulsant drugs that are used to treat psychomotor seizures, tonic-clonic seizures, and status epilepticus

ischemia—reduced blood flow resulting from narrowing or blockage of an artery or other causes

myoclonic seizures—sudden forceful contractions of the muscles of the trunk, neck, and extremities

neuromuscular-blocking drugs—drugs that relax skeletal muscles by disrupting the transmission of nerve impulses at the motor end plate

nondepolarizing blocking drugs—a class of neuromuscular-blocking drugs that prevent muscle contractions by blocking acetylcholine at receptor sites of the skeletal muscle membrane; also referred to as *competitive* or *stabilizing drugs*

parasympathetic nervous system—the part of the autonomic nervous system that's concerned with conserving body energy

paresthesia—an abnormal sensation such as numbness, tingling, prickling, or heightened sensitivity

psychomotor seizures—seizures that most often occur in children younger than three years of age through adolescence; may involve an aura with perceptual alterations, such as hallucinations or a strong sense of fear; also referred to as *temporal lobe seizures*

skeletal muscle relaxants—drugs that relieve musculoskeletal pain or spasm and severe musculoskeletal spasticity

somnolence—prolonged drowsiness; sleepiness

status epilepticus—a continuous seizure state requiring emergency intervention

temporal lobe seizures—see *psychomotor seizures*

tonic-clonic seizures—seizures involving the alternate contraction and relaxation of muscles, along with loss of consciousness and abnormal behavior

triptans—a group of drugs that are the treatment of choice for moderate to severe migraines; also known as 5-HT$_1$ receptor agonists

vasoconstriction—the narrowing of blood vessels

vasodilation—an increase in the size of blood vessels, primarily small arteries and arterioles

---

There are several classes of neurologic (related to the nervous system) and neuromuscular drugs. These drugs have a variety of uses. In this chapter, you'll learn about muscle relaxants that depress the central nervous system (CNS)—the division of the nervous system that consists of the brain and spinal cord—and others that act directly on the muscles themselves. You'll also learn about drugs that relax muscles by blocking the transmission of nerve impulses to the muscle fibers. Finally, you'll learn about drugs that are used in the treatment of Parkinson disease, seizures disorders, and migraine headaches.

SKELETAL MUSCLE RELAXANTS

Skeletal muscle relaxants are used to relieve musculoskeletal pain or spasm, as well as severe musculoskeletal spasticity, or stiff, awkward movements. These symptoms can be associated with a number of conditions, including:

- multiple sclerosis (MS), a progressive disease that causes widespread neurologic dysfunction (impaired or abnormal functioning)
- cerebral palsy, a motor (movement or motion) disorder caused by neurologic damage
- stroke, a sudden reduction in or loss of consciousness, sensation, or voluntary motion resulting from reduced oxygen supply to the brain
- spinal cord injuries that can result in paralysis or death

There are two main classes of skeletal muscle relaxants—centrally acting and direct-acting.

Centrally Acting Skeletal Muscle Relaxants

Severe cold, lack of blood flow to a muscle, overexertion, or other trauma can send sensory impulses from a muscle to nerve fibers in the spinal cord and to higher levels of the CNS. These impulses can trigger an involuntary muscle contraction or spasm. The contraction further stimulates spinal cord or CNS receptors to a more intense contraction, establishing a cycle. **Centrally acting skeletal muscle relaxants** are believed to break this cycle by acting as CNS depressants.

The process by which these drugs work is unknown. They don't relax skeletal muscles directly. They also don't depress neuron conduction, neuromuscular transmission, or muscle excitability. Their results may be related to their sedative effects.

Centrally acting skeletal muscle relaxants are used to treat spasms resulting from conditions such as:

- anxiety
- inflammation
- pain
- trauma
- other acute musculoskeletal conditions

They're usually prescribed along with rest and physical therapy.

The centrally acting skeletal muscle relaxants interact with other CNS depressants, including alcohol, narcotics, barbiturates, anticonvulsants, tricyclic antidepressants, and antianxiety drugs. The result can be increased sedation, impaired motor function, and respiratory depression. Some of these drugs have other interactions as well. The interactions of specific centrally acting skeletal muscle relaxants are included with the discussion of those drugs below.

 T I P Centrally acting skeletal muscle relaxants take 30 to 60 minutes to take effect. Remind patients that relief takes time.

⚠ PROCEED WITH CAUTION

Adverse Reactions to Centrally Acting Skeletal Muscle Relaxants

A patient can become physically and psychologically dependent on centrally acting skeletal muscle relaxants after long-term use. Abruptly stopping any of these drugs can cause severe withdrawal symptoms. Other adverse reactions also can occur.

The most common adverse reactions to these drugs are dizziness and drowsiness. Occasional adverse reactions include:

- abdominal distress
- ataxia (loss of control of voluntary movements)
- constipation
- diarrhea
- heartburn
- nausea and vomiting

More severe reactions include:

- allergic reactions
- arrhythmia (irregular heartbeat)
- bradycardia

Baclofen

Baclofen comes in a tablet that can be swallowed. For patients with severe spasticity who don't respond to or cannot take oral drugs, an injectable form (Lioresal Intrathecal) is available.

This drug is usually prescribed to treat patients with intermittent or chronic spasms. It produces less sedation than diazepam and less peripheral muscle weakness than dantrolene. (Both of these drugs will be discussed.) This makes it the drug of choice to treat spasticity.

Baclofen's main use is in the treatment of paraplegic or quadriplegic patients with spinal cord lesions most commonly caused by MS or trauma. The drug significantly reduces the number and severity of painful muscle spasms. However, it does not improve manual dexterity, muscle function, or stiff gait.

In addition to the adverse reactions generally associated with this class of drugs, baclofen may cause:

- fatigue
- muscle weakness
- depression
- headache

Injections of baclofen should not be discontinued abruptly. Doing so may result in high fever, altered mental status, and an exaggerated rebound in muscle spasms and spasticity that has, in rare cases, resulted in multiple organ system failure and death.

There are several drug interactions associated with baclofen:

- When taken with another CNS depressant, including alcohol, an increase in CNS depression will likely result.
- When fentanyl and baclofen are given together, prolonged analgesia (relief from pain) can result.
- Taking lithium carbonate and baclofen together can aggravate hyperkinesia (an abnormal increase in motor function or activity).
- When baclofen is taken with tricyclic antidepressants, increased muscle relaxation can result.

Carisoprodol

Carisoprodol (Soma) is used to treat acute muscle spasms. It is available in tablet form and is taken by mouth. Although this drug is not classified as a controlled substance by the FDA, it is commonly abused, and therefore, pharmacy technicians should exercise caution while dispensing.

Chlorzoxazone

Chlorzoxazone (Parafon Forte DSC, Relax DS) comes only in tablet form. A patient with acute muscle spasms may receive this drug. An adverse reaction to chlorzoxazone, which is not seen with most of the other drugs in its class, is a rash.

Cyclobenzaprine

Cyclobenzaprine (Fexmid, Flexeril, Amrix) comes in the form of tablets and extended-release capsules and is administered by mouth. A patient with acute muscle spasms may receive this drug, but use for longer than two to three weeks is not recommended.

Cyclobenzaprine interacts with monoamine oxidase inhibitors (MAOIs) and can result in a high body temperature, excitation, and seizures. It also can decrease the antihypertensive effects of the blood pressure-lowering drugs guanethidine and clonidine. Cyclobenzaprine sometimes enhances the effects of cholinergic-blocking drugs.

Diazepam

Diazepam (Diastat, Diazepam Intensol, Valium) is a Schedule IV controlled substance. It is available as tablets, concentrated oral solution, regular oral solution, an injectable form, and in rectal gel twin packs. A patient with intermittent or chronic spasms may receive this drug. However, diazepam is primarily used as an antianxiety drug. It relieves anxiety, muscle spasms, and seizures, and it induces calmness and sleep.

Diazepam is helpful to patients with spinal cord lesions and occasionally is given to patients with cerebral palsy. It's also useful in treating patients with painful continuous muscle spasms who aren't overly susceptible to its sedative effects. However, its use is limited by its CNS effects and by the tolerance for the drug that develops with prolonged use.

Metaxalone and Methocarbamol

A patient with acute muscle spasms may receive metaxalone (Skelaxin), which is available in tablet form, or methocarbamol (Robaxin), which may be administered by mouth or by IM or IV administration. Methocarbamol can antagonize the cholinergic effects of the anticholinesterase drugs used to treat myasthenia gravis.

Orphenadrine

Orphenadrine (Norflex) is available in tablet, powder, or injectable forms. A patient with acute muscle spasms may receive this drug.

AT THE COUNTER

Dealing with Diazepam

When receiving a prescription or medication order for diazepam, can you assume it is being used as a skeletal muscle relaxant?

No. diazepam is used to treat acute muscle spasms and spasticity caused by chronic disease, but it is also used to treat anxiety, alcohol withdrawal, and seizures. Do not make any assumptions about why the patient is taking it.

Orphenadrine sometimes enhances the effects of cholinergic-blocking drugs. It also can reduce the effects of phenothiazines. Orphenadrine and propoxyphene taken together can cause additional CNS effects, including mental confusion, anxiety, and tremors.

Tizanidine

Tizanidine (Zanaflex) comes in capsule and tablet form and is taken by mouth. A patient with intermittent, chronic, or acute muscle spasms may receive this drug. Tizanidine combined with diuretics, central alpha-adrenergic agonists, or antihypertensives may increase hypotensive drug effects.

The use of tizanidine with CNS depressants may cause additive CNS depression. Hormonal contraceptives may hinder the clearance of tizanidine, therefore requiring a reduction in tizanidine dosage.

Direct-Acting Skeletal Muscle Relaxants

The most common **direct-acting skeletal muscle relaxant** is dantrolene sodium (Dantrium). This drug, an essential on the anesthesia cart, helps manage all types of spasticity, although it seems most effective for spasticity that has a cerebral (or brain) origin. It is most effective in treating patients with:

- cerebral palsy
- MS
- spinal cord injury
- stroke

Dantrolene is available in capsules of various strengths and in a liquid form for use with IV solutions.

Malignant Hyperthermia

Dantrolene is also used to treat and prevent malignant hyperthermia. This is a rare but possibly fatal complication of anesthesia that is characterized by high fever and rigidity of the skeletal muscles. By promoting muscle relaxation, dantrolene prevents or reduces the rigidity that contributes to life-threatening body temperatures.

Mechanism of Action

Dantrolene is chemically and pharmacologically unrelated to other skeletal muscle relaxants. It has a therapeutic effect similar to that of centrally acting drugs. However, it works through a different mechanism of action (see *How Dantrolene Works*). Because its major effect is on the muscle, it has a lower incidence of adverse CNS effects. However, because it produces muscle weakness, it's of questionable benefit for patients whose strength is already weakened. At therapeutic levels, dantrolene has little effect on cardiac or intestinal smooth muscle.

Dantrolene's peak concentration occurs within about five hours after it is given. Its elimination half-life in healthy adults is about nine hours. Because the drug is metabolized in the liver, its half-life may be longer in patients who have impaired liver function. A patient taking dantrolene may not notice a therapeutic benefit for a week or more.

Drug Interactions

Be aware of the following drug interactions involving dantrolene:

- Dantrolene's depressive effects can increase when it's taken with CNS depressants. Sedation, lack of coordination, and respiratory distress can result.
- The risk of liver toxicity increases when estrogens are taken with dantrolene.
- Verapamil (Isoptin) should not be administered intravenously with dantrolene. Cardiovascular collapse may result if the two drugs are given together.
- Alcohol may increase CNS depression when used with dantrolene.
- Sun exposure may increase photosensitivity in patients taking dantrolene.

 PROCEED WITH CAUTION

Adverse Reactions to Dantrolene

Common adverse reactions to dantrolene include:

- drowsiness
- vertigo
- malaise (a general feeling of ill health)
- fatigue
- weakness

More serious adverse reactions include:

- seizures
- hepatitis

High doses of dantrolene are toxic to the liver, and long-term use risks damaging the liver. The drug should be discontinued if benefits aren't seen in 45 days.

 HOW IT WORKS

How Dantrolene Works

Dantrolene works by acting on the muscles itself. It decreases the release of calcium ions from the sarcoplasmic reticulum. The sarcoplasmic reticulum is a structure in muscle cells that is involved in muscle contraction and relaxation by storing and releasing calcium. Lowering the calcium level in the muscle plasma or myoplasm means that less energy will be produced when calcium prompts the muscle's actin and myosin filaments to interact. This interaction produces a contraction of the muscle. Less calcium and less energy result in a weaker contraction.

NEUROMUSCULAR-BLOCKING DRUGS

Neuromuscular-blocking drugs relax skeletal muscles by disrupting the transmission of nerve impulses at the motor end plate. (See *Motor End Plates.*) These drugs have three major uses:

- to relax skeletal muscles during surgery
- to reduce the severity of muscle spasms in electrically or drug-induced seizures
- to manage patients who are fighting a ventilator to help them breathe

Some neuromuscular-blocking drugs are naturally occurring substances. Others are synthetic and are manufactured in a lab. There are two main classes of neuromuscular-blocking drugs:

- nondepolarizing blocking drugs
- depolarizing blocking drugs

Nondepolarizing Blocking Drugs

Nondepolarizing blocking drugs are also called **competitive** or **stabilizing drugs**. They are derived from curare alkaloids and similar synthetic compounds.

These drugs are used for intermediate or long-term muscle relaxation. Here are some situations in which nondepolarizing blocking drugs might be used:

- to ease the passage of an endotracheal (ET) tube
- to paralyze patients who need breathing support but who fight the ET tube and ventilation
- to facilitate the realignment of broken bones and dislocated joints
- to decrease the amount of anesthetic required during surgery
- to prevent muscle injury during electroconvulsive therapy, a process in which an electric current is passed through the brain to treat depression. Using a nondepolarizing blocking drug reduces the intensity of the patient's muscle spasms.

Nondepolarizing blockers are absorbed poorly from the GI tract. For this reason, they're given parenterally. The IV route is preferred because the action is more predictable. The drug competes with the neurotransmitter acetylcholine at the cholinergic receptor sites of the skeletal muscle membrane. This blocks acetylcholine's action, which prevents the muscle from contracting.

TIP A neurotransmitter is a chemical substance that is released at nerve endings to help transmit nerve impulses.

The initial muscle weakness produced by these drugs quickly changes to a flaccid (losing muscle tone) paralysis that affects the muscles in a specific sequence:

- First, the muscles of the eyes, face, and neck are the first to become paralyzed.
- Next, the limb, abdomen, and trunk muscles become flaccid.
- Finally, the intercostal muscles (between the ribs) and diaphragm (the breathing muscle) are paralyzed.

Recovery from paralysis usually occurs in the reverse order.

Because nondepolarizing blockers don't cross the blood-brain barrier, patients receiving these drugs will remain conscious. They will also be able to feel pain. Patients

HOW IT WORKS

Motor End Plates

The motor nerve axon divides to form several branching terminals called *motor end plates* (figure 3-1). These motor end plates are enfolded in muscle fibers. However, the synaptic cleft separates the motor end plates from the fibers.

A stimulus to the nerve causes acetylcholine to be released into the synaptic cleft. There, acetylcholine occupies receptor sites on the muscle cell membrane, depolarizing the membrane and causing muscle contraction. Neuromuscular-blocking agents act at the motor end plate by competing with acetylcholine for the receptor sites or by blocking depolarization.

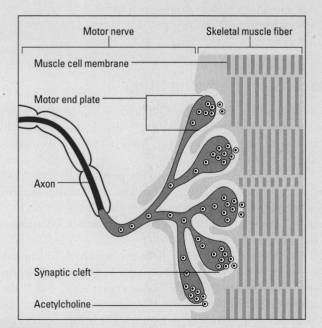

FIGURE 3-1 Motor end plate. (From *Clinical Pharmacology Made Incredibly Easy.* 2nd Ed. Philadelphia, PA: Lippincott Williams & Wilkins; 2005.)

will be aware of what is happening, but will be paralyzed and unable to communicate. They may experience extreme anxiety. For this reason, an analgesic or antianxiety drug is often administered with a neuromuscular blocker.

The effects of nondepolarizing blockers can be counteracted by anticholinesterase drugs such as neostigmine, pyridostigmine, and edrophonium. These drugs act as antidotes by inhibiting the action of acetylcholinesterase, the enzyme that destroys acetylcholine. Certain other drugs also alter the effects of nondepolarizing neuromuscular blockers:

- Aminoglycoside antibiotics and anesthetics increase the neuromuscular blockade.
- Drugs that decrease the neuromuscular blockade when taken with a nondepolarizing blocker include carbamazepine, hydantoins, ranitidine, and theophylline.
- Drugs that increase the intensity and duration of paralysis when taken with a nondepolarizing blocker include inhalation anesthetics, aminoglycosides, clindamycin, polymyxin, verapamil, quinine derivatives, ketamine, lithium, nitrates, thiazide diuretics, tetracyclines, and magnesium salts.
- Drugs that alter the levels of the electrolytes calcium, magnesium, or potassium in the blood also alter the effects of nondepolarizing blockers.
- Use of corticosteroids with nondepolarizing neuromuscular blockers may result in prolonged muscle weakness.

Atracurium

Atracurium is a solution that is usually given by rapid IV bolus injection. It can also be given by intermittent or continuous infusion. It is used to help with ET intubation and to relax patients' skeletal muscles during surgery.

Cisatracurium

Cisatracurium (Nimbex) is a solution that is administered by IV injection. Similar to atracurium, it is used to facilitate ET intubation and to relax skeletal muscles during surgery.

 TIP Vials should be inspected before cisatracurium is administered to a patient. If the solution is unclear or if it contains visible particles, it should not be used.

! PROCEED WITH CAUTION

Adverse Reactions to Nondepolarizing Blockers

Adverse reactions to all drugs in this class may include:

- apnea (interrupted breathing)
- hypotension
- skin reactions
- bronchospasm
- excessive bronchial and salivary secretions

Mivacurium

Mivacurium (Mivacron) is also administered by IV injection. It shares the same therapeutic usefulness as atracurium and cisatracurium. Among other reactions common to nondepolarizing blocking drugs, an additional common adverse reaction to mivacurium is flushing.

Pancuronium

Pancuronium is administered by IV injection. It is given in addition to anesthesia to relax skeletal muscle and to help with intubation.

In addition to the adverse reactions caused by all nondepolarizing blockers, pancuronium may also cause:

- tachycardia (rapid heart rate)
- cardiac arrhythmias
- hypertension

Rocuronium

Rocuronium (Zemuron) is a solution that may be given by rapid IV injection or continuous infusion. Like many other drugs in this class, it's administered to help with ET intubation and to relax skeletal muscles during surgery.

Vecuronium

Vecuronium is given by injection into IV lines. It is used to facilitate ET intubation. This drug is also administered to relax skeletal muscles during surgery.

Serious adverse effects associated with vecuronium include:

- prolonged muscle weakness
- unusually fast or slow heart rate
- dizziness
- fever

Depolarizing Blocking Drugs

Succinylcholine (Anectine, Quelicin) is the only therapeutic depolarizing blocking drug. It's the drug of choice for short-term muscle relaxation, such as during intubation and electroconvulsive therapy.

Succinylcholine is similar to the nondepolarizing blockers in its therapeutic effects. Also, like the nondepolarizing blockers, it isn't absorbed well from the GI tract, so it too is usually administered by IV injection. However, IM administration is possible if necessary.

The biggest difference between succinylcholine and the nondepolarizing blockers is in how succinylcholine works. Succinylcholine acts like acetylcholine, but it isn't inactivated by cholinesterase. It is rapidly metabolized, but at a slower rate than acetylcholine. Therefore, it remains attached to receptor sites on the skeletal muscle membrane for a longer period of time. This prevents repolarization of the motor end plate and results in muscle paralysis.

A number of anesthetics and antibiotics affect the action of succinylcholine. In addition, anticholinesterases

PROCEED WITH CAUTION

Adverse Reactions to Succinylcholine

The main adverse reactions to succinylcholine are:

- prolonged apnea
- hypotension

The risks associated with succinylcholine increase with patients who are genetically predisposed to certain conditions, such as:

- a low pseudocholinesterase level
- a tendency to develop malignant hyperthermia

---

have an effect on succinylcholine that is opposite to the effect they have on nondepolarizing blockers. Anticholinesterases reverse the effects of nondepolarizing blockers. However, when combined with succinylcholine, anticholinesterase drugs increase the neuromuscular blockade.

ANTIPARKINSONIAN DRUGS

Drug therapy is an important part of the treatment of Parkinson disease. Parkinson disease is a progressive neurological disorder that is characterized by four main features:

- muscle rigidity (inflexibility)
- akinesia (loss of muscle movement)
- tremors at rest
- disturbances of posture and balance

Parkinson disease affects the extrapyramidal system—the system that influences movement. This system includes the corpus striatum, globus pallidus, and substantia nigra of the brain.

In Parkinson disease, a dopamine deficiency occurs in the basal ganglia, the dopamine-releasing pathway that connects the substantia nigra to the corpus striatum. Less dopamine in the corpus striatum upsets the balance between the two neurotransmitters, acetylcholine and dopamine. The result is an excess of acetylcholine. The excessive excitation caused by cholinergic activity creates the movement disorders that characterize Parkinson disease.

Anticholinergic Drugs

As you learned in Chapter 2, anticholinergic drugs are sometimes called parasympatholytic drugs. This is because they restrict the action of acetylcholine at special receptors in the **parasympathetic nervous system**. This is the part of the **autonomic nervous system** that's concerned with conserving body energy—for example, slowing the heart rate

and digesting food. The autonomic nervous system is the part of the peripheral nervous system that's concerned with the automatic functions essential to life, such as maintaining blood pressure and heart rate.

High acetylcholine levels excite the CNS, which can cause a parkinsonian tremor. Patients with Parkinson disease take anticholinergics to inhibit the action of acetylcholine at receptor sites in the CNS and autonomic nervous system.

Although anticholinergics are used to treat all forms of Parkinson disease, they're most commonly used in its early stages when symptoms are mild and don't have a major effect on the person's lifestyle. Anticholinergics effectively control sialorrhea (excessive saliva flow). They are also about 20 percent effective in reducing the occurrence and severity of akinesia and rigidity.

Anticholinergics can be given alone or with certain dopaminergic drugs. (You'll read about dopaminergic drugs later in this chapter.) For example, anticholinergic drugs can be used with amantadine during the early stages of Parkinson disease. These drugs may also be given with levodopa during the disease's later stages to relieve symptoms further.

Interactions may take place when certain other medications are taken with anticholinergic drugs:

- Amantadine can increase the adverse effects of anticholinergics.
- The absorption of levodopa can be decreased, which can lead to a worsening of the signs and symptoms of Parkinson disease.
- Taking antipsychotics and anticholinergics together decreases the effectiveness of both classes of drugs. Antipsychotics also increase the incidence of adverse effects associated with anticholinergic drugs.
- Over-the-counter cough or cold medicines, diet aids, and analeptics (drugs used to keep a person awake) increase the effects of anticholinergics.
- Consuming alcohol with anticholinergic drugs increases CNS depression.

Benztropine

Benztropine (Cogentin) is classified as a synthetic tertiary amine. It is used as adjunct therapy in the treatment of Parkinson disease. Benztropine is produced as a tablet for oral administration and as a liquid that may be given by IM or IV injection.

Trihexyphenidyl

Trihexyphenidyl, which comes in oral tablet and liquid forms, is also classified as a tertiary amine. This drug is used as an adjunct in the treatment of Parkinson disease.

Diphenhydramine

Antihistamines such as diphenhydramine (Benadryl) have anticholinergic properties and are also effective in treating the symptoms of Parkinson disease. Diphenhydramine may

PROCEED WITH CAUTION

Adverse Reactions to Anticholinergics

Mild adverse reactions are seen in 30 percent to 50 percent of patients who take anticholinergic drugs, depending on the size of the dose.

Common adverse reactions may include:

- confusion
- restlessness
- agitation and excitement
- drowsiness or insomnia
- tachycardia and heart palpitations
- nausea and vomiting
- urine retention
- constipation
- increased intraocular pressure, blurred vision, pupil dilation, and photophobia (sensitivity to light)

Sensitivity-related reactions may include:

- hives
- allergic rash

Reactions in patients aged 60 years and older may include:

- increased confusion
- heightened agitation
- hallucinations
- possible psychotic symptoms

---

be administered by mouth, in tablet or capsule forms, or by IM or IV injection.

Dopaminergic Drugs

Dopaminergic drugs act in the brain to improve motor function in one of two ways:

- by increasing the concentration of dopamine, a naturally occurring substance in the brain
- by enhancing neurotransmission of dopamine

Dopaminergic drugs include several drugs that are chemically unrelated:

- levodopa, the metabolic precursor to dopamine
- carbidopa-levodopa, a combination drug composed of carbidopa and levodopa
- amantadine, an antiviral drug with dopaminergic activity
- bromocriptine and pergolide, ergot-type dopamine agonists
- ropinirole and pramipexole, two non–ergot-type dopamine agonists
- selegiline, a type B MAOI

These drugs are usually used to treat patients with severe Parkinson disease who don't respond to anticholinergic drugs alone.

A number of drug interactions are related to dopaminergic drugs. Some of these reactions can be fatal.

- Levodopa's effectiveness may be reduced when used along with pyridoxine (vitamin B_6), phenytoin, benzodiazepines, reserpine, or papaverine.
- Levodopa also can produce a significant interaction with food in some patients. Dietary amino acids can decrease levodopa's effectiveness by competing with it for absorption in the intestines, thereby slowing its transport to the brain.
- MAOIs such as tranylcypromine increase the risk of a hypertensive crisis.
- Antipsychotics such as phenothiazines, thiothixene, haloperidol, and loxapine can reduce the effectiveness of levodopa and pergolide.
- Amantadine may increase the adverse effects, such as confusion and hallucinations, of anticholinergic drugs and reduce the absorption of levodopa.
- Meperidine taken with selegiline at higher than recommended doses can cause a fatal reaction.

In addition, the dosage of some dopaminergic drugs such as amantadine, levodopa, pramipexole, and bromocriptine must be gradually tapered to avoid causing a parkinsonian crisis—a sudden marked clinical deterioration. Otherwise, possibly life-threatening complications, including muscle rigidity, elevated body temperature, tachycardia, mental changes, and increased serum creatine kinase (resembling neuroleptic malignant syndrome), may result.

Levodopa

Levodopa is the most effective and commonly used drug for treating Parkinson disease. However, it loses its effectiveness after three to five years. Single-ingredient products are no longer available, although levodopa is commonly prescribed in combination with carbidopa.

When a patient's response fluctuates, the dosage and frequency with which the drug is taken may be increased. Another approach is adjunctive therapy in which amantadine, selegiline, dopamine agonists, or catechol-O-methyltransferase (COMT) inhibitors may be added. Controlled-release forms of carbidopa-levodopa may also be helpful in managing the wearing-off effect (when levodopa's effects don't last as long as they used to) or in managing delayed-onset motor fluctuations.

Adverse reactions to levodopa may include:

- nausea and vomiting
- orthostatic hypotension
- anorexia
- neuroleptic malignant syndrome
- arrhythmias
- irritability
- confusion

T I P Levodopa is controversial—some physicians believe its use should begin at diagnosis, while others don't prescribe it until symptoms become severe, and still others believe its use may speed the advance of Parkinson disease.

Carbidopa-Levodopa

Carbidopa-levodopa (Sinemet, Sinemet CR, Parcopa) is available as a standard tablet, controlled-release tablet, or in dissolving tablet form. Levodopa is almost always combined with carbidopa as the standard therapy for Parkinson disease.

Levodopa is metabolized in large amounts in the stomach and during the first pass through the liver. Carbidopa isn't metabolized as extensively. Levodopa is inactive until it crosses the blood-brain barrier and is converted to dopamine by enzymes in the brain to increase dopamine concentrations in the basal ganglia. Because of its slower rate of metabolism, carbidopa enhances levodopa's effectiveness by blocking its conversion elsewhere outside the brain. This permits increased levels of levodopa to reach the brain.

T I P Carbidopa-levodopa comes in several different strengths: 10/100, 25/100, and 25/250. The sustained release formula comes in 25/100 and 50/200. Always double-check whether the prescription or medication order is for the regular tablet or the sustained-release (Sinemet CR) formula. This is important because both dosage forms come in a 25/100 strength.

Amantadine

Amantadine (Symmetrel) is available in capsule, tablet, or oral solution form. It is sometimes prescribed to treat the symptoms of early Parkinson disease or in combination with levodopa when that drug becomes less effective.

Amantadine's exact mechanism of action is not known. It's believed to release dopamine from intact neurons, but it may have nondopaminergic mechanisms as well.

Adverse reactions to amantadine may include orthostatic hypotension and constipation.

Bromocriptine

Bromocriptine (Parlodel) is produced as capsules and tablets. It stimulates dopamine receptors in the brain and produces effects that are similar to dopamine's effects. For this reason, bromocriptine is used to treat Parkinson disease and neuroleptic malignant syndrome.

Possible adverse reactions to bromocriptine may include:

- persistent orthostatic hypotension
- ventricular tachycardia
- bradycardia
- worsening angina

Ropinirole

Ropinirole (Requip, Requip XL) is available in tablet form in both regular and extended-release form. Its effect is similar to that of bromocriptine. This drug is used to treat Parkinson disease and moderate to severe restless leg syndrome.

Adverse reactions to ropinirole may include:

- orthostatic hypotension
- dizziness
- confusion
- insomnia

Pramipexole

Pramipexole (Mirapex) is produced only in tablet form. It has the same effect as bromocriptine and ropinirole. Likewise, it's used to treat the signs and symptoms of Parkinson disease.

Pramipexole has been known to cause the same adverse reactions as ropinirole.

Pergolide

Pergolide is available as an oral tablet. The drug directly stimulates postsynaptic receptors in the CNS. Pergolide is used as an adjunct treatment with carbidopa-levodopa in managing the signs and symptoms of Parkinson disease.

Adverse reactions to pergolide may include:

- confusion
- dyskinesia (jerky movements)
- hallucinations
- nausea

Selegiline

Selegiline (Eldepryl, EMSAM, Zelapar) is produced as a capsule, tablet, orally disintegrating tablet, and 24-hour transdermal patch. This drug can increase dopaminergic activity by inhibiting type B MAOI activity or by other mechanisms. It is used to prolong the duration of levodopa's therapeutic action by blocking its breakdown. The effect of selegiline on MAOI activity also makes it useful as an antidepressant when administered in patch form. Finally, selegiline has been used in the early stages of Parkinson disease because of its neuroprotective properties and potential to slow the progression of the disease.

COMT Inhibitors

COMT inhibitors are used in addition to carbidopa-levodopa therapy. These drugs are used to treat patients who experience the wearing-off effect at the end of the dosing interval or random "on-off" fluctuations in response to carbidopa-levodopa.

COMT inhibitors have no antiparkinsonian effect when used alone and should always be combined with carbidopa-levodopa. Adding a COMT inhibitor often requires reducing the carbidopa-levodopa dose, especially for patients whose levodopa dose is more than 800 mg.

COMT is the major metabolizing enzyme for levodopa in situations in which a decarboxylase inhibitor such as carbidopa is present. Inhibiting COMT alters the pharmacokinetics of levodopa, leading to sustained plasma levels of the drug. This result is more sustained dopaminergic stimulation in the brain and improvement in the signs and symptoms of Parkinson disease.

Rapid withdrawal from a COMT inhibitor may lead to parkinsonian crisis and may cause a syndrome with the following symptoms:

- muscle rigidity
- high fever
- tachycardia
- elevated serum creatine kinase
- confusion

Specific schedules for gradually reducing COMT inhibitors haven't been evaluated. However, a slow tapering of the dose is best.

The following drug interactions may occur if COMT inhibitors are administered with certain drugs:

- COMT inhibitors shouldn't be used along with type A MAOIs. However, they may be used with selegiline (a type B MAOI).
- COMT inhibitors shouldn't be used with linezolid because of MAO inhibition.
- When COMT inhibitors are combined with catecholine drugs (dopamine, dobutamine, epinephrine, methyldopa, or norepinephrine), significant arrhythmias or other cardiac effects may result.
- Using COMT inhibitors with CNS depressants (benzodiazepines, tricyclic antidepressants, antipsychotics, ethanol, opioid analgesics, and other sedative hypnotics) may cause additive CNS effects.
- Use of COMT inhibitors may increase the risk of orthostatic hypotension in patients receiving dopaminergic therapy.

! PROCEED WITH CAUTION

Adverse Reactions to COMT Inhibitors

Common adverse reactions to COMT inhibitors may include:

- nausea
- dyskinesia (impairment of voluntary movement)
- diarrhea
- hyperkinesia (excessive muscle activity)
- hypokinesia (decreased muscle activity)

COMT inhibitors can also be toxic to the liver—a potentially life-threatening adverse reaction.

Tolcapone

Tolcapone (Tasmar) is manufactured in tablet form. This drug is used as adjunct therapy to carbidopa and levodopa for treating the signs and symptoms of Parkinson disease. It is prescribed for patients who are experiencing fluctuation in their symptoms or who haven't responded to other adjunctive treatment.

Tolcapone may produce acute liver failure. For this reason, tolcapone should be used only with patients who are experiencing fluctuations in levodopa response and aren't responding to—or aren't appropriate candidates for—other adjunctive therapies. In addition, tolcapone should never be used with patients who have liver disease or whose alanine aminotransferase level or aspartate aminotransferase level is above the normal limit on two occasions.

Baseline liver function tests should be performed before tolcapone therapy is started. The tests should be repeated every two weeks during the 12 months of therapy, every four weeks for months 13 to 15, and every eight weeks thereafter. Patients also must be advised of the risks of liver injury and provide written informed consent before receiving tolcapone.

Entacapone

The drug entacapone (Comtan) is available only as a tablet. Like tolcapone, it is used as adjunctive therapy to carbidopa and levodopa. This drug is used to treat Parkinson disease in patients who are experiencing the wearing-off effect at the end of a dosing interval.

In addition to the adverse reactions caused by COMT inhibitors, entacapone may also cause brownish-orange urine discoloration.

The following drug interactions may occur with entacapone use:

- The use of entacapone with bromocriptine or pergolide may cause fibrotic complications.

AT THE COUNTER

Parkinsonian Precautions

A patient with Parkinson disease is currently taking carbidopa-levodopa, amantadine, and benztropine. The patient's caregiver has noticed that the patient often complains about dry mouth. Recently, the patient seems to be experiencing episodes of confusion and agitation. These symptoms are most likely being caused by which drug(s)?

Dry mouth is a common adverse reaction of anticholinergics. Confusion and agitation are adverse reactions often seen in patients older than 60 years of age. The anticholinergic drug this patient is taking is benztropine. However, the combination of amantadine and benztropine (or any anticholinergic) can result in increased adverse reactions related to the anticholinergic drugs.

■ The elimination of entacapone may be decreased if the patient is also taking drugs that interfere with glucuronidation (erythromycin, rifampin, cholestyramine, and probenecid).

TIP Both tolcapone and entacapone are selective and reversible inhibitors of COMT.

ANTICONVULSANT DRUGS

Anticonvulsant drugs inhibit neuromuscular transmission. They're used for:

- long-term management of the recurring seizures of chronic epilepsy
- short-term management of isolated acute seizures not caused by epilepsy, such as seizures occurring after trauma or brain surgery
- emergency treatment of **status epilepticus**, a continuous seizure state

The drug used in treatment depends on seizure type, drug characteristics, and patient preferences. The newer seizure medications are more seizure specific. For example, treatment of epilepsy typically begins with a single drug. The dosage is increased until seizures are controlled or until adverse reactions become a problem for the patient. Generally, a second single drug is tried before combination therapy is considered.

Anticonvulsants fall into several major classes:

- hydantoins
- barbiturates
- iminostilbenes
- benzodiazepines
- carboxylic acid derivative
- 1-(aminomethyl) cyclohexane-acetic acid
- phenyltriazines
- carboxamides
- sulfamate-substituted monosaccharides
- succinimides
- sulfonamides

Hydantoins

In most cases, the hydantoin anticonvulsants stabilize nerve cells to keep them from getting overexcited. **Hydantoins** (particularly phenytoin and fosphenytoin) are the long-acting anticonvulsants of choice to treat status epilepticus after initial benzodiazepines have been administered intravenously.

Hydantoin anticonvulsants decrease the effects of the following drugs:

- oral anticoagulants
- levodopa
- amiodarone

- corticosteroids
- doxycycline
- methadone
- metyrapone
- quinidine
- theophylline
- thyroid hormone
- hormonal contraceptives
- valproic acid
- cyclosporine
- carbamazepine

Phenytoin and Phenytoin Sodium

Phenytoin and phenytoin sodium (Dilantin, Dilantin Infatabs, Phenytek) are available as a capsule, extended-release capsule, chewable tablet, oral suspension, and injectable liquid.

Phenytoin seems to work in the motor cortex of the brain, where it stops the spread of seizure activity. Its effectiveness and relatively low toxicity make it the most commonly prescribed anticonvulsant. It's one of the drugs of choice used to treat:

- complex partial seizures, also called **psychomotor** or **temporal lobe seizures**
- **tonic-clonic seizures**—seizures involving the alternate contraction (the tonic phase) and relaxation (the clonic phase) of muscles, along with loss of consciousness and abnormal behavior

TIP Phenytoin and phenytoin sodium are the most commonly prescribed anticonvulsant drugs.

! PROCEED WITH CAUTION

Adverse Reactions to Hydantoins

Adverse reactions to hydantoins include:

- drowsiness
- ataxia (inability to coordinate voluntary muscle movements)
- irritability
- headache
- nystagmus (rapid involuntary oscillation of the eyeballs)
- dizziness and vertigo
- dysarthria (a difficulty in speaking)
- nausea and vomiting
- anorexia
- depressed atrial and ventricular conduction
- ventricular fibrillation (in toxic states)
- bradycardia, hypotension, and cardiac arrest (with IV administration)
- hypersensitivity reactions

Phenytoin is also used as an antiarrhythmic drug to control irregular heart rhythms. It has properties similar to those of quinidine or procainamide.

Phenytoin's effect is *decreased* when it is taken with:

- phenobarbital
- diazoxide
- theophylline
- carbamazepine
- rifampin
- antacids
- sucralfate

Phenytoin's effect and potential for toxicity *increase* when it's taken with:

- cimetidine
- disulfiram
- fluconazole
- isoniazid
- omeprazole
- sulfonamides
- oral anticoagulants
- chloramphenicol
- valproic acid
- amiodarone

Enteral tube feedings may interfere with the absorption of oral phenytoin. Tube feedings should be stopped for two hours before and after phenytoin is administered.

Fosphenytoin

Fosphenytoin (Cerebyx) can be given by IM or IV injection for short-term administration. Along with phenytoin, it's the long-acting drug of choice to treat status epilepticus after initial benzodiazepines are given intravenously.

Ethotoin

Ethotoin (Peganone) is available in tablet form. It is sometimes prescribed in combination with other anticonvulsants for partial and tonic-clonic seizures in patients who are intolerant of or resistant to other anticonvulsants.

Barbiturates

Barbiturates are effective alternative therapy for treating:

- partial seizures
- tonic-clonic seizures
- febrile seizures

However, barbiturates are ineffective in treating **absence seizures**. Formerly called petit mal seizures, these are seizures characterized by a brief loss of consciousness during which physical activity ceases. They may last a few seconds and happen many times per day.

Barbiturates elevate the seizure threshold by decreasing postsynaptic excitation. They can be used alone or with other anticonvulsants. They are effective at lower doses than those that produce hypnotic effects. For this reason,

PROCEED WITH CAUTION

Adverse Reactions to Barbiturates

Possible adverse reactions to barbiturates include:

- hypersensitivity rash and other rashes
- an inflammatory disorder known as lupus erythematosus-like syndrome
- enlarged lymph nodes

they usually don't cause addiction when they are used to treat epilepsy.

Here are some important general drug interactions with barbiturates:

- The effects of barbiturates can be reduced when they're taken with rifampin.
- Barbiturate use can decrease the effects of many drugs, including beta-adrenergic blockers, corticosteroids, digoxin, estrogens, doxycycline, oral anticoagulants, hormonal contraceptives, quinidine, phenothiazine, metronidazole, tricyclic antidepressants, theophylline, cyclosporine, carbamazepine, felodipine, and verapamil.
- The risk of adverse reactions to tricyclic antidepressants increases when they're taken with barbiturates.
- The use of evening primrose oil may increase the dosage requirement of anticonvulsant drugs.

Phenobarbital

The long-acting barbiturate phenobarbital (Luminal) was once one of the most widely used anticonvulsant drugs. It is now used less frequently because of its sedative effects.

Phenobarbital is sometimes used for long-term treatment of epilepsy. It is sometimes given by IV injection to treat status epilepticus if hydantoins are ineffective. Its major disadvantage for this use is that it has a delayed onset of action when an immediate response is needed. It is also available in tablet form and as an oral solution.

In addition to the reactions common to drugs in the barbiturate class, adverse reactions to phenobarbital may also include:

- drowsiness, lethargy, and dizziness
- nystagmus, confusion, and ataxia (with large doses)
- laryngospasm, respiratory depression, and hypotension (when administered intravenously)

The risk of toxicity increases when phenobarbital is taken with CNS depressants, valproic acid, chloramphenicol, felbamate, cimetidine, or phenytoin. The metabolism of corticosteroids, digoxin, and estrogens may be enhanced by phenobarbital, which may reduce the effectiveness of these drugs. Phenobarbital is a Schedule IV controlled substance.

Mephobarbital

Mephobarbital (Mebaral) is another long-acting barbiturate that is sometimes used as an anticonvulsant. It has no advantage over phenobarbital, but it is used when the patient can't tolerate the adverse effects of phenobarbital. This drug is taken by mouth in tablet form.

Adverse reactions to mephobarbital are the same as those for phenobarbital. Mephobarbital is a Schedule IV controlled substance.

Primidone

Primidone (Mysoline) is closely related chemically to barbiturates. It is taken orally in tablet form and is used to treat chronic epilepsy. However, because of monitoring, costs, and dosing frequency, phenobarbital is usually tried before primidone. This drug may be effective for patients who do not respond to phenobarbital.

In addition to the CNS and GI reactions caused by phenobarbital, patients taking primidone may experience the following adverse reactions:

- hair loss
- impotence
- osteomalacia (softening of the bones)
- acute psychosis

Iminostilbenes

Carbamazepine (Carbatrol, Epitol, Equetro, Tegretol, Tegretol XR) is the most commonly used iminostilbene. It's available in the form of tablets, extended-release tablets, chewable tablets, extended-release capsules, and oral suspension. Carbamazepine is the drug of choice for:

- simple and complex partial seizures
- generalized tonic-clonic seizures

It's also effective in treating:

- partial tonic-clonic seizures
- mixed seizure types

T I P Don't confuse Tegretol, a brand name for carbamazepine, with Toradol, a brand name for ketorolac.

Carbamazepine may worsen absence seizures or **myoclonic seizures**—sudden forceful contractions of the muscles of the trunk, neck, and extremities. However, it relieves pain when used to treat a form of trigeminal neuralgia known as tic douloureux, which is characterized by intense facial pain along the trigeminal nerve. It also may be useful in treating certain psychiatric disorders.

The drug's anticonvulsant effect is similar to that of phenytoin. Its anticonvulsant action results from its ability to limit the spread of seizure activity or neuromuscular transmission in general.

Carbamazepine can reduce the effects of several other drugs, including:

- haloperidol
- bupropion
- lamotrigine
- tricyclic antidepressants
- oral anticoagulants
- hormonal contraceptives (such as birth control pills or patches)
- doxycycline
- felbamate
- theophylline
- valproic acid

Increased carbamazepine levels and toxicity can occur when a patient is also taking any of the following drugs:

- cimetidine
- danazol
- diltiazem
- erythromycin
- isoniazid
- selective serotonin reuptake inhibitors (SSRIs)
- propoxyphene
- troleandomycin
- ketoconazole
- valproic acid
- verapamil

Other drug interactions also may occur.

- Carbamazepine and lithium taken together increase the risk of neurologic effects.
- Carbamazepine levels may be decreased when taken with barbiturates, felbamate, or phenytoin.
- Carbamazepine is primarily metabolized in the liver by a cytochrome P-450 enzyme (CYP450) and is excreted in the urine. Patients with liver dysfunction should be monitored closely, because carbamazepine induces its own metabolism, which leads to a variable half-life. Many interactions are seen among drugs that are metabolized by CYP450. As a pharmacy technician, you should be aware of these drugs because they may interact with other medications that a patient is taking.
- Plantain, an herbal medication that some people use for treating coughs and chronic bronchitis, may block the absorption of carbamazepine in the GI tract.

! PROCEED WITH CAUTION

Adverse Reactions to Carbamazepine

- Rash is the most common hypersensitivity response.
- Hives and Stevens-Johnson syndrome (a potentially fatal inflammatory disease) can also occur.
- Occasionally, serious hematologic toxicity occurs.
- Because this drug is structurally related to the tricyclic antidepressants, it can cause similar toxicities and affect emotions and behaviors.

Benzodiazepines

Benzodiazepine drugs, which are classified as Schedule IV controlled substances, have several uses. They act as anticonvulsants, antianxiety agents, sedative-hypnotics, and muscle relaxants. Patients can receive benzodiazepines orally, parenterally, and sometimes rectally. The mechanism of action of these drugs is poorly understood.

The depressant effects of benzodiazepines are increased when they are taken with:

- CNS depressants
- hormonal contraceptives
- cimetidine

The results can be excessive sedation, CNS depression, and respiratory depression. Death may even occur at high does.

Four of these drugs provide anticonvulsant effects. Each is discussed below.

Clonazepam

Clonazepam (Klonopin, Klonopin Wafer) is the only benzodiazepine recommended for long-term treatment of epilepsy. It is used to treat the following types of seizures:

- absence (petit mal)
- atypical absence (Lennox-Gastaut syndrome)
- atonic
- myoclonic

Clonazepam tablets are generally swallowed by the patient. Another form of the tablet disintegrates in the mouth.

Diazepam

Only parenteral forms of diazepam (Diastat, Diazepam Intensol, Valium) are used as anticonvulsants. Diazepam isn't recommended for long-term treatment because of the amount of the drug required to control seizures and also because it can be addictive.

When given by IV injection, diazepam is used to control status epilepticus. Because it has only a short-term effect (less than one hour), the patient must also receive a long-acting anticonvulsant such as phenytoin or phenobarbital. The rectal gel is approved for treatment of repetitive seizures and has reduced the incidence of recurrent seizures in children.

TIP When filling a prescription for diazepam or other benzodiazepines, remember that they are Schedule IV controlled substances. Use of these drugs is regulated by the Controlled Substances Act.

Lorazepam and Clorazepate

Lorazepam (Ativan, Lorazepam Intensol) is available as tablets, concentrated oral solution, or an injectable solution. Intravenous lorazepam is currently considered the benzodiazepine of choice in treating status epilepticus. When preparing lorazepam in IV form, remember that the drug should be placed in a glass bottle because it is less stable in the standard via-flex IV bags.

Clorazepate (Tranxene-SD, Tranxene-T) is produced as standard tablets and as extended-release tablets. It is used with other drugs to prevent partial seizures.

Carboxylic Acid Derivative

Valproic acid, the most widely used carboxylic acid derivative, is unrelated structurally to other anticonvulsants. It is marketed in capsule and oral solution form under the trade names Depakene and Stavzor and is also available as:

- valproate (Depacon)—an injectable solution
- divalproex (Depakote, Depakote ER, Depakote Sprinkles)—standard tablets, extended-release tablets, or capsules

Valproate is rapidly converted to valproic acid in the stomach. Divalproex is a precursor of valproic acid and separates into valproic acid in the GI tract. The mechanism by which valproic acid works is unknown. It is believed to increase the levels of gamma-aminobutyric acid (GABA), an inhibitory neurotransmitter, and to have a direct membrane-stabilizing effect.

Valproic acid is prescribed for the long-term treatment of:

- absence seizures
- myoclonic seizures
- tonic-clonic seizures
- partial seizures

It may also be useful in treating neonatal seizures.

Valproic acid should be used with caution in patients who have liver disease. Extreme caution is needed for use in children under two years old, especially if they:

PROCEED WITH CAUTION

Adverse Reactions to Benzodiazepines

The most common adverse reactions to benzodiazepines include:

- drowsiness
- confusion
- ataxia
- weakness
- dizziness
- nystagmus
- vertigo
- fainting
- dysarthria
- headache
- tremor
- glassy-eyed appearance

- are receiving multiple anticonvulsants
- have congenital metabolic disorders, severe seizures with mental retardation, or organic brain disease

In such patients, this drug carries a risk of potentially fatal liver toxicity, especially during the first six months of treatment.

> **TIP** Valproic acid's hepatic risks limit its use in treating seizure disorders, but the risk decreases with age.

Here are the most important drug interactions associated with valproic acid:

- Cimetidine, aspirin, erythromycin, and felbamate may increase valproic acid levels in the body.
- Carbamazepine, lamotrigine, phenobarbital, primidone, phenytoin, and rifampin may decrease levels of valproic acid.
- Valproic acid may decrease the effects of felbamate, lamotrigine, phenobarbital, primidone, benzodiazepines, CNS depressants, warfarin, and zidovudine.

1-(Aminomethyl) Cyclohexane-Acetic Acid

The drug gabapentin (Neurontin) is part of the 1-(aminomethyl) cyclohexane-acetic acid class. This drug was designed to be a GABA agonist, but the exact means by which it works is not known. It doesn't seem to act at the GABA receptor, affect GABA uptake, or interfere with GABA transaminase. Instead, it seems to bind to a carrier protein and act as a unique receptor in the brain, resulting in increased GABA levels in the brain.

Gabapentin is available in capsules and tablets of various strengths. It is used in conjunction with other therapies

PROCEED WITH CAUTION

Adverse Reactions to Valproic Acid

Most adverse reactions to valproic acid are tolerable and dose related. They include:

- nausea and vomiting
- diarrhea
- constipation
- sedation
- dizziness
- ataxia
- headache
- muscle weakness
- increased blood ammonia level

In addition, rare but deadly liver toxicity has occurred with valproic acid. This drug should be used with caution in patients with a history of liver disease. There's a high risk of liver toxicity in children under two years of age.

PROCEED WITH CAUTION

Adverse Reactions to Gabapentin

Common adverse reactions to gabapentin may include:

- fatigue
- **somnolence** (prolonged drowsiness, sleepiness)
- dizziness
- ataxia
- leucopenia (abnormally low white blood cell count)

against partial and secondary generalized seizures in adults and children aged three years and older. It also seems to be an effective therapy by itself, although it isn't approved by the FDA for that purpose.

Gabapentin doesn't induce or inhibit liver enzymes, so it causes very few drug interactions and doesn't affect the metabolism of other anticonvulsants. However, antacids and cimetidine may affect gabapentin concentration. In addition, patients with renal impairment (creatinine clearance less than 60 mL/min) will require a dosage reduction.

Finally, like carbamazepine, gabapentin may worsen myoclonic seizures.

Phenyltriazines

The phenyltriazine drug lamotrigine (Lamictal) is chemically unrelated to other anticonvulsants. It is available in tablet, chewable tablet, and orally disintegrating form and is approved by the FDA for use with other drugs in treating:

- adults who have partial seizures
- children over age two years who have generalized seizures or Lennox-Gastaut syndrome

Additionally, lamotrigine seems to be effective for many types of generalized seizures, although it can worsen myoclonic seizures. The drug may also lead to improvement of the patient's mood.

Lamotrigine's exact mechanism of action is not known. It is believed to block voltage-sensitive sodium channels, thus inhibiting the release of the excitatory neurotransmitters glutamate and aspirate.

Several drugs interact with lamotrigine to alter its effects:

- Lamotrigine's effects may be decreased if the drug is given with carbamazepine, phenytoin, phenobarbital, primidone, or acetaminophen.
- Valproic acid may decrease the clearance and increase the effects and steady-state level of lamotrigine.
- Lamotrigine may produce additive effects when combined with folate inhibitors.

! PROCEED WITH CAUTION

Adverse Reactions to Lamotrigine

Common adverse reactions to lamotrigine may include:

- dizziness
- ataxia
- somnolence
- headache
- **diplopia** (double vision)
- nausea
- vomiting
- rash

Several types of rash, including Stevens-Johnson syndrome, may occur with this drug. A generalized, red, measles-like rash may appear in the first three to four weeks of therapy. It's usually mild to moderate, but it may be severe. The risk of rash may be increased by starting at high doses, rapidly increasing doses, or using valproate at the same time.

Lamotrigine now carries a "black box" warning regarding the rash, and the manufacturer recommends discontinuing the drug at the first sign of rash.

Carboxamides

Oxcarbazepine (Trileptal) is used alone or as adjunctive therapy for adults with partial seizures. It's also used as adjunctive therapy for children over four years old who have partial seizures.

This drug is administered orally, in tablet or oral suspension form. It is chemically similar to the iminostilbene anticonvulsant carbamazepine. Its exact mechanism of action (and that of its metabolite 10-hydroxycarbazepine, or MHD) is not known. However, it is believed to prevent

! PROCEED WITH CAUTION

Adverse Reactions to Oxcarbazepine

Common reactions to oxcarbazepine may include:

- somnolence
- dizziness
- diplopia
- ataxia
- nausea and vomiting
- abnormal gait
- tremor
- aggravated seizures
- rectal bleeding

About 20 percent to 30 percent of patients who have had an allergic reaction to carbamazepine will have an allergic reaction to oxcarbazepine.

seizures by blocking sodium-sensitive channels, which prevents seizure spread in the brain. Like carbamazepine, it's also effective for generalized seizures, but may worsen myoclonic and absence seizures.

Here are some other issues to consider:

- Carbamazepine, phenytoin, phenobarbital, valproic acid, and verapamil may decrease levels of oxcarbazepine's active metabolite MHD.
- Oxcarbazepine may decrease the effectiveness of hormonal contraceptives and felodipine.
- Oxcarbazepine is secreted in breast milk.
- Dosage reductions are necessary for patients with kidney impairment (creatinine clearance less than 30 mL/min) and for those at risk for kidney impairment, such as older adult patients.

Sulfamate-Substituted Monosaccharides

Topiramate (Topamax, Topamax Sprinkle) is one of the newer anticonvulsant drugs available. Administered orally in tablet or capsule form, it is believed to act by blocking voltage-dependent sodium channels, enhancing activity of the GABA receptors, and antagonizing glutamate receptors.

This drug is approved as adjunctive therapy for partial and primary generalized tonic-clonic seizures in adults and children older than two years of age. Topiramate is also used for migraine headache therapy and to treat children with Lennox-Gastaut syndrome. It may prove beneficial for other types of seizures as well and as monotherapy (used alone, without other drugs).

! PROCEED WITH CAUTION

Adverse Reactions to Topiramate

The following common reactions may require stopping use of the drug. Low starting doses and slow dosage titration may minimize these effects:

- psychomotor slowing
- word-finding difficulty
- impaired concentration
- memory impairment

Other common adverse reactions to topiramate may include:

- drowsiness
- dizziness
- headache
- ataxia
- nervousness
- confusion
- **paresthesia** (a prickling or tingling sensation on the skin)
- weight gain
- diplopia

Drug interactions with topiramate and other considerations regarding its use are as follows:

- Carbamazepine, phenytoin, and valproic acid may cause decreased topiramate levels.
- Topiramate may decrease the effectiveness of hormonal contraceptives and decrease valproic acid levels.
- Combining CNS depressants and topiramate may cause added CNS effects.
- For kidney-impaired patients (creatinine clearance less than 70 mL/min), the topiramate dose should be cut in half.

Succinimides

The succinimides ethosuximide (Zarontin) and methsuximide (Celontin) are used to manage absence seizures. Ethosuximide, which is administered orally in capsule, solution, or syrup form, is the drug of choice for this therapy. Its exact mechanism of action is unknown, but it's believed to inhibit an enzyme necessary for the formation of gamma-hydroxyburate, which has been associated with the induction of absence seizures.

Ethosuximide isn't protein-bound, so displacement reactions can't occur. Carbamazepine may induce the metabolism of ethosuximide. Valproic acid may inhibit ethosuximide, but only if the metabolism is near saturation.

TIP Ethosuximide is used in combination with valproic acid for hard-to-control absence seizures.

Sulfonamides

One sulfonamide, zonisamide (Zonegran), which comes in capsule form only, is approved as adjunctive treatment for partial seizures in adults. This drug is not approved for other uses. However, it seems to have a broad spectrum of activity for other types of seizures, including infantile spasms and myoclonic, generalized, and atypical absence seizures.

PROCEED WITH CAUTION

Adverse Reactions to Succinimides

Ethosuximide is generally well tolerated. The most common adverse reactions, which occur in up to 40 percent of patients, are nausea and vomiting. Other common adverse reactions include:

- drowsiness and fatigue
- lethargy
- dizziness
- hiccups
- headaches
- mood changes

PROCEED WITH CAUTION

Adverse Reactions to Sulfonamides

Common adverse reactions to zonisamide include:

- somnolence
- dizziness
- confusion
- anorexia
- nausea
- diarrhea
- weight loss
- rash

These effects may be eased by slow titration of dosage and by taking the medication with meals.

Zonisamide's mechanism of action is unknown. However, it's believed to involve stabilization of neuronal membranes and suppression of neuronal hypersensitivity.

Drugs that induce liver enzymes, such as phenytoin, carbamazepine, and phenobarbital, increase the metabolism and decrease the half-life of zonisamide. Use of zonisamide with drugs that inhibit or induce CYP3A4 enzymes in the liver may increase or decrease the serum concentration of zonisamide. This drug isn't an inducer of CYP3A4, so it's unlikely to affect other drugs metabolized by this system.

Zonisamide is contraindicated in patients with an allergy to sulfonamides. Low doses should be initiated in older adult patients because of the possibility of kidney impairment in this population.

ANTIMIGRAINE DRUGS

Migraine is one of the most common primary headache disorders, affecting roughly 24 million people in the United States. It produces a unilateral pain that's described as pounding, pulsing, or throbbing. It may be preceded by perception of an aura. Other common symptoms are:

- sensitivity to light or sound
- nausea and vomiting
- constipation
- diarrhea

Researchers believe that migraine symptoms are primarily caused by cranial **vasodilation**—an increase in the size of blood vessels (primarily small arteries and arterioles)—or by the release of vasoactive and proinflammatory substances from nerves in an activated trigeminal system. (Trigeminy is an irregular pulse rate consisting of three beats followed by a pause before the next three beats.) Migraines can also be triggered in some patients by certain foods, hormones, and smells.

Treatment of migraines aims to either prevent an attack (called prophylactic therapy) or to alter an attack once it's underway (called abortive or symptomatic treatment). The choice of therapy depends on the severity, duration, and frequency of the headaches; on the degree of disability that the headache creates in the patient; and on patient characteristics.

Prophylactic therapy may include:

- beta-adrenergic blockers
- tricyclic antidepressants
- valproic acid
- nonsteroidal anti-inflammatory drugs (NSAIDs)

Abortive treatments, however, may include:

- analgesics (aspirin and acetaminophen)
- NSAIDs
- ergotamine preparations
- various miscellaneous drugs such as isometheptene combinations, intranasal butorphanol, metoclopramide, and corticosteroids
- 5-hydroxytryptaminergic (5-HT$_1$) receptor agonists

The 5-HT$_1$ receptor agonists, commonly known as the **triptans**, are the treatment of choice for moderate to severe migraines.

Triptans

Triptans are serotonin 5-HT$_1$ receptor agonists. They act by:

- constricting the cranial blood vessels
- inhibiting neuropeptide release
- reducing neurologic inflammatory process transmission along the trigeminal pathway

These actions may abort the headache or provide relief from migraine symptoms. Aside from relieving pain, triptans are also effective in controlling the nausea and vomiting associated with migraines.

The choice of a triptan generally depends on three factors:

- the patient's preference for dosage form (for example, a patient experiencing nausea and vomiting may prefer a drug that comes in an injectable or intranasal form)
- the drug's onset and duration of action
- presence of recurrent migraines

When comparing the triptans, the key pharmacokinetic features are onset of action and duration of action. Generally, triptans with a longer half-life have a delayed onset of effect.

Triptans have many contraindications. They aren't for use in a number of situations or for patients with certain conditions.

- The safety of treating more than three migraine attacks in a 30-day period with triptans hasn't been established.

- A triptan shouldn't be taken within 24 hours of taking another 5-HT$_1$ receptor agonist.
- Ergotamine-containing and ergot-type drugs, such as methysergide and dihydroergotamine, shouldn't be given within 24 hours of a 5-HT$_1$ receptor agonist because prolonged vasospastic reactions (contractions of the blood vessels) may occur.
- In rare cases, certain SSRIs, such as citalopram, fluoxetine, fluvoxamine, paroxetine, and sertraline, have caused weakness, hyperreflexia, and loss of coordination when administered with a triptan. (This reaction has also been reported when the appetite suppressant sibutramine is used with a triptan.) Patients should be closely monitored if treatment with a triptan and an SSRI is required.

Triptans are contraindicated for patients with ischemic heart disease—such as angina pectoris, a past myocardial infarction, or documented silent **ischemia** (reduced blood flow)—or who present symptoms or findings consistent with ischemic heart disease. Patients with coronary artery vasospasm (including Prinzmetal variant angina) or other significant underlying cardiovascular conditions also should not be treated with triptans.

Triptans also aren't recommended for patients with risk factors for coronary artery disease (CAD), unless a cardiovascular evaluation shows the patient is relatively free from underlying CAD. These risk factors include:

- hypertension
- hypercholesterolemia (high blood cholesterol levels)
- smoking
- obesity
- diabetes
- strong family history of CAD
- female with surgical or physiological menopause
- male over age 40

 PROCEED WITH CAUTION

Adverse Reactions to Triptans

Adverse reactions to triptans may include:

- tingling, warm or hot sensation, flushing
- nasal and throat discomfort
- vision disturbances
- paresthesia
- dizziness
- fatigue or somnolence
- chest or jaw pain or pressure
- neck or throat pain
- weakness
- dry mouth
- indigestion, nausea, sweating
- injection site reaction (subcutaneous sumatriptan)
- taste disturbances (intranasal sumatriptan)

If a triptan is used in these circumstances, the first dose should be given in a physician's office or some other medically staffed and equipped facility.

Finally, triptans shouldn't be prescribed for patients with cerebrovascular syndromes such as strokes or transient ischemic attacks (TIAs). These drugs also are contraindicated in patients with peripheral vascular disease, including ischemic bowel disease. Additionally, triptans shouldn't be given to patients with uncontrolled hypertension or with certain types of migraines, such as those accompanied by hemiplegia (one-sided paralysis).

Almotriptan

Almotriptan (Axert) is taken orally as a tablet. It is used to treat acute migraine attacks. This drug has a rapid onset of action and a half-life of three to four hours. Almotriptan should not be used with or within two weeks of discontinuing an MAOI.

Eletriptan

Like almotriptan, eletriptan (Relpax) is also used to treat acute migraine attacks. It is administered orally in tablet form. Also like almotriptan, eletriptan has a half-life of three to four hours and a rapid onset of action.

In terms of drug interactions, propranolol increases the bioavailability of eletriptan. This drug also shouldn't be taken within at least 72 hours of these potent CYP3A4 inhibitors: ketoconazole, itraconazole, nefazodone, troleandomycin, clarithromycin, ritonavir, nelfinavir, or any other drugs that demonstrate potent CYP3A4 inhibition, as described in their labeling.

Frovatriptan

Frovatriptan (Frova) comes in tablet form and is taken orally to treat acute migraine attacks. This drug has the most delayed onset of action and a half-life of 25 hours.

For patients who are also taking hormonal contraceptives, the bioavailability of frovatriptan is 30 percent greater. Propranolol also increases the bioavailability of this drug.

Naratriptan

The drug naratriptan (Amerge) is administered orally as a tablet. Like the triptans mentioned previously, naratriptan is used to treat acute migraine attacks. This drug has a half-life of about six hours.

Rizatriptan

Rizatriptan (Maxalt, Maxalt MLT) comes in two forms: it can be taken orally as a tablet or an orally disintegrating tablet. Rizatriptan is used to treat acute migraine headaches. This drug has a half-life of approximately two hours.

In terms of drug interactions, rizatriptan should not be used with or within two weeks of discontinuing an MAOI. Also, the bioavailability of this drug is increased when it's taken with propranolol.

Sumatriptan

Sumatriptan (Imitrex) is used to treat acute migraine attacks. This drug is available in several forms, including:

- tablets
- nasal spray
- injection

Sumatriptan has a half-life of approximately two hours. Like almotriptan and rizatriptan, it should not be used with or within two weeks of discontinuing an MAOI.

Zolmitriptan

The drug zolmitriptan (Zomig, Zomig ZMT) may be administered in one of three ways according to the different forms of the drug available:

- oral tablets
- orally disintegrating tablets
- nasal spray

It is used to treat acute migraine headaches and has a half-life of about two hours. Like several other triptans, zolmitriptan should not be used with or within two weeks of discontinuing an MAOI.

TIP When filling prescriptions for triptans, always be sure to check: the initial dose (how many tablets), when the second dose may be taken, and the maximum daily dose.

Ergotamine Preparations

Ergotamine and its derivatives may be used as abortive or symptomatic therapy for migraines. These drugs are used to prevent or treat vascular headaches, such as migraines, migraine variant, and cluster headaches.

The antimigraine effects of ergotamine derivatives are believed to result from the blockade of neurogenic inflammation. These drugs also act as partial agonists or antagonists at serotonin, dopaminergic, and alpha-adrenergic receptors, depending on their site. They often need to be prescribed with antiemetic (antivomiting) preparations when used for migraines.

There are a number of drug interactions to be aware of when a patient is taking an ergotamine preparation:

- Propranolol and other beta-adrenergic blocking drugs block the natural pathway for vasodilation in patients receiving ergotamine preparations. This can result in excessive **vasoconstriction** (a narrowing of blood vessels) and cold extremities.
- There may be an increased risk of weakness, hyperflexion, and lack of coordination when using ergotamine preparations with SSRIs.
- Sumatriptan may cause an additive effect and increase the risk of coronary vasospasm. Ergotamine preparations and triptans should not be taken within 24 hours of each other.

PROCEED WITH CAUTION

Adverse Reactions to Ergotamine Derivatives

Possible adverse reactions to ergotamine derivatives may include:

- nausea and vomiting
- numbness
- tingling
- muscle pain
- leg weakness
- itching

Prolonged use of ergotamine derivatives may result in gangrene and rebound headaches.

- Vasoconstrictors may cause an additive effect when taken with ergotamine preparations. This increases the risk of high blood pressure.
- Drugs that inhibit certain CYP450 enzymes (such as erythromycin, clarithromycin, troleandomycin, ritonavir, nelfinavir, indinavir, and azole-derivative antifungal agents) may alter the metabolism of ergotamine. This increases the risk of vasospasm and cerebral or peripheral ischemia. These drugs shouldn't be taken together.

Ergotamine and Dihydroergotamine

Ergotamine (Ergomar) is used as therapy to abort or prevent migraine headaches. This drug is available in sublingual tablet form.

Dihydroergotamine (D.H.E. 45, Migranal) is available in injectable and intranasal forms. This drug is a hydrogenated form of ergotamine. It differs mainly in degree of activity. It has much less vasoconstrictive action than ergotamine and much less potential to cause vomiting. Dihydroergotamine is used when rapid control of migraine is desired or when other routes are undesirable.

QUICK QUIZ

Answer the following multiple-choice questions.

1. Which skeletal muscle relaxant is marketed under the brand name Valium?
   a. baclofen
   b. diazepam
   c. methocarbamol
   d. phenobarbital
2. Which of these skeletal muscle relaxants is *not* a centrally acting skeletal muscle relaxant?
   a. baclofen
   b. carisoprodol
   c. dantrolene
   d. tizanidine

3. Which of the following pairs *incorrectly* matches an antiparkinsonian drug with its brand name?
   a. procyclidine (Kemadrin)
   b. benztropine (Cogentin)
   c. ropinirole (Requip)
   d. entacapone (Alavert)
4. In what situation would the use of the drug succinylcholine be indicated?
   a. when inserting an endotracheal tube to provide breathing support
   b. to manage chronic epileptic seizures
   c. to relieve the symptoms of a migraine headache or to prevent its occurrence
   d. in treating someone who has suffered a stroke
5. Which route of administration is *not* commonly used when taking antimigraine drugs?
   a. orally in tablet form
   b. by nasal spray
   c. by injection
   d. rectally by suppository or gel

Please answer each of the following questions in one to three sentences.

1. Why is baclofen usually a better choice for treating spasticity than diazepam or dantrolene?

   _____

   _____

2. Contrast the mechanism of action of nondepolarizing and depolarizing blocking drugs.

   _____

   _____

3. Why is carbidopa usually added to the drug levodopa when levodopa is prescribed to treat Parkinson disease?

   _____

   _____

4. Identify the three major uses for anticonvulsant drugs.

   _____

   _____

5. What cardiovascular and cerebrovascular conditions in a patient would contraindicate the use of a triptan in treating migraines?

   _____

   _____

Answer the following questions as either true or false.

1. ___ Long-term use can cause patients to become physically and psychologically dependent on centrally acting skeletal muscle relaxants.
2. ___ Skeletal muscle relaxants and neuromuscular-blocking drugs are both used to treat muscle spasms.

3. ___ The most common adverse reaction to skeletal muscle relaxants is a potentially dangerous elevation in the body's liver enzymes.

4. ___ A COMT inhibitor would be the type of drug to use when treating seizures.

5. ___ The commonly used antimigraine drug sumatriptan is sold under the brand name Imitrex.

Match the generic name of each anticonvulsant drug in the left column with its classification from the right column.

1. carbamazepine	a. barbiturate
2. clonazepam	b. benzodiazepine
3. ethosuximide	c. hydantoin
4. fosphenytoin	d. iminostilbene
5. phenobarbital	e. succinimide

DRUG CLASSIFICATION TABLE

Classification	Generic Name	Trade Name(s)
Skeletal muscle relaxants	baclofen *bak'-loe-fen*	*tablets:* (no longer marketed under trade name) *injection:* Lioresal Intrathecal
	carisoprodol *ker-eye-soe-proe'-dol*	*tablets:* Soma
	carisoprodol and aspirin *ker-eye-soe-proe'-dol, ass'-purr-in*	*tablets:* (no longer marketed under trade name)
	carisoprodol, aspirin, and codeine *ker-eye-soe-proe'-dol ass'-purr-in koe'-deen*	*tablets:* (no longer marketed under trade name)
	chlorzoxazone *klor-zox'-a-zone*	*tablets:* Parafon Forte DSC, Relax DS
	cyclobenzaprine *sye-kloe-ben'-za-preen*	*tablets:* Fexmid, Flexeril *extended-release capsules:* Amrix
	diazepam *dye-az'-e-pam*	*tablets:* Valium *rectal gel:* Diastat *concentrated oral solution:* Diazepam Intensol *oral solution:* (no longer marketed under trade name) *injection:* (no longer marketed under trade name)
	metaxalone *me-taks'-a'lone*	*tablets:* Skelaxin
	methocarbamol *meth-oh-kar'-ba-mol*	*tablets:* Robaxin *injection:* Robaxin
	orphenadrine *or-fen'-a-dreen*	*tablets:* (no longer marketed under trade name) *extended release tablets:* Norflex *injection:* Norflex
	orphenadrine, aspirin, and caffeine *or-fen'-a-dreen ass'-purr-in kaf-een'*	*tablets:* (no longer marketed under trade name)
	tizanidine *tye-zan'-i-deen*	*capsules:* Zanaflex *tablets:* Zanaflex
	dantrolene *dan'-troe-leen*	*capsules:* Dantrium *injection:* Dantrium
Neuromuscular-blocking drugs	atracurium *a-tra-kyoo'-ree-um*	*injection:* (no longer marketed under trade name)
	cisatracurium *sis-a-tra-kyoo'-ree-um*	*injection:* Nimbex
	mivacurium *mye-va-kyoo'-ree-um*	*injection:* Mivacron
	pancuronium *pan-kyoo-roe'-nee-um*	*injection:* (no longer marketed under trade name)

continued

DRUG CLASSIFICATION TABLE *(continued)*

Classification	Generic Name	Trade Name(s)
Neuromuscular-blocking drugs *(continued)*	rocuronium *roe-kyoor-oh'-nee-um*	*injection:* Zemuron
	vecuronium *vek-ue-roe'-nee-um*	*injection:* (no longer marketed under trade name)
	succinylcholine *suks-in-il-koe'-leen*	*injection:* Anectine, Quelicin
Antiparkinsonian drugs	benztropine *benz'-tro-peen*	*tablets:* (no longer marketed under trade name) *injection:* Cogentin
	trihexyphenidyl *trye-hex-ee-fen'-i-dill*	*tablets:* (no longer marketed under trade name) *oral solution:* (no longer marketed under trade name)
	diphenhydramine *dye-fen-hye'-dra-meen*	*tablets:* Benadryl *capsules:* Benadryl *injection:* (no longer marketed under trade name)
	carbidopa-levodopa *kar'-bi-doe-pa lee'-voe-doe-pa*	*tablets:* Sinemet *controlled-release tablets:* Sinemet CR *orally disintegrating tablets:* Parcopa
	carbidopa, entacapone, and levodopa *kar'-bi-doe-pa en-tah-kap'-own lee'-voe-doe-pa*	*tablets:* Stalevo
	amantadine *a-man'-ta-deen*	*tablets:* Symmetrel *oral solution:* (no longer marketed under trade name) *capsules:* (no longer marketed under trade name)
	bromocriptine *broe-moe-krip'-tine*	*tablets:* Parlodel Snap Tabs *capsules:* Parlodel
	ropinirole *roe-pin'-o-role*	*tablets:* Requip *extended-release tablets:* Requip XL
	pramipexole *pram-ah-pex'-ole*	*tablets:* Mirapex
	pergolide *per'-goe-lide*	*tablets:* (no longer marketed under trade name)
	selegiline *sell-eh'-geh-leen*	*capsules:* Eldepryl *tablets:* (no longer marketed under trade name) *orally disintegrating tablets:* Zelapar *transdermal patch:* EMSAM
	tolcapone *toll-kap'-own*	*tablets:* Tasmar
	entacapone *en-tah-kap'-own*	*tablets:* Comtan
Antimigraine drugs	phenytoin *fen'-i-toe-in*	*suspension:* Dilantin *chewable tablets:* Dilantin Infatabs *extended-release capsules:* Dilantin, Phenytek *injection:* (no longer marketed under trade name)

continued

DRUG CLASSIFICATION TABLE *(continued)*

Classification	Generic Name	Trade Name(s)
Antimigraine drugs *(continued)*	fosphenytoin *fos'-fen-i-toyn*	*injection:* Cerebyx
	ethotoin *eth'-i-toe-in*	*tablets:* Peganone
	phenobarbital *fee-noe-bar'-bi-tal*	*injection:* Luminal *tablets:* (no longer marketed under trade name) *oral solution:* (no longer marketed under trade name)
	mephobarbital *me-foe-bar'-bi-tal*	*tablets:* Mebaral
	primidone *pri'-mi-done*	*tablets:* Mysoline
	carbamazepine *kar-ba-maz'-e-peen*	*tablets:* Epitol, Tegretol *extended-release tablets:* Tegretol XR *chewable tablets:* Tegretol *extended-release capsules:* Equetro, Carbatrol *suspension:* Tegretol
	clonazepam *clo-nay'-zeh-pam*	*tablets:* Klonopin *orally disintegrating tablets:* Klonopin Wafer
	diazepam *dye-az'-e-pam*	*tablets:* Valium *concentrated oral solution:* Diazepam Intensol *oral solution:* (no longer marketed under trade name) *rectal gel:* Diastat *injection:* (no longer marketed under trade name)
	lorazepam *lor-a'-ze-pam*	*tablets:* Ativan *injection:* Ativan *concentrated oral solution:* Lorazepam Intensol
	clorazepate *klor-az'-e-pate*	*tablets:* Tranxene-T *extended-release tablets:* Tranxene-SD
	valproic acid *val-proe'-ik*	*capsules:* Depakene, Stavzor *oral solution:* Depakene
	valproate *val-proe'-ate*	*injection:* Depacon
	divalproex *dye-val-proe'-ex*	*tablets:* Depakote *extended release tablets:* Depakote ER *capsules:* Depakote Sprinkles
	gabapentin *gab-ah-pen'-tin*	*tablets:* Neurontin *capsules:* Neurontin *oral solution:* Neurontin
	lamotrigine *la-mo'-tri-geen*	*tablets:* Lamictal *chewable tablets:* Lamictal CD *orally disintegrating tablets:* Lamictal ODT
	oxcarbazepine *ox-car-baz'-e-peen*	*tablets:* Trileptal *oral suspension:* Trileptal
	topiramate *toe-pyre'-a-mate*	*tablets:* Topamax *capsules:* Topamax Sprinkle

continued

DRUG CLASSIFICATION TABLE (continued)

Classification	Generic Name	Trade Name(s)
Antimigraine drugs (continued)	ethosuximide *eth-oh-sux'-i-mide*	*capsules:* Zarontin *oral syrup:* Zarontin *oral solution:* (no longer marketed under trade name)
	methsuximide *meth-sux'-i-mide*	*capsules:* Celontin
	zonisamide *zoh-niss'-ah-mide*	*capsules:* Zonegran
Anticonvulsant drugs	almotriptan *al-moh-trip'-tan*	*tablets:* Axert
	eletriptan *el-e-trip'-tan*	*tablets:* Relpax
	frovatriptan *froe-va-trip'-tan*	*tablets:* Frova
	naratriptan *nar'-a-trip-tan*	*tablets:* Amerge
	rizatriptan *rye-za-trip'-tan*	*tablets:* Maxalt *orally disintegrating tablets:* Maxalt MLT
	sumatriptan *soo'-ma-trip'-tan*	*tablets:* Imitrex *nasal spray:* Imitrex *injection:* Imitrex
	zolmitriptan *zohl-mi-trip'-tan*	*tablets:* Zomig *nasal spray:* Zomig *orally disintegrating tablets:* Zomig ZMT
	ergotamine *er-got'-a-meen*	*sublingual tablets:* Ergomar
	ergotamine and caffeine *er-got'-a-meen kaf-een'*	*tablets:* Cafergot *rectal suppositories:* Migergot
	dihydroergotamine *dye-hye-droe-er-got'-a-meen*	*nasal spray:* Migranal *injection:* D.H.E. 45

CHAPTER 4

Drugs for Pain, Fever, and Inflammation

CHAPTER OBJECTIVES

- Match brand and generic names of commonly used drugs for pain, fever, and inflammation
- Identify the classification of commonly used drugs for pain, fever, and inflammation
- Recognize commonly used drugs for pain, fever, and inflammation as prescription or over-the-counter drugs
- Describe the different uses of aspirin
- Compare and contrast the mechanisms of action for salicylates, acetaminophen, and NSAIDs
- List common adverse reactions of commonly used drugs for pain, fever, and inflammation
- Match common drug interactions of commonly used drugs for pain, fever, and inflammation with the appropriate drug and category
- Match brand and generic names of opioid agonists, mixed agonist-antagonists, and antagonists with the appropriate category
- Identify commonly used inhalation anesthetics
- Identify commonly used injection anesthetics

KEY TERMS

acetaminophen—an OTC drug that has analgesic and antipyretic properties

analgesic—a drug used to control or relieve pain without causing the patient to lose consciousness

anesthetic drugs—drugs that block the perception or cause a loss of feeling, allowing the patient to undergo medical procedures without distress and pain

angioedema—swelling of the mucosal tissues beneath the skin resulting in welts

antipyretic—a drug that lowers an elevated body temperature

ataxia—a loss of control of voluntary movements, especially producing an unsteady gait

black box warning—a warning required by the FDA for certain drugs that lists any serious or life-threatening adverse reactions

competitive inhibition—process in which an antagonist drug stops an agonist drug from acting by filling up the receptor cells

endorphins—naturally occurring opiates that are part of the body's pain relief system

epidural block—a type of anesthesia administered during childbirth in which a drug is injected into the outer lining of the spinal cord (epidural space)

inhalation anesthetics—anesthetic drugs that are brought into the body through the lungs

intravenous anesthetics—anesthetic drugs that are administered directly into a vein

leukopenia—an abnormal decrease in a specific type of white blood cell, or leukocytes

local anesthetics—drugs that block pain and other sensations in a specific body part

mixed opioid agonist-antagonists—drugs that act like agonists and antagonists by relieving pain and reducing the risk of adverse reactions

myasthenia gravis—a disease that causes fatigue of skeletal muscles because of the lack of acetylcholine released at the nerve endings of parasympathetic nerve fibers

narcotic agonists—see *opioid agonists*

neurotoxicity—condition involving damage to the nerves or nervous tissue

nonsteroidal anti-inflammatory drugs (NSAIDs)—a class of drugs that act to reduce pain, fever, and inflammation by stopping the body from producing prostaglandins

opioids—derivatives of the opium plant or synthetic drugs that imitate natural narcotics

opioid agonists—controlled substances used to relieve or decrease pain without causing loss of consciousness in the patient

opioid antagonists—drugs that work against opioid agonists to block their effects and reverse adverse reactions; also known as *narcotic agonists*

osteoarthritis—a chronic disease that involves wear and deterioration of joints in the body, causing inflammation

phenazopyridine hydrochloride—dye used in commercial coloring that helps relieve symptoms associated with urinary tract infections

phlebitis—inflammation of a vein

prostaglandin—a chemical found in most body fluids and tissues that makes nerve cells sensitive to pain

pruritus—itching

Reye syndrome—a potentially life-threatening disorder that affects children by damaging the brain and liver

rheumatic fever—a disease associated with a delayed response to a previous streptococcal infection in the body and characterized by fever and pain in the joints

rheumatoid arthritis—a chronic inflammatory disease of the peripheral joints

salicylates—a commonly used class of drugs for controlling pain, fever, and inflammation

thrombocytopenia—an abnormal decrease in the number of platelets circulating in the blood

tinnitus—a sensation of ringing or buzzing in the ears

topical anesthetics—drugs that are applied to the skin and mucous membranes to block pain and other sensations in a specific area of the body

urticaria—a skin condition commonly known as hives that involves red, itchy, or swollen areas of the skin

volatility—a property of liquids that causes them to evaporate and become gas when exposed to air

A wide range of drugs are used to control pain. They range from mild over-the-counter (OTC) drugs, such as aspirin and acetaminophen, to strong general anesthetics. Drugs that relieve pain often reduce fever and inflammation (swelling), too. In this chapter, you'll learn about drugs for pain, fever, and inflammation that are used to treat conditions such as:

- mild to moderate pain caused by injury or surgery
- fever, headaches, and painful menstruation
- **rheumatoid arthritis** (a chronic inflammatory disease of the peripheral joints)
- **osteoarthritis** (a chronic disease that involves wear and deterioration of joints in the body, causing inflammation)
- chronic pain associated with cancer, AIDS, multiple sclerosis, or sickle cell disease

T I P Acute pain lasts for short periods of time, often less than three months. Chronic pain may last for years.

NONOPIOID ANALGESICS, ANTIPYRETICS, AND NONSTEROIDAL ANTI-INFLAMMATORY DRUGS

Drugs that control pain without causing the patient to lose consciousness are referred to as **analgesics**.

- Nonopioid analgesic drugs are drugs that are not derived from the opium plant. They do not cause physical dependence in patients.
- Opioid analgesic drugs are synthetic (human made) or are made from the opium plant. These drugs may cause physical dependence.

Nonsteroidal anti-inflammatory drugs are better known as **NSAIDs**. The body's natural response to injury, irritation, or infection is inflammation. Signs of inflammation include redness, swelling, pain, and heat. Anti-inflammatory drugs reduce the swelling and pain of inflammation.

Nonopioid analgesics and NSAIDs affect the body in similar ways. When nonopioid analgesics and NSAIDs enter the body, they stop the body from producing **prostaglandin**. Prostaglandin is a chemical that makes nerve cells sensitive to pain. It is found in almost all body fluids and tissues. Preventing the body from making prostaglandin may have two main effects:

- *Analgesic effect.* When prostaglandin is released, the body becomes sensitive to pain. By stopping the body from producing prostaglandin, nonopioid analgesics and NSAIDs reduce the pain response.
- *Anti-inflammatory effect.* Stopping prostaglandin is also believed to reduce the pain and swelling of the body's inflammatory response. However, only some nonopioid analgesics have an anti-inflammatory effect.

Nonopioid analgesic drugs and NSAIDs are also **antipyretics**, meaning they can reduce body temperature to control fever. These drugs reduce fever by stimulating a gland called the hypothalamus. With the hypothalamus (a region of the brain that regulates temperature and other body processes) in action, peripheral blood vessels (in the feet, legs, arms, lower abdomen, neck, or head) enlarge, and sweating increases. This results in the body's loss of heat through the skin and cooling by evaporation.

There are four main groups of nonopioid analgesic and antipyretic drugs:

- salicylates
- nonsalicylate analgesics
- NSAIDs
- the urinary tract analgesic phenazopyridine hydrochloride

T I P Because nonopioid analgesic drugs and NSAIDs are often taken with other medications, patients need to be aware of possible drug interactions.

Salicylates

Salicylates are among the most commonly used medications for controlling pain, fever, and inflammation. They are available over the counter or by prescription and usually cost less than other analgesics. Salicylates are mainly used for the following:

- relieving mild to moderate pain
- reducing fever
- reducing inflammation from **rheumatic fever** (a disease characterized by fever and pain in the joints), rheumatoid arthritis, and osteoarthritis

Salicylates relieve headache and muscle aches at the same time. They can provide considerable relief in 24 hours for the inflammation of arthritis. However, they are not effective for relieving pain of the organs or smooth muscles. They are also not effective for controlling severe pain from trauma.

The various forms of salicylates have different ways of acting on the body and producing effects. They relieve pain by stopping the body from producing prostaglandin. Stopping prostaglandin production may reduce inflammation. Because prostaglandin E increases body temperature, this also reduces fever. Although salicylates will bring down a higher-than-normal body temperature, they won't decrease the temperature below normal.

Salicylates are taken orally or rectally. Some salicylates are given rectally using suppositories. This form is absorbed slowly and in an unpredictable way. Most salicylates are given by mouth.

T I P Food or antacids in the stomach will slow down the body's absorption of salicylates.

Salicylates have specific interactions with several types of drugs. Patients need to be aware of the following interactions:

- Oral anticoagulants, heparin, methotrexate, oral antidiabetic agents, and insulin have increased effects or an increased risk of toxicity when taken with salicylates.
- Probenecid, sulfinpyrazone, and spironolactone may have decreased efficacy when taken with salicylates.
- Corticosteroids may decrease the levels of salicylates in plasma (the liquid part of blood). This may increase the risk of ulcers.
- Alkalinizing drugs and antacids may reduce levels of salicylates in the body.
- The antihypertensive effect of angiotensin-converting enzyme (ACE) inhibitors and beta-adrenergic blockers may be reduced when these drugs are combined with salicylates.
- NSAIDs may be less effective when taken with salicylates. Taking NSAIDs and salicylates together may also increase the risk of gastrointestinal effects.

! PROCEED WITH CAUTION

Adverse Reactions to Salicylates

Adverse reactions for salicylates vary from drug to drug. The most common adverse reactions include:

- gastric distress
- nausea
- vomiting
- bleeding tendencies

Acetylsalicylic Acid

Acetylsalicylic acid is better known as ASA or aspirin. It's used to treat mild to moderate pain, fever, and inflammation. It may also be used to reduce the risk of heart attack or to prevent blood from clotting. ASA is available over the counter in several dosage forms and many trade names. The most common dosage forms and trade names are:

- chewing gum (Aspergum)
- chewable tablets (Bayer Children's Aspirin, St. Joseph Adult Chewable Aspirin)
- tablets (Bayer)
- enteric-coated tablets (Ecotrin, Halfprin)
- delayed-release tablets Bayer
- extended-release tablets (Extended Release Bayer 8-Hour)

By prescription, ASA is available as tablets (ZORprin, Easprin).

T I P Aspirin interferes with the ability of blood platelets to gather and form clots. For this reason, physicians often recommend a dose between 75 and 100 mg of aspirin daily to reduce the chance of heart attack or angina.

In tablet form, ASA may be enteric-coated to reduce gastric irritation. In delayed-release forms, the ASA is formulated so that it takes longer to begin acting, which reduces gastric irritation. Extended-release forms are formulated so the effects last for longer periods of time.

ASA is also available over the counter in buffered forms. Buffered aspirin (Ascriptin, Bufferin) contains small amounts of antacids to decrease GI irritation. Buffered forms of aspirin have similar dosages as other tablet forms of aspirin. Because they are absorbed more slowly, they are often used for the treatment of long-term conditions, such as arthritis.

ASA may have adverse effects that are not found with other salicylates:

- **leukopenia** (decrease in white blood cells)
- prolonged bleeding time
- **thrombocytopenia** (decrease in blood platelets)

Choline Magnesium Trisalicylate

Choline magnesium trisalicylate is available by prescription. It's used to treat osteoarthritis, rheumatoid arthritis, and acute painful shoulder syndrome. This drug is administered by mouth in tablet or oral liquid form.

Diflunisal and Salsalate

Diflunisal (Dolobid) is used to treat osteoarthritis and rheumatoid arthritis. It may also be used to relieve mild to

moderate pain. It is not used to reduce fever. Diflunisal is available by prescription in an oral tablet form. It is usually taken with food, water, or milk. This drug may greatly increase levels of acetaminophen and other NSAIDs. Patients should be advised not to use these drugs while taking diflunisal.

Salsalate (Argesic-SA) is used to treat mild pain and to reduce fever. It may also be used to treat pain and inflammation caused by arthritis. Salsalate comes in tablet form to be taken by mouth.

Acetaminophen

Acetaminophen belongs to a group of drugs called para-aminophenol (APAP) derivatives. Acetaminophen is an OTC drug that has analgesic (pain-relieving) and anti-pyretic (fever-reducing) properties. Similar to salicylates, acetaminophen affects the central nervous system. Although the way it works is not completely known, it is believed to stop the body from making prostaglandin. It relieves fever by acting on the hypothalamus.

Unlike salicylates, acetaminophen does not have an anti-inflammatory effect. It also does not affect the way blood platelets work to form clots. Acetaminophen is used to treat the following:

- fever
- headache
- muscle ache
- general pain

Acetaminophen is also the preferred drug for treating fever and flu-like symptoms in children. The American Arthritis Association notes that acetaminophen is an effective pain reliever for some types of arthritis.

Acetaminophen can interact with several other drugs. Patients should be aware of the following interactions:

- The effects of oral anticoagulants and thrombolytic drugs such as warfarin may be slightly increased when taken with acetaminophen.
- The risk of liver toxicity is increased when acetaminophen is combined with long-term alcohol use, phenytoin, barbiturates, carbamazepine, or isoniazid. Therefore, dosages should be monitored in long-term use, and the maximum daily dose of acetaminophen for adults is four grams.
- The effects of some drugs may be reduced when taken with acetaminophen. These drugs include lamotrigine, loop diuretics, and zidovudine.

T I P Beware of acetaminophen in disguise! Many OTC and prescription medications contain acetaminophen in combination with other drugs. Patients need to take this into account when they manage their total daily dose.

Acetaminophen is absorbed quickly from the GI tract (when taken orally) or from the mucous layer of the rectum (when administered rectally). Forms and common trade names of acetaminophen include:

- tablets (Aspirin Free Anacin, Tylenol)
- chewable tablets
- delayed-release tablets (Tylenol)
- orally dissolving tablets (Tylenol)
- elixir
- drops (Tylenol)
- rectal suppositories (Acephen, Feverall)
- oral suspension (Tylenol)
- oral solution (Comtrex, Tylenol)
- capsules

Oral liquid forms such as drops or elixir are used for children and patients who have difficulty swallowing. It is important to note that infant formulations (concentrated drops) are highly concentrated; therefore, the amount of medication that must be swallowed is less than the equivalent of an oral liquid. This is helpful for caregivers who are administering acetaminophen to infants, who have difficulty swallowing a great deal of liquid at a time.

For example, when administering 80 mg of Tylenol Infants' Drops, the infant would receive one dropper, which is 0.8 mL. The equivalent dose of Children's Tylenol liquid would be 1/2 teaspoon, or 2.5 mL. If the liquid dose of the concentrated drops were given instead, the infant would receive 200 mg, which is indicated for an infant weighing twice as much. Clarifying the difference between concentrated drops and liquid forms of acetaminophen is key in helping prevent an infant from receiving an overdose.

Children should not receive more than five doses of acetaminophen in a 24-hour period. In adults who have a history of alcohol abuse, their use of this drug should be limited to two grams per day. The maximum daily dose for long-term therapy is four grams, unless the patient is closely monitored by a health care provider.

T I P Doses of APAP higher than four grams per day can cause liver toxicity, so you will need to check the dosing on all APAP prescriptions that you receive. If a patient is receiving a prescription medication with APAP, you'll need to pay close attention to any other prescription or OTC medications the patient consumes at the same time, to see if they contain additional APAP.

Nonsteroidal Anti-Inflammatory Drugs

NSAIDs are typically used to combat inflammation. Their anti-inflammatory effect is equal to aspirin. Similar to salicylates, NSAIDs have analgesic and antipyretic effects. NSAIDs may affect blood platelets, but unlike aspirin, their effects are temporary. Some NSAIDs are available over the counter, and others are available only by prescription.

NSAIDs have been useful in treating the following conditions:

- ankylosing spondylitis (an inflammatory joint disease that affects the spine)
- moderate to severe rheumatoid arthritis (an inflammatory disease of the peripheral joints)
- osteoarthritis (a degenerative joint disease) in the hip, shoulder, or other large joints
- acute gouty arthritis (urate deposits in the joints)
- dysmenorrhea (severe pain and cramping during menstruation)
- migraine headaches
- bursitis and tendonitis
- mild to moderate pain

All NSAIDs are absorbed through the GI tract. They're mostly metabolized in the liver and are excreted primarily by the kidneys. NSAIDs work by acting on enzymes known as cyclooxygenase-1 (COX-1) and cyclooxygenase-2 (COX-2). Enzymes are special proteins that trigger chemical reactions in the body. COX-1 and COX-2 enzymes convert arachidonic acid, one of the essential fatty acids, into prostaglandins. The prostaglandin made by COX-1 maintains the stomach lining. Prostaglandin produced by COX-2, however, causes inflammation. When NSAIDs stop COX-1 and COX-2 from making prostaglandins, they reduce inflammation.

There are two types of NSAIDs:

- Nonselective NSAIDS block both COX-1 and COX-2. Because COX-1 makes prostaglandins that maintain the stomach lining, nonselective NSAIDs may cause adverse GI effects.
- Selective NSAIDs are sometimes called COX-2 inhibitors. They block only the prostaglandins made by COX-2. They relieve pain and inflammation without causing significant GI effects.

People who take NSAIDs may have a higher risk of having a heart attack or a stroke than people who don't take these medications. Manufacturers of NSAIDs typically include warnings about the risk of cardiac effects on the labels. This risk may be greater for patients who take NSAIDs over long periods of time or for patients with cardiovascular conditions. NSAIDs also stop the body from making renal prostaglandins and may affect kidney function. Patients with kidney, heart, or liver conditions are at higher risk for kidney damage when taking NSAIDs.

Nonselective Nonsteroidal Anti-Inflammatory Drugs

Many nonselective NSAIDs are available over the counter. They are used to treat the pain and inflammation of osteoarthritis and rheumatoid arthritis.

Nonselective NSAIDs may interact with other medications. Patients need to be aware of the following interactions:

- Nonselective NSAIDs may decrease the antihypertensive effects of ACE inhibitors.

- Taking antacids with nonselective NSAIDs may reduce the level of NSAIDs in the body.
- Nonselective NSAIDs taken with aspirin may increase the patient's risk of developing ulcers. Patients need to be monitored for signs of gastrointestinal bleeding.
- Taking lithium with some nonselective NSAIDs may increase lithium levels in the body.
- Nonselective NSAIDs taken with warfarin or anticoagulants may increase bleeding complications.
- Nonselective NSAIDs may increase levels of methotrexate, digoxin, and cyclosporine, leading to toxicity.

T I P Remind patients to follow package/prescription directions about the dose and duration of treatment of NSAIDs, especially since there are potential cardiovascular and GI risks involved.

Diclofenac

Diclofenac sodium (Voltaren, Voltaren XR, Solaraze) and diclofenac potassium (Cataflam) are used in the treatment of:

- ankylosing spondylitis
- actinic keratosis
- osteoarthritis
- rheumatoid arthritis
- dysmenorrhea
- pain

! PROCEED WITH CAUTION

Adverse Reactions to Nonselective Nonsteroidal Anti-Inflammatory Drugs

Because nonselective NSAIDs inhibit COX-1 and COX-2 enzymes, they may also cause unwanted GI effects, such as bleeding or increased risk of ulcers.

There are also many other adverse reactions associated with NSAIDs. However, most patients experience few adverse effects. The adverse reactions to nonselective NSAIDs include:

- constipation
- diarrhea
- dizziness
- drowsiness
- GI upset or pain
- GI bleeding
- ulcers
- headache
- nausea
- rash
- visual disturbances
- vomiting

Diclofenac is available by prescription. It comes in tablets to be taken by mouth. The tablets are available in delayed-release or extended-release forms. This drug is also available as a topical gel and ophthalmic solution.

Etodolac, Fenoprofen, and Flurbiprofen

Etodolac is available by prescription for managing the pain and inflammation of osteoarthritis and rheumatoid arthritis, as well as for acute pain. It is available in capsule, tablet, and extended-release tablet forms.

Fenoprofen (Nalfon) is used for long-term management of mild to moderate pain. It's also used in the treatment of rheumatoid arthritis and osteoarthritis. This drug is available by prescription as capsules or tablets.

Flurbiprofen is used in treating the signs and symptoms of rheumatoid arthritis and osteoarthritis. It is also prescribed for treating ankylosing spondylitis. It is available by prescription in tablet form and ophthalmic solution.

Ibuprofen

Ibuprofen is commonly used to control fever in adults and children. It's also used to treat mild to moderate pain and menstrual pain, in addition to treating symptoms of osteoarthritis and rheumatoid arthritis. Ibuprofen is available by prescription and over the counter in several different forms:

- tablets (Advil, Motrin IB, Midol Cramps and Body Aches Formula)
- prescription-strength tablets (Motrin)
- chewable tablets (Advil, Motrin)
- caplets (Motrin IB, Advil)
- liquid-gel capsules (Advil, Motrin IB)
- gelcaps (Motrin IB)
- drops (Advil, Motrin)
- oral suspension (Advil, Motrin)

T I P You need to know which NSAIDs are prescription and which are over the counter. Some NSAIDs are available in prescription and nonprescription strengths. Know the labeling and dosing differences. For example, nonprescription ibuprofen is 200 mg, but the prescription forms of this drug come in 400-mg, 600-mg, and 800-mg strengths.

Indomethacin

Indomethacin (Indocin) is available by prescription. It is used to relieve moderate to severe pain for several different chronic conditions, including:

- osteoarthritis
- rheumatoid arthritis
- ankylosing spondylitis
- gouty arthritis
- acute painful shoulder syndrome (bursitis or tendonitis)

Indomethacin may also be prescribed in the treatment of patent ductus arteriosus in newborn babies. This is a heart problem involving abnormal blood circulation. In babies, indomethacin is given by IV injection. For other conditions, the drug is available in several different forms:

- capsules
- sustained-release capsules
- oral suspension
- suppositories

Dosages vary with the form of the drug. Capsules, sustained-release capsules, and oral suspensions should be taken with food, milk, or antacids to prevent GI upset.

Like other NSAIDs, indomethacin may interact with many other drugs. In addition to the interactions that may affect all drugs in this class, you need to be aware of the following possible interactions for indomethacin:

- Indomethacin taken with bisphosphonates may increase the patient's risk of GI ulcer formation.
- Taking diflunisal or probenecid with indomethacin may increase levels of indomethacin.
- Indomethacin may increase levels of penicillamine, increasing the risk of toxic effects.
- Taking indomethacin with triamterene may cause damage to the kidneys. This combination should be avoided.

Ketoprofen, Ketorolac, and Meloxicam

Prescription ketoprofen is used to treat pain and inflammation from osteoarthritis and rheumatoid arthritis. It may also be prescribed to treat painful menstruation. It is available in capsules and extended-release capsules.

Ketorolac is prescribed for short-term management of severe, acute pain. It may be administered as a single-dose treatment by mouth or by IM or IV injection. Ketorolac may also be given as a multiple-dose treatment in the form of tablets, injection, or ophthalmic solution. Ketorolac stops platelets from gathering to form clots. In addition to the adverse reactions that are typical of other nonselective NSAIDs, patients taking ketorolac have an increased risk of prolonged bleeding time for up to 48 hours after taking the drug.

Meloxicam (Mobic) may be used in treating juvenile rheumatoid arthritis as well as osteoarthritis and rheumatoid arthritis. It is available by prescription. Meloxicam is taken by mouth as an oral suspension or as tablets.

Nabumetone

Nabumetone is available by prescription in tablet form. Fewer adverse reactions are associated with nabumetone than with many other NSAIDs. Nabumetone also has fewer reported interactions with other drugs than the other NSAIDs in this class. You should be aware of the following drug interactions:

- Taking nabumetone with diuretics may decrease the effectiveness of the diuretics.

- Nabumetone may cause adverse reactions when taken with warfarin or other highly protein-bound drugs.

Naproxen

Naproxen and naproxen sodium are used to treat osteoarthritis and rheumatoid arthritis as well as many other conditions, including:

- ankylosing spondylitis
- painful menstruation
- tendonitis
- bursitis
- juvenile arthritis
- acute gout
- mild to moderate pain

Naproxen is available by prescription in several different forms, including:

- extended-release tablets (EC-Naprosyn)
- tablets (Naprosyn)
- oral suspension (Naprosyn)

Over the counter, naproxen sodium is available in the form of tablets, caplets, and gelcaps (Aleve) and extended-release tablets (Midol Extended Relief). Naproxen sodium is also available by prescription. This drug comes in the form of tablets (Anaprox) and extended-release tablets (Naprelan).

T I P Similar to aspirin, naproxen may protect the heart by preventing blood from clotting.

In addition to the adverse reactions typical of other drugs in this class, patients using naproxen may have an increased risk of the following:

- edema
- prolonged bleeding time
- palpitations
- **tinnitus** (ringing in the ears)

Taking probenecid with naproxen may decrease the body's ability to eliminate naproxen. This increases the risk of toxicity.

T I P Most NSAIDs should be taken with food or milk to protect the stomach. When filling prescriptions for these drugs, be sure to place a "Take with food" auxiliary label on the vial.

Oxaprozin, Piroxicam, and Sulindac

Oxaprozin (Daypro) is used to treat osteoarthritis and rheumatoid arthritis in adults and juvenile arthritis in children older than six years of age. It is available by prescription in tablet form.

Piroxicam (Feldene) is available by prescription for treating symptoms of osteoarthritis and rheumatoid arthritis. It's administered by mouth as a capsule. In addition to

Concerns About Nonselective Nonsteroidal Anti-Inflammatory Drugs

Before distributing nonsteroidal anti-inflammatory drugs, you need to be aware of some concerns for special groups:

- *Children.* Some nonselective NSAIDs are not recommended for use in children. However, ibuprofen is commonly used for reducing fever in children.
- *Elderly patients.* The risk of ulcers increases with age.
- *Pregnant women.* Some nonselective NSAIDs are pregnancy risk category B drugs, meaning there is no evidence of risk in humans. These include diclofenac, ketoprofen, and naproxen. Other nonselective NSAIDs are classified as pregnancy risk category C drugs, such as etodolac, ketorolac, meloxicam, nabumetone, oxaprozin, and piroxicam. Most NSAIDs appear in breast milk. It is best to advise patients who are breastfeeding not to use these drugs.

the adverse reactions of other drugs in this class, patients using piroxicam may have an increased risk of prolonged bleeding.

Sulindac (Clinoril) is used in the treatment of bursitis, tendonitis, and acute gouty arthritis, as well as for symptoms of osteoarthritis and rheumatoid arthritis. It's available by prescription in tablet form.

Misoprostol

Misoprostol (Cytotec) is available in tablet form and is manufactured alone or in combination with nonselective NSAIDs to help protect the stomach from NSAID-induced gastric ulcers. Because this drug can cause abortion, premature birth, or birth defects, it should not be taken by pregnant women to reduce the risk of NSAID-induced ulcers.

Selective Nonsteroidal Anti-Inflammatory Drugs

Selective NSAIDs are better known as COX-2 inhibitors, because they block only the prostaglandins made by COX-2 enzymes. This reduces the possibility of some adverse GI effects, such as ulcers, compared to nonselective NSAIDs.

The only COX-2 inhibitor currently available is celecoxib (Celebrex). This drug is used to relieve pain and inflammation associated with the following:

- osteoarthritis
- rheumatoid arthritis
- ankylosing spondylitis

Celecoxib is also effective for relieving pain associated with dysmenorrhea and as part of the treatment program for familial adenomatous polyposis (an inherited condition in which small polyps form in the colon). Celecoxib is available by prescription only and comes in capsule form. Celecoxib should always include the use of a **black box warning**.

(A black box warning lists any serious or life-threatening adverse reactions to the drug.)

In recent years, several COX-2 inhibitors have been withdrawn from the market. Because prostaglandins are involved in regulating blood pressure, COX-2 inhibitors may cause adverse cardiovascular effects. The use of COX-2 inhibitors also increases the risk of serious GI bleeding.

COX-2 inhibitors are classified as pregnancy risk category C drugs; most appear in breast milk. They are not recommended for women who are breastfeeding.

Similar to nonselective NSAIDs, COX-2 inhibitors may interact with other drugs. Some drug interactions that you should be aware of include the following:

- Taking COX-2 inhibitors with ACE inhibitors may lead to blood pressure difficulties.
- Antacids containing aluminum and magnesium may decrease the level of COX-2 inhibitors. These medications should be taken at separate times.
- Taking COX-2 inhibitors with aspirin leads to an increased risk of ulcers. Patients need to be monitored for GI bleeding.
- Fluconazole may have the effect of increasing the level of COX-2 inhibitors.
- Furosemide and thiazides taken with COX-2 inhibitors may increase sodium retention. This results in a higher risk of swelling and increased blood pressure.
- Taking lithium with COX-2 inhibitors may increase lithium levels.
- COX-2 inhibitors taken with warfarin increases anticoagulant effects and may lead to bleeding complications.

Phenazopyridine Hydrochloride

Phenazopyridine hydrochloride is a dye used in commercial coloring that helps relieve symptoms associated with urinary tract infections, including:

Adverse Reactions to COX-2 Inhibitors

COX-2 inhibitors may cause the following adverse reactions:

- dyspepsia
- nausea
- vomiting
- GI ulcers (to a lesser degree than with nonselective NSAIDs)
- hypertension
- fluid retention
- peripheral edema
- dizziness
- headache

AT THE COUNTER

Stain Savvy

A patient picks up two prescriptions for a urinary tract infection: SMZ-TMP and phenazopyridine. The patient remembers that one of the medications will change the color of her urine, but she cannot remember which one. What should you tell her?

Tell the patient that phenazopyridine turns urine an orange or brownish color. Remind her that the urine will stain anything it touches, including clothing and possibly the toilet seat.

- pain
- burning
- urgency
- frequency

Taken orally, only 35 percent of phenazopyridine is metabolized by the liver. The rest is excreted unchanged in the urine. This causes the patient's urine to turn an orange or brown color.

Phenazopyridine is available over the counter (Azo-Gesic, Azo-Standard) and by prescription (Pyridium). It comes as a tablet to be taken by mouth. Phenazopyridine is usually taken three times a day after meals with a full glass of water. Phenazopyridine should not be taken for more than two days.

Phenazopyridine is sometimes included in combination with other drugs and does not cause any significant food or drug interactions. However, patients need to be aware of the following possible adverse reactions:

- If this drug builds up in the body, the patient's skin and sclera (whites of the eyes) may take on a yellow tinge. If this occurs, the patient may need to discontinue use of the drug.
- Acute renal or hepatic failure may occur.

OPIOID AGONIST AND ANTAGONIST DRUGS

The word **opioid** refers to derivatives of the opium plant (also known as opiates) or to synthetic drugs that imitate natural narcotics.

- **Opioid agonists** are controlled substances used to relieve or decrease pain without causing the patient to lose consciousness. These drugs are sometimes called **narcotic agonists**.
- **Opioid antagonists** are drugs that work against opioid agonists to block their effects and reverse adverse reactions, such as respiratory and CNS depression, produced by those drugs.

Some drugs are classified as **mixed opioid agonist-antagonists**. These drugs act like agonists *and* antagonists by relieving pain and reducing the risk of adverse reactions.

Opioids are typically used in treating moderate to severe acute pain and in treating chronic pain resulting from cancer and other diseases.

Opioid Agonists

Opioid agonists are mainly used to manage moderate to severe acute and chronic pain. They work by binding with opiate receptors in the central and peripheral nervous systems. When these drugs stimulate the receptors, they mimic the effects of **endorphins**. Endorphins are naturally occurring opiates that are part of the body's pain relief system. In binding with the receptors, opioid agonists provide pain control. The binding process also has the following effects on the body:

- antidiarrheal action (controlling diarrhea)
- contraction of the bladder and ureters (causing the urge to urinate more frequently)
- constriction of the bronchial muscles (reducing respiration rate)
- dilation of blood vessels, especially in the face, head, and neck
- slowing of intestinal peristalsis, or the contractions that move food along the digestive tract (resulting in constipation)
- suppression of the cough center in the brain

Opioid agonists may be administered in many different ways. Opioid agonists administered by IV injection provide the most rapid and immediate pain relief. Subcutaneous and intramuscular injections may delay the absorption of the drug, especially in patients with poor circulation. Also, many of these opioids are available as bulk powders for compounding purposes. Because opioid agonists are metabolized in the liver, the levels of the drug in the body may build up in patients with liver failure. This can cause an increased risk of **neurotoxicity** (damage to the nervous system) and seizures.

Opioid agonists have specific interactions with other drugs. Patients need to be aware of the following:

- Opioid agonists decrease breathing rate and depth. The use of opioid agonists with other drugs that also decrease respiration, such as alcohol, sedatives, hypnotics, and anesthetics, increases the patient's risk of severe respiratory depression, which can be fatal.
- Taking tricyclic antidepressants, phenothiazines, or anticholinergics with opioid agonists may cause severe constipation or urine retention.
- Drugs that may affect the analgesic effect of opioid agonists include amitriptyline, diazepam, phenytoin, protease inhibitors, and rifampin.
- Drugs that may be affected by opioid analgesics include carbamazepine, warfarin, beta-adrenergic blockers, and calcium-channel blockers.

PROCEED WITH CAUTION

Adverse Reactions to Opioid Agonists

One of the most common adverse reactions to opioid agonists is decreased rate and depth of breathing that worsens as the dose of the opioid is increased. This may cause periodic, irregular breathing or may trigger asthmatic attacks in susceptible patients. Other adverse reactions include:

- constipation
- flushing
- orthostatic hypotension
- pupil constriction

Codeine

Codeine is a Schedule II controlled substance, which indicates that it has a high potential for abuse and dependence. Codeine phosphate is available as a subcutaneous injection. Codeine sulfate is available in tablet form. Codeine is also available in combination with other drugs, such as codeine with acetaminophen (Tylenol with Codeine), which is a Schedule III controlled substance. Because codeine acts directly on the cough center in the brain, it can suppress the cough reflex. Cough medications that contain codeine, such as promethazine and guaifenesin, are Schedule V controlled substances. Depending on state law, Schedule V controlled substances may or may not require a prescription. This drug is also used for relief of mild to moderate pain. Taking oral doses of codeine with food or milk can reduce potential GI discomfort.

In addition to the drug interactions that occur with all opioid agonists in this class, codeine may also cause the following interactions:

- Taking codeine with cimetidine or sodium oxybate (GHB) increases the risk of drowsiness, breathing difficulties, and seizures.
- Naltrexone or quinidine may reduce the effects of codeine.

TIP You need to know which pain medications are controlled substances and which are not. Always double-check controlled substances when dispensing to make sure no errors are made. You can also circle and initial the quantity on the label and the hard copy to help prevent errors and keep patients from seeking additional medication when it isn't necessary.

Fentanyl Citrate

Fentanyl citrate is also a Schedule II controlled substance. This drug is prescribed to manage moderate to severe chronic pain. Administration of fentanyl citrate may be

transmucosal (in which the drug is placed in the mouth between the cheek and gum for absorption), transdermal, or by injection.

- For transmucosal administration, fentanyl comes as buccal tablets to be inserted between the cheek and gum (Fentora) or as a flavored lozenge on a stick (Actiq). Transmucosal fentanyl is typically used for treating breakthrough cancer pain.
- For transdermal administration, fentanyl (Duragesic) comes as a patch to be applied to the skin. Transdermal fentanyl is generally used to manage moderate to severe chronic pain in patients who need 24-hour pain control. The patch is worn for 72 hours before it should be removed.

In addition to the adverse effects noted for all opioid agonists in this class, fentanyl may result in muscle rigidity or paralysis.

Hydrocodone

Similar to codeine and fentanyl, hydrocodone is a Schedule II controlled substance, although it is classified as Schedule III substance when in combination form. Aside from a bulk powder for compounding, this drug is currently available only in combination with other drugs to treat coughs and acute pain. Although hydrocodone may be combined with NSAIDs, these drug combinations are not typically used to treat osteoarthritis, rheumatoid arthritis, or other chronic conditions. The dosage form of hydrocodone depends on the drug combination.

- The combination drug hydrocodone and acetaminophen (DuoCet, Lorcet, Lortab, Norco, Xodol, Co-Gesic, Lorcet Plus, Maxidone, Vicodin, Vicodin ES, Vicodin HP, Zydone, Hycet, Liquicet, Zamicet Dolorex Forte, Margesic H, Stagesic) is available in the form of tablets, capsules, oral solution, and elixir.
- Hydrocodone and ibuprofen (Reprexain, Vicoprofen) are available as coated tablets.

These drug combinations generally have interactions with drugs that affect either or both drugs in the combina-

ON THE FRONTLINE

Understanding Orders

You receive an order in the pharmacy for hydrocodone/APAP. You notice that the order also includes a stool softener. Why?

Opioid agonists like hydrocodone slow intestinal peristalsis, the action of the intestinal muscles during digestion. Long-term use of hydrocodone will result in constipation. Increasing fiber in the diet or taking a stool softener will help prevent constipation.

HOW IT WORKS

How Opioid Agonists Control Pain

Opioid agonists, such as meperidine, block pain by mimicking the way the body naturally controls pain (figure 4-1).

In the spinal cord, pain neurons from the limbs and trunk meet the neurons of the CNS (first panel of figure). At the synapse (the junction where the signal is passed from one neuron to another), the pain neuron releases substance P (a pain neurotransmitter). Substance P helps transfer pain impulses to the CNS neurons. The CNS neurons carry those impulses to the brain.

Neurons in the spine release natural opiates. When a natural opiate in the body binds to the pain neuron, it stops the pain neuron from releasing substance P. This slows the movement of the pain impulse to the CNS neuron and the brain (second panel of figure).

Synthetic opiates or opioid agonists add to this pain-blocking effect by binding with open opiate receptors. This stops the release of substance P and slows the transmission of the pain impulse (third panel of figure). Opioid agonists also alter a patient's consciousness of pain, but how this mechanism works remains unknown.

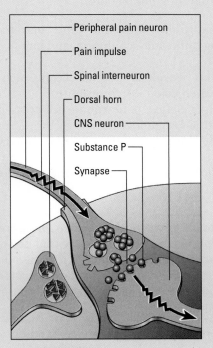
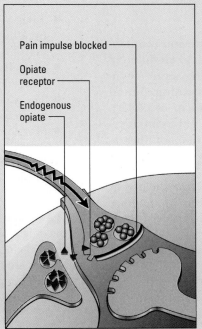
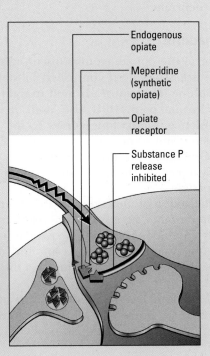

FIGURE 4-1 How opioid agonists control pain. (From *Clinical Pharmacology Made Incredibly Easy.* 2nd Ed. Philadelphia, PA: Lippincott Williams & Wilkins; 2005.)

tion. For example, taking a hydrocodone and aspirin combination drug with warfarin increases the risk of gastric bleeding.

TIP Hydrocodone/APAP comes in a variety of strengths. Always triple-check the prescription with the product from the shelf to make sure the appropriate product has been pulled.

Hydromorphone

Hydromorphone is also a Schedule II controlled substance. Hydromorphone (Dilaudid) is used in treating moderate to severe pain and cough. It is available in several forms, including:

- oral tablets
- oral solution
- injection
- rectal suppositories

Levorphanol

Levorphanol (Levo-Dromoran) is prescribed for relieving moderate to severe pain. This drug is another Schedule II controlled substance. It is available as a tablet or as an injection. In addition to the adverse effects noted for all opioid agonists in this class, taking levorphanol increases the risk of visual disturbances, cardiovascular events, and effects on the central nervous system (for example, nervousness or abnormal dreams).

Meperidine

Meperidine (Demerol, Meperitab) is a Schedule II controlled substance. This drug is available by prescription for the treatment of moderate to severe pain. It may also be used as an adjunct to anesthesia or before surgery.

Meperidine can be given by mouth, as a tablet or oral solution, and by injection. This drug is less effective when given orally. Dosage is adjusted depending on the needs of the patient.

In addition to the adverse effects typical of drugs in this class, other adverse reactions to meperidine may include:

- tremors
- palpitations
- tachycardia
- delirium

Methadone

Similar to the opioid agonists discussed previously, methadone is a Schedule II controlled substance. Methadone (Dolophine, Methadose) is used in treating severe acute and chronic pain. It is also used in treating opioid dependence. Methadone comes in the form of tablets, tablets for oral suspension, oral solution, and as an injection. Oral administration is less effective than administration by injection. Dosage is adjusted to meet the needs of each patient.

The action of methadone is different from the action of other opioid agonists. Pain relief from methadone usually does not occur until the patient has received treatment for three to five days. Respiratory effects of methadone last longer and occur later than the drug's analgesic effects.

Methadone has the following interactions with other drugs that are not typical of other opioid agonists in this class:

- Methadone therapy increases the level of desipramine in the blood.
- Patients who are taking opioid agonist-antagonists with methadone therapy may experience withdrawal symptoms.
- Taking rifampin with methadone may decrease levels of methadone in the body.

Morphine

Morphine is a Schedule II controlled substance. It is the most potent opioid analgesic. This drug relieves shortness of breath in patients with pulmonary edema (fluid in the lungs) and left-sided heart failure (a condition in which the heart can't pump enough blood to meet the needs of the body). The effects of other opioid agonists are often compared to morphine. Morphine dilates peripheral blood vessels. This keeps more blood in the parts of the body away from the spinal cord and brain and decreases the load on the heart.

Morphine comes in several different forms:

- tablets
- extended-release tablets (MS Contin, Oramorph)
- extended-release capsules (Avinza, Kadian)
- oral solution (Roxanol)
- injection (Astramorph, DepoDur, Duramorph PF, Infumorph PF)
- rectal suppositories

Patients should be aware that morphine in capsule form must be swallowed whole or sprinkled on applesauce. Chewing or crushing the capsules would allow a large dose of the drug to be released quickly into the body, causing serious adverse effects. In addition to the drug interactions that occur with all opioid agonists in this class, morphine may cause the following interactions:

- Taking morphine with cimetidine may result in breathing difficulties, confusion, and muscle twitching.
- The effects of skeletal muscle relaxants may be increased when taken with morphine.
- The analgesic effect of morphine is increased when taken with neostigmine.
- Morphine may increase the effects of anticoagulant drugs.
- Reserpine blocks the pain-relieving effect of morphine.

TIP Be sure to double-check abbreviations. The abbreviation for the drug morphine sulfate (MSO_4) can be confused with the abbreviation for magnesium sulfate ($MgSO_4$). Because these abbreviations are easily confused, many facilities do not use them. However, it's important to be familiar with these abbreviations in case you do see them.

Oxycodone

Oxycodone is also a Schedule II controlled substance. It is prescribed for the relief of moderate to severe pain. Oxycodone is administered in several different forms:

- capsules (OxyIR)
- concentrated solution (ETH-Oxydose, OxyFast, Roxicodone)
- tablets (Roxicodone)
- extended-release tablets (OxyContin)
- oral solution (Roxicodone)

The patient should be aware that oxycodone tablets are to be swallowed whole. Chewing or crushing the tablets can lead to toxicity. Extended-release tablets are used when around-the-clock pain relief is needed over a period of time.

Oxycodone also comes in combination with other drugs:

- oxycodone and acetaminophen (Percocet, Roxicet, Tylox, Magnacet, Endocet)
- oxycodone and aspirin (Percodan, Endodan)
- oxycodone and ibuprofen (Combunox)

These combinations also require a prescription.

Oxymorphone

Oxymorphone, another Schedule II controlled substance, is used in the treatment of moderate to severe pain. It comes as oral tablets (Opana), extended-release tablets (Opana ER), a solution for injection (Numorphan, Opana), and a rectal suppository (Numorphan). Oxymorphone tablets, both the immediate and extended-release formulations, must be swallowed whole, rather than chewed or crushed, to avoid administering a potentially fatal dose. In addition to the typical adverse reactions associated with other opioid agonists in this class, some patients experience **pruritus** (itching).

Propoxyphene

Propoxyphene is a Schedule IV controlled substance, meaning it has less potential for abuse than Schedule III drugs and limited potential for dependence. This drug is used to treat mild to moderate pain. Propoxyphene is administered orally in the form of tablets (Darvon, Darvon-N 100).

Propoxyphene is also included in combination with other drugs, such as propoxyphene and acetaminophen (Balacet 325, Darvocet A500, Darvocet-N 100, Darvocet-N 50). This combination drug relieves fever as well as pain.

Patients should be aware that taking propoxyphene with food or milk will minimize GI upset. In addition to drug interactions noted for other opioid agonists, propoxyphene may increase levels of carbamazepine when these two drugs are taken together.

Remifentanil

Remifentanil (Ultiva) is a Schedule II controlled substance. This drug is used in inducing and maintaining anesthesia during surgery. It's also used after surgery for pain management. Remifentanil is administered by IV injection only.

Sufentanil

Sufentanil (Sufenta), also a Schedule II controlled substance, is used for pain relief during administration of general anesthesia in patients who are intubated and ventilated. Additionally, sufentanil is used as an anesthetic in patients undergoing surgery or as an adjunct to anesthesia.

Epidural administration may be used in combination with a low dose of bupivacaine during labor and delivery. Sufentanil is given by IV injection only. In addition to the adverse reactions associated with other opioid agonists in this class, sufentanil may cause muscle rigidity. Giving benzodiazepines with sufentanil may lead to decreased arterial pressure.

Mixed Opioid Agonist-Antagonists

Mixed opioid agonist-antagonists relieve pain while reducing toxic effects and dependency. Similar to opioid agonists, mixed opioid agonist-antagonists affect the CNS. It is believed that these drugs act in two different ways at the same time:

- At some opiate receptor sites, mixed opioid agonist-antagonists bind with the receptor and produce a pain relief effect similar to other opioids.
- At other opiate receptor sites, these drugs block the agonist action, reducing the adverse effects.

Mixed opioid agonist-antagonists are used for pain relief during childbirth and after surgery. They are sometimes prescribed instead of opioid agonists because they have a lower risk of drug dependence. However, patients with a history of opioid abuse shouldn't take these drugs because they could cause symptoms of withdrawal.

Because mixed opioid agonist-antagonists affect the CNS, they may interact with other CNS depressants, such as barbiturates or alcohol.

Mixed opioid agonist-antagonists are listed as pregnancy risk category C drugs. Their safety and use in breast-feeding women haven't been established.

T I P Mixed opioid agonist-antagonists are less likely to cause respiratory depression and constipation than opioid agonists.

Buprenorphine

Buprenorphine is a Schedule III controlled substance, which indicates that it has less abuse potential than Schedule II drugs and a potential for moderate physical or psychological dependence. Buprenorphine is administered as a sublingual tablet (Subutex) to treat opioid dependence. The combination drug buprenorphine and naloxone (Suboxone) also comes in sublingual tablet form for the same

 PROCEED WITH CAUTION

Adverse Reactions to Mixed Opioid Agonist-Antagonists

The most common adverse reactions to mixed opioid agonist-antagonists are:

- euphoria
- lightheadedness
- nausea
- vomiting
- sedation

use. In addition, buprenorphine is available by injection (Buprenex) to relieve moderate to severe pain.

Buprenorphine may affect opiate receptors in the limbic system (the part of the brain involved in emotions). It seems to release slowly from receptor binding sites compared with other drugs in this class. That means the pain relief effects of buprenorphine last for longer periods of time.

Adverse reactions to buprenorphine include a decrease or increase in pulse rate and blood pressure. Buprenorphine may interact with several other drugs.

- Taking buprenorphine with diazepam may lead to respiratory and cardiovascular collapse.
- Administration of naloxone may not reverse buprenorphine's adverse respiratory effects as it does for other opioids.
- Drugs that block the action of CYP3A4 enzyme, such as erythromycin, azole antifungal agents, and protease inhibitors, may decrease the elimination of buprenorphine from the body.
- Rifampin, carbamazepine, and phenytoin may increase the clearance of buprenorphine.

Butorphanol and Nalbuphine

Butorphanol (Stadol), a Schedule IV controlled substance, is used to treat moderate to severe pain. It may also be used before surgery to supplement balanced anesthesia and for pain relief during childbirth. Butorphanol is administered by IM or IV injection. It's also available as a nasal spray.

Nalbuphine, which is not a controlled substance, is used to relieve moderate to severe pain. In addition, it's used before surgery to supplement balanced anesthesia and for pain relief during childbirth. Nalbuphine is administered by SubQ, IM, or IV injection.

Pentazocine

Pentazocine is a Schedule IV controlled substance. Pentazocine lactate injection (Talwin) is used to treat moderate to severe pain. It may be used before surgery or anesthesia and as a supplement to anesthesia during surgery. The injection can be given subcutaneously, intramuscularly, or intravenously.

Pentazocine is also available for oral administration in combination with other drugs. These combinations are:

- pentazocine and acetaminophen (Talacen)
- pentazocine and naloxone (Talwin NX)

Opioid Antagonists

Opioid antagonists counteract the effects of opioids. When the opioid antagonist enters the central nervous system, it has a strong attraction for opiate receptors. However, opioid antagonists don't stimulate those receptors. Instead, the antagonist fills up the receptor sites so that the opioid (natural or synthetic) can't bind with them. The antagonist may also take the place of the opioid that binds with them. This process, called **competitive inhibition**, stops the opioid receptors from acting and blocks their effects.

Naloxone

Naloxone is used to reverse the effects of opioids such as respiratory depression, sedation, and lowered blood pressure. In addition, it's used to treat opioid overdose. As you read earlier in this chapter, naloxone is available in combination with buprenorphine (Suboxone) to treat opioid dependence. This drug is also available in combination with pentazocine (Talwin NX) to treat moderate to severe pain.

Naloxone is given as a SubQ, IM, or IV injection and is not a controlled substance. It is also available in a bulk powder for compounding purposes. It works by competing for the receptor sites that are used by opioid agonists. You need to be aware of the following:

- Naloxone does not produce agonist effects such as depressed breathing, hallucinations and delusions, or constricted pupils.
- Naloxone may not be effective in reversing respiratory depression associated with the use of buprenorphine.
- Because naloxone may also reverse the analgesic effect of opioids, patients taking naloxone may complain of pain or withdrawal symptoms.
- Naloxone has no significant drug interactions.

The adverse effects of naloxone are different from those of other opioid antagonists. The most common adverse reactions are nausea and vomiting. Occasionally, patients may experience hypertension and tachycardia.

Naltrexone

Naltrexone is used to block the effects of opioids in patients with opioid dependence and in the treatment of alcohol dependence. When administered with morphine or other opioids, naltrexone blocks physical dependence on these opioids. Naltrexone is believed to work by competing for the receptor sites that are used by opioids. Naltrexone is available as tablets (ReVia) or as an extended-release injection (Vivitrol) and is not a controlled substance.

There have been no studies to test possible interactions between naltrexone and drugs other than opiates. Naltrexone should not be given to a patient who is receiving an opioid agonist or is an opioid addict.

Naltrexone may cause a variety of adverse reactions, including:

- edema, hypertension, palpitations, **phlebitis** (inflammation of a vein), or shortness of breath
- anxiety, depression, disorientation, dizziness, headache, mood changes, or nervousness
- anorexia, diarrhea, constipation, nausea, thirst, GI pain, cramps, or vomiting
- urinary frequency
- liver toxicity

ANESTHETIC DRUGS

Anesthetic drugs block the perception of pain or cause a loss of feeling. They allow an individual to undergo surgery or other medical procedures without distress and pain. There are three main groups of anesthetic drugs: general anesthetics, local anesthetics, and topical anesthetics. General anesthetic drugs are further subdivided into two main types: those given by inhalation and those given intravenously.

Inhalation Anesthetics

Inhalation anesthetics are used for surgery. They allow precise and quick control of the depth of the anesthesia. Most inhalation anesthetics are liquids at room temperature. Liquid anesthetics are **volatile**—they evaporate when exposed to air, changing into gas form. Liquid anesthetics require a vaporizer (a device that changes the liquid to a gas) and a special delivery system. As a gas, anesthetics are combined with oxygen. They usually enter the patient's body through a mask or tube.

Inhalation anesthetic drugs move from the lungs into the blood. The blood distributes the drug to other tissues. The drug will be distributed most rapidly to organs with high blood flow, such as the brain, liver, kidneys, and heart.

Inhalation anesthetics are mainly eliminated from the body by the lungs. Some inhalation anesthetics (enflurane, sevoflurane) are also eliminated by the liver. Metabolites are excreted in the urine.

Inhalation anesthetics work by depressing the CNS. The effects of inhalation anesthetics on the CNS are:

- loss of consciousness
- loss of responsiveness to sensory stimulation
- muscle relaxation

Inhalation anesthetics are contraindicated in the patient with a known hypersensitivity to the drug, a liver disorder, or malignant hyperthermia (a potentially fatal complication of anesthesia characterized by muscle rigidity and high fever).

Inhalation anesthetics may interact with other drugs that affect the cardiac, respiratory, or central nervous systems. These interactions may result in the following reactions:

- CNS depression
- cardiac arrhythmias
- depressed respirations

Some inhalation anesthetics, such as enflurane, increase the effects of nondepolarizing relaxants.

Desflurane

Desflurane (Suprane) is a volatile liquid used to induce or maintain anesthesia. This drug isn't recommended for inducing anesthesia in children because of the risk of adverse

PROCEED WITH CAUTION

Adverse Reactions to Inhalation Anesthetics

The most common adverse reaction to inhalation anesthetics is an exaggerated response to a normal dose. After surgery, patients may experience reactions similar to those seen with other CNS depressants, including:

- **ataxia** (loss of coordination)
- confusion
- depressed breathing and circulation
- hypothermia
- nausea
- sedation
- vomiting

effects related to the upper airway. However, desflurane can be used to maintain anesthesia in children. Desflurane is administered using a special vaporizer to avoid irritating the respiratory tract.

Desflurane may reduce the effectiveness of some neuromuscular blocking drugs, including atracurium, pancuronium, and succinylcholine.

Enflurane, Isoflurane, and Sevoflurane

Enflurane (Ethrane, Compound 347) is a volatile liquid used to induce and maintain general anesthesia. It may also be used to provide pain relief during childbirth. For delivery by Caesarean section, lower concentrations of enflurane are used to avoid increased uterine relaxation and uterine bleeding. Enflurane works quickly to induce anesthesia, and patients recover quickly.

Isoflurane (Terrell) is a volatile liquid inhalation anesthetic. It's used to induce and maintain general anesthesia.

Sevoflurane (Ultane) is used to induce and maintain general anesthesia in adults and children. It is used during inpatient and outpatient surgery. This drug can be inhaled using a mask and has a neutral odor.

Nitrous Oxide

Nitrous oxide is a commonly used anesthetic drug that is administered in the form of a gas. Nitrous oxide is used in dental surgery to reduce patient anxiety. In dentistry, the gas is administered using a mask placed over the nose. Because the anesthetic effects of nitrous oxide are weak, for medical surgery, nitrous oxide is typically used in combination with other anesthetic drugs. Nitrous oxide has anesthetic and analgesic effects. However, it doesn't result in muscle relaxation.

Intravenous Anesthetics

Intravenous anesthetics are typically used when the patient needs general anesthesia for a short period of time, such as during outpatient surgery. They're also used to help induce general anesthesia more rapidly or to supplement inhalation anesthetics.

Different types of drugs used as intravenous anesthetics include:

- barbiturates
- benzodiazepines
- dissociatives
- hypnotics
- opiates

Intravenous anesthetics work in different ways, depending on the type of drug.

Methohexital

Methohexital (Brevital) is a Schedule IV controlled substance. This drug is a barbiturate that is used as an anesthetic in several different situations, including:

- to induce anesthesia before other anesthetic drugs are administered
- as an adjunct to other inhalation anesthetic drugs for short surgical procedures
- with opioid analgesics, to supplement other inhalation anesthetics for longer surgical procedures
- to induce a hypnotic state (adults only)

Methohexital may be administered by IV injection, IV continuous drip, or IM injection. Methohexital sodium may be administered rectally for young children. Dosage concentration varies depending on the situation.

Taking methohexital over a long period of time will result in cumulative effects. Long-term administration of barbiturates or phenytoin before taking methohexital reduces the effectiveness of methohexital.

Thiopental

Thiopental (Pentothal), a Schedule III controlled substance, is a barbiturate that acts quickly on the CNS to induce hypnosis and anesthesia. Thiopental has several different uses:

- to provide anesthesia for short surgical procedures (15 minutes)
- to supplement regional anesthesia
- to provide hypnosis with other pain relievers or muscle relaxants
- to control convulsions during inhalation anesthesia

Thiopental is administered by IV injection only. Dosage varies depending on the patient and the situation. Using slow injection minimizes respiratory depression.

You should be aware of several drug interactions with thiopental:

- Probenecid taken with thiopental will result in longer than normal action of thiopental.
- Taking diazoxide and thiopental together leads to hypotension.

- Zimelidine and aminophylline reduce the effects of thiopental.
- Midazolam taken with thiopental may increase the effect of thiopental.

Adverse reactions associated with thiopental include:

- respiratory depression
- hiccups, coughing, and muscle twitching
- depressed cardiac function and peripheral dilation

Midazolam

Midazolam is a Schedule IV controlled substance. Midazolam is a benzodiazepine that works quickly to induce anesthesia. It's used to induce general anesthesia or is administered before other anesthetic drugs. Midazolam is also administered before or during diagnostic, therapeutic, or endoscopic procedures. Procedures during which midazolam is used include the following:

- bronchoscopy
- cystoscopy
- angiography
- oncology procedures
- radiology procedures
- sutures

Midazolam is administered by IM injection or by IV sedation before surgery. It also comes in the form of flavored syrup to be administered orally before inducing anesthesia in children. It should not be administered by rapid injection in neonates because of the risk of severe hypotension. Midazolam isn't used for epidural or intrathecal (injection into the spinal canal) administration.

Drug interactions specific to midazolam include the following:

- Taking midazolam with other CNS depressants increases the risk of hypoventilation, airway obstruction, or apnea.
- Midazolam taken with cimetidine, erythromycin, diltiazem, verapamil, ketoconazole, or itraconazole may result in longer than normal sedation effects.
- In neonates, taking midazolam with fentanyl increases the risk of severe hypotension.

Adverse reactions to midazolam may include:

- CNS and respiratory depression
- hypotension
- dizziness

Ketamine

Ketamine (Ketalar), a Schedule III controlled substance, is a dissociative drug. It is used before the administration of other general anesthetics and to supplement other low-potency anesthetics such as nitrous oxide. Ketamine is also used as an anesthetic for surgical procedures that don't require muscle relaxation. Some examples of procedures in which ketamine is used include:

- skin grafting and débridement
- procedures related to the eye, ear, nose, and mouth
- procedures of the pharynx, larynx, or bronchial tree
- sigmoidoscopy
- orthopedic procedures

Ketamine is well suited for use for short periods of time, but it can be used over longer periods by giving additional doses. Ketamine is administered by IV or IM injection. Slow administration of ketamine (over periods greater than 60 seconds) reduces the chance of respiratory depression or increased blood pressure.

Ketamine acts directly on the cortex and limbic system in the brain. As a result, it produces a sense of dissociation from the environment. Patients should not drive or operate machinery for 24 hours after taking ketamine.

Ketamine may cause the following interactions with other drugs:

- Administering ketamine together with halothane increases the risk of hypotension and reduces cardiac output (the amount of blood pumped by the heart each minute).
- Giving ketamine and nonpolarizing drugs together increases neuromuscular effects, resulting in prolonged respiratory depression.
- Using barbiturates or opioids with ketamine may prolong recovery time after anesthesia.
- Ketamine plus theophylline may promote seizures.
- Ketamine and thyroid hormones may cause hypertension and tachycardia (rapid heart rate).

Adverse reactions to ketamine may include:

- prolonged recovery
- irrational behavior
- excitement
- disorientation
- delirium, hallucinations
- increased heart rate
- hypertension

Etomidate

Etomidate (Amidate) is a hypnotic drug used to induce general anesthesia. It may also be used to supplement weak anesthetics, such as nitrous oxide, during short surgical procedures. Etomidate doesn't have analgesic effects.

In terms of drug interactions, the effects of etomidate are enhanced by verapamil, causing respiratory depression and apnea. Adverse reactions to etomidate may include hiccups, coughing, and muscle twitching.

Propofol

Propofol (Diprivan) is a hypnotic drug that is used to induce or maintain anesthesia in surgical procedures. It may also be used for sedation in the following situations:

- diagnostic procedures
- procedures that require a local anesthetic

- intubated or respiratory-controlled patients in intensive care centers

Propofol is not recommended for inducing anesthesia in patients under the age of three years or during pregnancy.

In addition to the adverse reactions associated with etomidate, propofol may also cause respiratory depression.

Fentanyl

Fentanyl (Sublimaze), a Schedule II controlled substance, is an opioid analgesic. (You read about this drug previously under opioid agonists.) Opiates work by binding with receptor cells scattered throughout the CNS. They stop the cells from sending signals to release neurotransmitters from sensory nerves entering the CNS. Fentanyl is used as an adjunct to general or regional anesthesia. It may also be used to maintain anesthesia and for postoperative pain and restlessness. Fentanyl may be used in combination with a neuroepileptic, such as droperidol, to produce a tranquilizing effect and pain relief for surgical procedures.

Fentanyl is administered by IM or IV injection. It has several drug interactions that are not found with other intravenous anesthetics.

- Tranquilizers such as droperidol used with fentanyl may result in decreases in blood pressure or, less commonly, increases in blood pressure.
- Diazepam with fentanyl may result in cardiovascular depression.
- The use of MAOIs with fentanyl increases the risk of hypertension.

Adverse reactions associated with fentanyl include:

- CNS and respiratory depression
- hypoventilation
- cardiac arrhythmias
- muscle rigidity

Sufentanil

Like fentanyl, sufentanil (Sufenta) is a Schedule II controlled substance and an opioid analgesic. It's used as an anesthetic in patients undergoing surgery or as an adjunct to anesthesia. It may also be used in epidural administration along with a low dose of bupivacaine during labor and delivery. Sufentanil is given by slow IV injection. In addition to the injection formulation, sufentanil is also available as a bulk powder for compounding purposes.

In terms of drug interactions, giving benzodiazepines with sufentanil may lead to decreased arterial pressure.

Local Anesthetics

Local anesthetics are administered to prevent or relieve pain in a specific area of the body. In addition, local anesthetic drugs are often used as an alternative to general anesthesia for elderly or debilitated patients.

There are two main groups of local anesthetics:

- "amide" drugs (with nitrogen in the molecular chain)
- "ester" drugs (with oxygen in the molecular chain)

The absorption of local anesthetics varies depending on the drug and the area of the body. However, distribution occurs throughout the body. Esters and amides are metabolized differently, but they both yield metabolites that are excreted in the urine.

Local anesthetics work by blocking nerve signals at the point where different nerves meet. As the local anesthetic accumulates, it causes the membrane of each nerve cell to expand. When the cell membrane expands, the nerve cell loses its ability to depolarize, which is necessary to send the nerve signal.

These drugs may be used:

- to prevent and relieve pain from medical procedures, disease, or injury
- to treat severe pain that topical anesthetics or analgesics can't relieve
- as an alternative to general anesthetics in surgery for older patients
- as an alternative to general anesthetics in surgery for patients with disorders that affect respiratory function, such as chronic obstructive pulmonary disease or **myasthenia gravis** (a disease that causes skeletal muscle fatigue)

For some procedures, a local anesthetic is combined with a drug that constricts blood vessels, such as epinephrine. Vasoconstriction helps control local bleeding and reduces absorption of the anesthetic. Reduced absorption prolongs the anesthetic's action at the site and limits its distribution and CNS effects.

PROCEED WITH CAUTION

Adverse Reactions to Local Anesthetics

Dose-related CNS reactions include:

- shivering
- positional headache
- pain

Dose-related reactions related to the cardiovascular system may include:

- bradycardia (slow heart rate)
- hypotension

Local anesthetic solutions that contain vasoconstrictors such as epinephrine can also produce CNS and cardiovascular reactions. These reactions include the following:

- anxiety
- restlessness
- palpitations
- tachycardia

Local anesthetics produce few significant interactions with other drugs. They can, however, produce adverse reactions.

"Amide" Drugs

In general, amide local anesthetics are less prone to allergic reactions than their ester cousins. However, some amide drugs, such as lidocaine and bupivacaine, contain preservatives that can cause allergic reactions.

It's important to be aware that the effects of amide drugs are additive.

Bupivacaine

Bupivacaine (Marcaine, Sensorcaine) is available as an injection to produce local anesthesia for dental procedures and oral surgery. It's also administered for medical surgery, diagnostic and therapeutic procedures, and, in lower concentrations, for obstetrical procedures. Bupivacaine is also available in formulations that contain epinephrine.

Lidocaine

Lidocaine (Xylocaine) is administered for local anesthesia by infiltration methods (where the drug is administered by SubQ injection near nerve endings) and as a nerve block, such as a caudal or **epidural block**. It may also be administered by IV injection to control cardiac arrhythmias. Lidocaine may be administered with or without epinephrine.

Lidocaine has the following interactions with other drugs:

- Administration of lidocaine with beta-blockers may result in increased levels of lidocaine.
- Cimetidine administered with lidocaine may increase the risk of lidocaine toxicity.
- Administration of procainamide with lidocaine may result in additive effects that may depress cardiovascular function.
- Administration of lidocaine with succinylcholine may prolong the neuromuscular effects of succinylcholine.

Mepivacaine

Mepivacaine (Carbocaine, Polocaine) is typically administered as a nerve block or by infiltration for dental procedures. Mepivacaine is also administered as a block in several other situations, including:

- for peripheral nerves
- during obstetrical procedures (for example, epidural block)
- for pain management

The concentration of the solution varies depending on the purpose of the block.

Prilocaine

Prilocaine (Citanest) is used in dental procedures. It's administered by injection as a nerve block or by infiltration.

Prilocaine may be administered with epinephrine for longer procedures or without epinephrine for shorter procedures (15 minutes or less).

Ropivacaine

Ropivacaine (Naropin) is administered through an IV infusion or bolus after surgery or labor to treat acute pain. Additionally, this drug is used as a local anesthetic for surgery, as an epidural block for Caesarean section, and as a major nerve block. Ropivacaine may also be administered by infiltration.

T I P You can recognize local anesthetics by their names: most end with the letters - *caine*.

"Ester" Drugs

Some "ester" types of local anesthetics are formulated with a preservative called aminobenzoic acid. Some examples of esters that include this preservative are procaine and tetracaine.

Ester drugs containing aminobenzoic acid should not be used if the patient is taking sulfonamide drugs. Aminobenzoic acid blocks the action of the sulfonamides and may lead to infection.

Chloroprocaine (Nesacaine) is used by infiltration and as a peripheral nerve block when formulated with the preservative methylparaben. Without the preservative, chloroprocaine is administered by infiltration and as peripheral and central nerve blocks.

Procaine (Novocain) is used for spinal anesthesia and for local anesthesia by local infiltration or peripheral nerve block methods. Appropriate concentrations vary. For spinal anesthesia, full anesthesia occurs about five minutes after administration.

Tetracaine (Pontocaine) is used to induce and maintain spinal anesthesia for procedures that last for long periods of time (two to three hours).

Topical Anesthetics

Topical anesthetics are applied directly to unbroken skin or mucous membranes to prevent or relieve minor pain. Some injectable local anesthetics, such as lidocaine and tetracaine, are also topically effective. In addition, some topical anesthetics, such as lidocaine, are combined in other products.

Most topical anesthetics produce little systemic absorption. However, systemic absorption may occur if the patient receives frequent or high-dose applications to the eye or large areas of burned or injured skin.

Many topical anesthetics work by blocking nerve signals. Like local anesthetics, topical anesthetic accumulates in the nerve cell membranes. This causes the cell membrane to expand and lose its ability to depolarize. When the nerve signals are blocked, the patient experiences a loss of feeling or analgesic effect in the area.

! PROCEED WITH CAUTION

Adverse Reactions to Topical Anesthetics

Topical anesthetics can cause a hypersensitivity reaction, which may include:

- a rash
- itching
- hives
- swelling of the mouth and throat
- breathing difficulty

Topical anesthetics aren't well absorbed into systemic circulation. As a result, topical anesthetics have few interactions with other drugs.

Lidocaine

Lidocaine is an amide anesthetic that comes in a variety of different dosage forms. It is available over the counter.

Topical forms of the drug include:

- spray
- cream
- gel
- liquid
- ointment
- pads
- swabs

For oral administration, lidocaine is available in the following dosage forms:

- spray
- cream
- gel
- liquid
- drops
- lozenges
- ointment
- paste
- swabs
- wax

Lidocaine is also available as a rectal ointment for treating hemorrhoids and as an otic solution for treating ear ache/pain.

Tetracaine

Tetracaine (Pontocaine, Viractin, TetraVisc) is used as an ophthalmic anesthesia for short procedures such as:

- cataract removal
- diagnostic procedures involving the eye
- removing sutures or foreign bodies from the eye

Benzocaine

Benzocaine is available over the counter to relieve topical pain and itching from minor cuts and scrapes, sunburn, and insect bites. It may also be used to numb mucosal tissues inside the nose, mouth, rectum, or vagina to reduce pain during minor medical procedures.

Benzocaine comes in a variety of different dosage forms and strengths. Different forms of the drug may have different uses.

- Some liquids, gels, or ointments are used to relieve pain from cold sores and fever blisters.
- Other liquids are in lotion form to relieve pain and itching from scrapes, cuts, insect bites, sunburn, or other skin irritations.
- Gels, sprays, or liquid forms of benzocaine are used to reduce mouth pain associated with teething or dental procedures.
- Some sprays are used for oral or mucosal anesthesia. They control pain and suppress the gag reflex.
- Other sprays are used for soothing minor skin irritations such as minor cuts and scrapes, insect bites, or sunburns.
- Several forms of benzocaine are designed to relieve pain and itching from hemorrhoids. These formulations are creams, ointments, or sprays.
- Benzocaine is used with other drugs in several ear preparations. For example, it's used with antipyrine in a drug that's used to treat ear infections.
- Benzocaine may also be formulated in combination with dextromethorphan in lozenges to relieve symptoms of the common cold, such as sore throat or cough.

Cocaine

Cocaine, a Schedule II controlled substance, is available as a topical solution or as a powder to mix as solution. Cocaine is also available as a bulk powder for compounding purposes. The solution can be administered in several different ways:

- using cotton applicators or packs
- dripped into a cavity
- as a spray

Topical cocaine shouldn't be used for ophthalmic procedures, because it can damage the cornea of the eye.

Dyclonine and Dibucaine

Dyclonine is used as a topical anesthetic for mucous membranes. It is available over the counter in lozenges or solution. It is commonly used in combination products as well.

Dibucaine (Nupercainal) is an amide anesthetic used for rectal anesthesia. It is available as an ointment for relief of pain and itching due to hemorrhoids. It is available over the counter.

Pramoxine

Pramoxine is available over the counter in several forms:

- cream (AmLactin AP, Prax, Tronothane, Sarna, Campho-Phenique)
- lotion (Prax, Sarn, Dermarest, Eczemaa)
- gel (PrameGel, Itch-X)
- spray (Itch-X)
- wipes (Bactine)
- aerosol foam (ProctoFoam) for hemorrhoids

Pramoxine creams, gels, lotions, sprays, and wipes are mainly used to relieve itching and pain for minor skin irritations and burns. Pramoxine lotion may also be used to cleanse the anogenital area after rectal surgery and to relieve pain and itching from hemorrhoids. Pramoxine for rectal use comes in the form of foam, creams, or ointments.

Pramoxine also comes in combination with hydrocortisone. This combination drug has anesthetic and anti-inflammatory effects. It is used to treat a variety of skin conditions.

Aromatic Compounds

Some topical anesthetics are aromatic compounds, such as benzyl alcohol and clove oil. These chemicals seem to stimulate nerve endings. This stimulation causes irritation that interferes with the perception of pain.

Benzyl alcohol can cause topical reactions such as skin irritation.

Clove oil contains eugenol, a substance that may have analgesic and antiseptic effects. Clove oil has been used in dental materials such as cements or fillers. When used topically, clove oil may have a mild anesthetic effect. Clove oil is sometimes combined with other pain-reducing products, such as lidocaine or prilocaine.

Cooling Effect

Other topical anesthetics produce a cooling effect. Ethyl chloride spray superficially freezes the tissue, stimulating the cold-sensation receptors and blocking the nerve endings in the frozen area. However, because ethyl chloride is a refrigerant, it may produce frostbite in areas where it has been applied.

Menthol selectively stimulates the sensory nerve endings for cold, causing a cool sensation and some local pain relief. Menthol is often used in combination with other topical anesthetics in OTC preparations to treat cold sores, cold symptoms, nasal congestion, itching, minor skin irritations, and minor aches and pains.

QUICK QUIZ

Answer the following multiple-choice questions.

1. Which of the following characteristics of acetylsalicylic acid allows it to protect the heart?
   a. antipyretic
   b. anti-inflammatory
   c. anticoagulant
   d. analgesic

2. Which of the following is *not* a possible drug interaction associated with nonselective NSAIDs?
   a. The antihypertensive effects of ACE inhibitors are decreased.
   b. There is an increased risk of bleeding complications with anticoagulants.
   c. Pramoxine may cause increased levels of NSAIDs in the body, resulting in hyperventilation.
   d. Antacids may reduce the level of NSAIDs in the body.
3. Which of the following is *not* a nonopioid analgesic drug?
   a. salsalate
   b. etodolac
   c. phenazopyridine hydrochloride
   d. sufentanil
4. Which of the following drugs can be administered to depress the CNS, resulting in loss of consciousness and muscle relaxation?
   a. naproxen
   b. oxaprozin
   c. isoflurane
   d. tetracaine
5. Which route of administration is commonly used for the drugs prilocaine and procaine?
   a. oral solution
   b. nerve block injection
   c. spray
   d. suppository

Please answer each of the following questions in one to three sentences.

1. What is the difference between selective and nonselective NSAIDs?

2. How do opioid agonists work in the body to relieve pain? Briefly describe their mechanism of action.

3. How do opioid antagonists counteract the effects of opioid agonists?

4. Briefly explain the differences between general anesthesia, local anesthesia, and topical anesthesia.

5. List three uses of topical anesthetic drugs.

Answer the following questions as either true or false.

1. ___ Similar to salicylates, acetaminophen has an anti-inflammatory effect.
2. ___ Opioid agonists like hydrocodone slow intestinal peristalsis.
3. ___ Enflurane is an inhalation anesthetic that may be used to provide pain relief during childbirth.
4. ___ A common adverse reaction to mixed opioid agonist-antagonists is fever.
5. ___ Topical anesthetics work by causing the membranes of cells to expand and depolarize.

Match the generic name of each drug in the left column with the correct trade name from the right column.

1. diflunisal   a. Pentothal
2. meperidine   b. Sublimaze
3. prilocaine   c. Dolobid
4. thiopental   d. Citanest
5. fentanyl   e. Demerol

DRUG CLASSIFICATION TABLE

Classification	Generic Name	Trade Name(s)
Salicylates	aspirin *ass'-purr-in*	*chewing gum (OTC):* Aspergum *tablets (OTC):* Bayer *chewable tablets (OTC):* Bayer Children's Aspirin, St. Joseph Adult Chewable Aspirin *delayed-release tablets (OTC):* Bayer *enteric-coated tablets (OTC):* Ecotrin, Halfprin *extended-release tablets (OTC):* Extended Release Bayer 8-Hour *extended-release tablets (Rx):* ZORprin *rectal suppositories (OTC):* (no longer marketed under trade name)
	buffered aspirin *ass'-purr-in*	*tablets:* Ascriptin, Aspir-Mox, Bufferin
	choline magnesium trisalicylate *co'-leenmag-nee'-see-um-trye-sal-ih'-sah-late*	*tablets:* (no longer marketed under trade name) *oral solution:* (no longer marketed under trade name)
	diflunisal *dye-floo'-ni-sal*	*tablets:* Dolobid
	salsalate *sal'-sa-late*	*tablets:* Argesic-SA
Nonsalicylates	acetaminophen *a-sea-tah-min'-oh-fen*	*chewable tablets:* (no longer marketed under trade name) *dissolving tablets:* Tylenol *elixir:* (no longer marketed under trade name) *drops:* Tylenol *rectal suppositories:* Acephen, Feverall, *oral suspension:* Tylenol *tablets:* Aspirin Free Anacin, Panadol, Tylenol *delayed-release tablets:* Tylenol 8 Hour, Tylenol Arthritis Pain *oral solution:* Comtrex Sore Throat, Tylenol *capsules:* (no longer marketed under trade name)
NSAIDs	diclofenac sodium *dye-kloe'-fen-ak*	*delayed-release tablets:* Voltaren *extended-release tablets:* Voltaren XR *topical gel:* Solaraze *ophthalmic solution:* Voltaren
	diclofenac potassium *dye-kloe-fen'-ak*	*tablets:* Cataflam
	etodolac *ee-toe-doe'-lak*	*capsules:* (no longer marketed under trade name) *tablets:* (no longer marketed under trade name) *extended-release tablets:* (no longer marketed under trade name)
	fenoprofen *fen-oh-proe'-fen*	*capsules:* Nalfon *tablets:* (no longer marketed under trade name)
	flurbiprofen *flure-bi'-proe-fen*	*tablets:* (no longer marketed under trade name) *ophthalmic solution:* Ocufen
	ibuprofen *eye'-byoo-proe-fen*	*chewable tablets:* Advil, Motrin *caplets:* Motrin IB, Advil *liquid-gel capsules:* Advil, Motrin IB

continued

DRUG CLASSIFICATION TABLE *(continued)*

Classification	Generic Name	Trade Name(s)
NSAIDs *(continued)*		*gelcaps:* Motrin IB *drops:* Advil, Motrin *oral suspension:* Advil, Motrin *tablets (Rx):* Motrin *tablets:* Advil, Motrin IB, Midol Cramps and Body Aches Formula
	indomethacin *in-doe-meth'-a-sin*	*injection:* Indocin *oral suspension:* Indocin *capsules:* (no longer marketed under trade name) *sustained-release capsules:* Indocin SR *rectal suppositories:* Indocin
	ketoprofen *kee-toe-proe'-fen*	*tablets:* (no longer marketed under trade name) *capsules:* (no longer marketed under trade name) *extended-release capsules:* (no longer marketed under trade name)
	ketorolac *ket-ór-o-lac*	*ophthalmic solution:* Acular *tablets:* (no longer marketed under trade name) *injection:* (no longer marketed under trade name)
	meloxicam *mel-ox'-i-kam*	*tablets:* Mobic *oral suspension:* Mobic
	nabumetone *nah-byew'-meh-tone*	*tablets:* (no longer marketed under trade name)
	naproxen *na-prox'-en*	*extended-release tablets:* EC-Naprosyn *tablets:* Naprosyn *oral suspension:* Naprosyn
	naproxen sodium *na-prox'-en*	*caplets (OTC):* Aleve *gelcaps (OTC):* Aleve *tablets (OTC):* Aleve *extended-release tablets (OTC):* Midol Extended Relief *tablets (Rx):* Anaprox *extended-release tablets:* Naprelan
	oxaprozin *oks-a-pro'zin*	*tablets:* Daypro
	piroxicam *peer-ox'-i-kam*	*capsules:* Feldene
	sulindac *sul-in'-dak*	*tablets:* Clinoril
	misoprostol *my'-so-prahst'-ole*	*tablets:* Cytotec
	misoprostol and diclofenac *my'-so-prahst'-ole dye-kloe'-fen-ak*	*delayed-release tablets:* Arthrotec
	celecoxib *sell-ah-cocx'-ib*	*capsules:* Celebrex
Other pain relievers	phenazopyridine hydrochloride *fen-az-oh-peer'-i-deen*	*tablets (Rx):* Pyridium *tablets (OTC):* Azo-Gesic, Azo-Standard
Opioid agonists	codeine *koe'-deen*	*injection:* (no longer marketed under trade name) *tablets:* (no longer marketed under trade name)

continued

DRUG CLASSIFICATION TABLE (continued)

Classification	Generic Name	Trade Name(s)
Opioid agonists (continued)	codeine and acetaminophen koe'-deen a-sea-tah-min'-oh-fen	elixir: (no longer marketed under trade name) oral solution: (no longer marketed under trade name) oral suspension: Capital and Codeine tablets: Tylenol #3, Tylenol #4
	fentanyl citrate fen'-ta-nil	lollipops/lozenges: Actiq extended-release transdermal patch: Duragesic buccal tablets: Fentora injection (IV anesthetic): Sublimaze
	hydrocodone and acetaminophen hy-droe-coe-done a-sea-tah-min'-oh-fen	tablets: DuoCet, Lorcet, Lortab, Norco, Xodol, Co-Gesic, Lorcet Plus, Maxidone, Vicodin, Vicodin ES, Vicodin HP, Zydone oral solution: Hycet, Liquicet, Zamicet capsules: Dolorex Forte, Margesic H, Stagesic elixir: Lortab
	hydrocodone and ibuprofen hy-droe-coe-done eye'-byoo-proe-fen	tablets: Reprexain, Vicoprofen
	hydromorphone hy-droe-mor'-fone	injection: Dilaudid tablets: Dilaudid oral solution: Dilaudid rectal suppositories: (no longer marketed under trade name)
	levorphanol lee-vor'-fa-nole	tablets: (no longer marketed under trade name) injection: Levo-Dromoran
	meperidine me-per-i'-deen	injection: Demerol oral solution: (no longer marketed under trade name) tablets: Demerol, Meperitab
	methadone meth'-a-doan	oral solution: Methadose injection: (no longer marketed under trade name) tablets: Dolophine, Methadose tablet for oral suspension: (no longer marketed under trade name)
	morphine mor'-feen	extended-release capsules: Kadian, Avinza extended-release tablets: MS Contin, Oramorph injection: Astramorph, DepoDur, Infumorph PF, Duramorph PF oral solution: Roxanol tablets: (no longer marketed under trade name) suppositories: (no longer marketed under trade name)
	oxycodone ox-ee-koe'-done	capsules: OxyIR concentrated solution: ETH-Oxydose, OxyFast, Roxicodone tablets: Roxicodone extended-release tablets: OxyContin solution: Roxicodone

continued

DRUG CLASSIFICATION TABLE (continued)

Classification	Generic Name	Trade Name(s)
Opioid agonists (continued)	oxycodone and acetaminophen *ox-ee-koe'-done a-sea-tah-min'-oh-fen*	*capsules:* Tylox *oral solution:* Roxicet *tablets:* Percocet, Roxicet, Perloxx, Narvox, Magnacet, Endocet
	oxycodone and aspirin *ox-ee-koe'-done ass'-purr-in*	*tablets:* Percodan, Endodan
	oxycodone and ibuprofen *ox-ee-koe'-done eye'-byoo-proe-fen*	*tablets:* Combunox
	oxymorphone *ox-ee-mor'-phone*	*injection:* Numorphan, Opana *rectal suppositories:* Numorphan *tablets:* Opana *extended-release tablets:* Opana ER
	propoxyphene *proe-pox'-i-feen*	*tablets:* Darvon-N 100 *capsules:* Darvon
	propoxyphene and acetaminophen *proe-pox'-i-feen a-sea-tah-min'-oh-fen*	*tablets:* Balacet 325, Darvocet A500, Darvocet-N 100, Darvocet-N 50
	remifentanil *reh-mih-fen'-tah'-nil*	*injection:* Ultiva
	sufentanil *soo-fen'-ta-nil*	*injection:* Sufenta
Mixed opioid agonist-antagonists	buprenorphine *byoo-pren-nor'-feen*	*injection:* Buprenex *sublingual tablets:* Subutex
	buprenorphine and naloxone *byoo-pren-nor'-feen nal-ox'-ohn*	*sublingual tablets:* Suboxone
	butorphanol *byoo-to'-fa-nole*	*injection:* Stadol *nasal spray:* (no longer marketed under trade name)
	nalbuphine *nal'-byoo-feen*	*injection:* (no longer marketed under trade name)
	pentazocine *pen-taz'-oh-seen*	*injection:* Talwin
	pentazocine and acetaminophen *pen-taz'-oh-seen a-sea-tah-min'-oh-fen*	*tablets:* Talacen
	pentazocine and naloxone *pen-taz'-oh-seen nal-ox'-ohn*	*tablets:* Talwin NX
Opioid antagonists	naloxone *nal-ox'-ohn*	*injection:* (no longer marketed under trade name)
	naltrexone *nal-trex'-ohn*	*tablets:* ReVia *injection:* Vivitrol
Inhalation anesthetics	desflurane *des'-floo-rane*	*inhalation liquid:* Suprane
	enflurane *en'-floo-rane*	*inhalation liquid:* Compound 347, Ethrane
	nitrous oxide *nye'-trus*	*inhalation gas:* (no longer marketed under trade name)
	sevoflurane *see-vo-floo'-rane*	*inhalation liquid:* Ultane
Intravenous anesthetics	methohexital *meth-oh-hex'-i-tal*	*injection:* Brevital
	thiopental *thye-oh-pen'-tal*	*injection:* Pentothal

continued

DRUG CLASSIFICATION TABLE (continued)

Classification	Generic Name	Trade Name(s)
Intravenous anesthetics (continued)	midazolam *med-zool'-ham*	*injection:* (no longer marketed under trade name) *syrup:* (no longer marketed under trade name)
	ketamine *keet'-a'-meen*	*injection:* Ketalar
	etomidate *e-tom'-i-date*	*injection:* Amidate
	propofol *proe'-po-fole*	*injection:* Diprivan
	fentanyl *fen'-ta-nil*	*injection:* Sublimaze *lollipops/lozenges (pain):* Actiq *extended-release transdermal patch (pain):* Duragesic *buccal tablets (pain):* Fentora
	sufentanil *soo-fen'-ta-nil*	*injection:* Sufenta
Local anesthetics	bupivacaine *byoo-piv'-a-kane*	*injection:* Marcaine, Sensorcaine
	lidocaine *lye'-doe-kane*	*injection:* Xylocaine
	mepivacaine *me-piv'-a-kane*	*injection:* Carbocaine, Polocaine
	prilocaine *pril'-oh-kane*	*injection:* Citanest
	ropivacaine *roe-piv'-a-kane*	*injection:* Naropin
	chloroprocaine *klor-oh-proe'-kane*	*injection:* Nesacaine
	procaine *proe'-kane*	*injection:* Novocain
	tetracaine *tet'-ra-kane*	*injection:* Pontocaine
Topical anesthetics	lidocaine *lye'-doe-kane*	(available in many different dosage forms under a variety of trade names)
	tetracaine *tet'-ra-kane*	*injection:* Pontocaine *topical solution:* Pontocaine *topical gel:* Viractin *ophthalmic solutions:* TetraVisc
	benzocaine *ben'-zoe-kane*	(available in many different dosage forms under a variety of trade names)
	antipyrine and benzocaine *an-tee-pye'-reen ben'-zoe-kane*	*otic solution/drops:* A/B Otic, Aurodex, Dolotic, OtoCare, Otoalgan, Pro-Otic
	cocaine *ko'-kane*	*topical solution:* (no longer marketed under trade name)
	dyclonine *dye'-clone-een*	(marketed under a large number of trade names, including combination products)
	pramoxine *pra-mox'-een*	*cream:* AmLactin AP, Prax, Tronothane, Sarna, Campho-Phenique *lotion:* Prax, Sarna, Dermarest Eczema *gel:* PrameGel, Itch-X *spray:* Itch-X *wipes:* Bactine *aerosol foam:* ProctoFoam

continued

DRUG CLASSIFICATION TABLE (continued)

Classification	Generic Name	Trade Name(s)
Topical anesthetics (continued)	pramoxine and hydrocortisone *pra-mox'-een*	*cream:* Analpram HC, Pramosone *lotion:* Analpram HC *ointment:* Pramosone *gel:* Novacort *rectal foam:* Proctofoam HC *topical foam:* Epifoam
	dibucaine *dye-byoo'-kane*	*ointment:* Nupercainal
	benzyl alcohol *ben'-zil al-ko-hal*	(marketed under a large number of trade names, including combination products)
	clove oil *klov oil*	
	ethyl chloride spray *eth'-ill klor'-ide*	
	menthol *men'-thol*	(marketed under a large number of trade names, including combination products)

CHAPTER 5

Cardiovascular Drugs

CHAPTER OBJECTIVES

- Match brand and generic names of commonly used drugs for heart failure, arrhythmias, angina, hypertension, and high cholesterol
- Identify the classification of commonly used drugs for heart failure, arrhythmias, angina, hypertension, and high cholesterol
- List the applications of commonly used drugs for heart failure, arrhythmias, angina, hypertension, and high cholesterol
- Describe dosing parameters for digoxin, including the loading dose and the therapeutic dose
- Match antiarrhythmics to the correct class (IA, B, IC, II, III, and IV)
- Describe the mechanism of action and dosing parameters for nitroglycerin
- Compare the mechanisms of action of drugs used to treat hypertension
- Explain the rationale for using multiple antihypertensive drugs to regulate blood pressure
- Define LDL, HDL, and total cholesterol, and desirable levels of each
- Compare the mechanisms of action for antilipemic drugs

KEY TERMS

antianginal drugs—drugs that treat angina by reducing the amount of oxygen the heart needs and/or by increasing the supply of oxygen to the heart

antiarrhythmic drugs—a group of drugs used to treat cardiac arrhythmias

antilipemic drugs—drugs used to lower abnormally high blood levels of fats such as triglycerides and cholesterol

arrhythmia—disturbance of normal heart function characterized by irregularities in rate, rhythm, or both

atherosclerosis—a disorder in which lipid deposits accumulate on the lining of the blood vessels, eventually producing degenerative changes and obstruction of blood flow

atrial fibrillation (atrial fib or AF)—a common irregular rhythm that causes the atria to contract abnormally

atrial flutter—regular, rapid contractions of the heart's atria (the upper chambers of the heart)

cardiac glycosides—a group of drugs derived from digitalis, a substance that occurs naturally in foxglove plants and in certain kinds of toads

congestive heart failure—a condition in which a weakened heart cannot pump enough blood to meet the body's needs; often called "heart failure"

coronary artery disease (CAD)—a condition in which coronary arteries (vessels supplying blood and oxygen to the heart) are narrowed or blocked with fatty deposits

diuretics—drugs used to promote the excretion of water and electrolytes by the kidneys

heart block—a delay or complete block of the electrical impulse as it travels from the heart's sinus node to the ventricles, causing an irregular or slower heartbeat

hypertensive crisis—a condition of impending organ damage from severely high blood pressure

inotropic—affecting the force or energy of muscle contractions

negative chronotropic effect—the slowing of the heart's rate of contraction (or beating) through the use of cardiotonic drugs

negative dromotropic effect—the slowing of the conduction of the electrical impulses that cause the heart to beat through the use of cardiotonic drugs

neurotransmitters—chemical substances that are released at nerve endings to help transmit nerve impulses; also called neurohormones

paroxysmal atrial tachycardia (PAT)—an arrhythmia marked by alternating brief periods of tachycardia and normal sinus rhythm

paroxysmal supraventricular tachycardia (PSVT)—a rapid heart rate, usually with a regular rhythm, that originates above the ventricles

phosphodiesterase (PDE) inhibitors—a class of drugs used for short-term management of heart failure or long-term management in patients awaiting transplant surgery

positive inotropic effect—the increased force in the contraction of the heart muscle (myocardium) through the use of cardiotonic drugs

premature atrial contractions (PACs)—usually harmless extra beats that originate in the atria

premature ventricular contractions (PVCs)—usually harmless skipped heartbeats

statins—the common name for HMG-CoA reductase inhibitors, a class of drugs that are used to treat high cholesterol

supraventricular arrhythmias—abnormal heart rhythms that originate above the bundle branches of the heart's conduction system

sympathetic nervous system—the branch of the autonomic nervous system that regulates the expenditure of energy and has key effects in stressful situations

ventricular fibrillation (V-fib)—a disorganized firing of electrical impulses from the ventricles that causes the ventricles to quiver and to be unable to contract or pump blood to the body

ventricular tachycardia (V-tach)—a rapid rhythm originating from the ventricles (the lower chambers of the heart) that prevents the heart from adequately filling with blood and pumping enough blood to the body

---

The body's cardiovascular system provides life-supporting oxygen and nutrients, removes metabolic waste products, and carries hormones from one part of the body to another. Because this system serves such vital functions, problems in the cardiovascular system can seriously affect a person's health. Many drugs have been developed to treat these problems. In this chapter you'll learn about the classes of drugs that treat cardiovascular disorders, how these drugs are used, their mechanisms of action, and their interactions and adverse reactions with other drugs.

THE CARDIOVASCULAR SYSTEM

The cardiovascular system consists of the heart and blood vessels that transport blood throughout the body. There are three main types of blood vessels:

■ Arteries (except for pulmonary arteries) carry blood away from the heart and toward the tissues.

■ Capillaries are tiny, thin-walled vessels. These structures receive blood from the arteries and help transport nutrition to the body's cells.

■ Veins (except for pulmonary veins) carry blood from the body's tissues to the heart.

The Healthy Heart

Here's how a healthy heart works:

1. The right atrium receives deoxygenated blood returning from the body tissues. The blood travels into the right ventricle, which pumps it into the pulmonary arteries. These arteries carry the blood to the lungs to become oxygenated. The left atrium receives blood high in oxygen content as it returns from the lungs in pulmonary veins. The left ventricle pumps oxygenated blood to all parts of the body. This blood goes first into the aorta and then into the systemic arteries that take blood to the tissues.

2. The systemic arteries carry oxygenated blood throughout the body. The thin walls of the capillaries allow oxygen and nutrients to diffuse into the cells of the body tissues. The veins then carry this deoxygenated blood back to the heart's right atrium. There, the process of returning the blood to the lungs to become oxygenated starts again.

3. The heart's pumping action is due to contractions of the heart muscle, which is stimulated to contract by electrical impulses. The rate of these contractions, or "beats," is the heart's rhythm. It can be felt on the body's surface as the pulse.

4. The heart's beating and rhythm is controlled by the sinoatrial (SA) node, which is located in the right atrium. Because the SA node generates the impulse that begins the heartbeat, it is sometimes referred to as the heart's "pacemaker." The impulse travels from the SA node to the atrioventricular (AV) node, through the bundle of His, and then throughout the ventricular walls by means of the bundle branches and Purkinje fibers. As a safety measure, a region of the conduction system other than the SA node can generate a heartbeat even if the SA node fails, but it does so at a slower rate.

Heart Failure

Congestive heart failure (often just called heart failure or CHF) is a condition in which a weakened heart cannot pump enough blood to meet the body's needs. It can be the result of old age or caused by any number of disorders, including hypertension (high blood pressure) and ischemic heart disease, in which blood flow is reduced by a narrowing or blockage of the arteries.

The most common cause of ischemic heart disease is **coronary artery disease (CAD)**—also called **atherosclerosis** or "hardening of the arteries." CAD occurs when the coronary arteries, which supply blood and oxygen to the heart, are narrowed or blocked with fatty deposits called plaque.

Arrhythmias

A cardiac **arrhythmia** is a disturbance or irregularity in the rate or rhythm of the heart's contractions or "beats." An arrhythmia can occur as a result of heart disease or from a disorder that affects the functioning of the cardiovascular system as a whole. Conditions such as hypoxia (low oxygen levels), an electrolyte imbalance in the body, or emotional distress can also trigger arrhythmias.

There are many types of arrhythmias. Some of the more common types are:

- **atrial fibrillation** (atrial fib or AF)
- **premature atrial contractions** (PACs)
- **ventricular tachycardia** (V-tach)
- **ventricular fibrillation** (V-fib)
- **paroxysmal supraventricular tachycardia** (PSVT)
- **premature ventricular contractions** (PVCs)
- bradycardia
- **heart block**
- **paroxysmal atrial tachycardia** (PAT)
- **supraventricular arrhythmias**
- **atrial flutter**

INOTROPICS

Inotropic drugs, such as cardiac glycosides and phosphodiesterase inhibitors, increase the force of the heart's contractions. This is called a **positive inotropic effect**.

Cardiac glycosides also slow the heart rate; this is called a **negative chronotropic effect**. In addition, they slow the transmission of electrical impulses through the specialized bundle of nerve fibers that forms the conduction system of the heart. This is called a **negative dromotropic effect**.

Cardiac Glycosides

Cardiac glycosides are a group of drugs derived from digitalis, a substance that occurs naturally in foxglove plants and in certain kinds of toads. The most common cardiac glycoside is digoxin (Digitek, Lanoxin). It is used to treat heart failure and certain cardiac arrhythmias.

Digoxin is used to treat heart failure because it strengthens the contraction of the ventricles by boosting intracellular calcium at the cell membrane. It may enhance the movement of calcium into the cells of the myocardium, a muscle layer of the heart wall. It also may stimulate the release or block the reuptake of the norepinephrine neurotransmitter at the adrenergic nerve terminal.

Digoxin also acts on the central nervous system (CNS) to slow the heart rate. This mechanism of action makes it useful for treating paroxysmal atrial tachycardia (PAT) and supraventricular arrhythmias.

The drug also increases the refractory period—the period when the cells of the conduction system can't conduct an impulse. Digoxin is available in tablet form, oral solution, and injectable solution.

Because digoxin has a long half-life, a loading dose is given by capsule or injection to patients who need an immediate effect from the drug—for example, if a patient is having a dangerous arrhythmia. Giving a larger initial dose allows a minimum effective concentration of the drug in the blood to be obtained faster. However, to avoid toxicity loading doses are generally not given to patients with heart failure.

T I P Digoxin may be prescribed using either milligrams (mg) or micrograms (mcg). There are 1,000 micrograms in a milligram. Always double-check the unit in which it is prescribed. Reading "mcg" as "mg" would result in an overdose for the patient that would almost certainly be fatal.

Drug Interactions with Digoxin

The following are examples of drugs that interact poorly with digoxin:

- Antacids, barbiturates, cholestyramine resin, kaolin and pectin, neomycin, metoclopramide, rifampin, and sulfasalazine reduce digoxin's therapeutic effects.
- Calcium preparations, quinidine, verapamil, cyclosporine, tetracycline, clarithromycin, propafenone, amiodarone, spironolactone, hydroxychloroquine, erythromycin, itraconazole, and omeprazole increase the risk of digoxin toxicity.
- Amphotericin B, potassium-wasting diuretics, and steroids taken with digoxin may cause hypokalemia (low potassium levels) and increase the risk of digoxin toxicity.
- Beta-adrenergic blockers (commonly called "beta blockers") and calcium channel blockers may cause an excessively slow heart rate and arrhythmias.
- Succinylcholine and thyroid preparations increase the risk of arrhythmias.
- St. John's wort, an herbal preparation, can raise digoxin levels and increase the risk of toxicity.

Toxicity Alert

Because cardiac glycosides have a narrow therapeutic index, or margin of safety, they may produce digoxin toxicity. To prevent this, patients taking digoxin must be monitored closely by health care professionals and have their blood tested regularly to monitor drug levels.

PROCEED WITH CAUTION

Adverse Reactions to Digoxin

Signs and symptoms of digoxin toxicity include:

- nausea, abdominal pain, vomiting, diarrhea
- headache, irritability, depression, insomnia, confusion, vision changes
- arrhythmias, complete heart block

AT THE COUNTER

Digoxin

A patient is admitted to the hospital and diagnosed with a supra-ventricular arrhythmia. The physician orders a loading dose of digoxin ASAP. Why?

Digoxin has a long half-life, so a loading dose is given to patients who require immediate drug effects. The larger dose results in a minimum effective concentration of drug in the blood faster than the regular daily dose.

Later you receive an order for the same patient, but the digoxin is now dosed 0.125 mg PO QD. You also notice a "dig level" QAM has been ordered. What does this mean?

The physician is now ordering a daily oral dose of digoxin 0.125 mg. Because cardiac glycosides have a narrow therapeutic index, they may produce digoxin toxicity. To prevent toxicity, the patient's dose should be individualized based on the patient's serum digoxin concentration ("dig level"). Therefore, the patient's serum digoxin concentration will be checked every morning to ensure that the level remains within the therapeutic index.

Phosphodiesterase Inhibitors

Phosphodiesterase (PDE) inhibitors are typically used for short-term management of heart failure and long-term management in patients who are waiting for heart transplants.

These drugs improve cardiac output by strengthening contractions. They are thought to help move calcium into cardiac cells or to increase calcium storage in the sarcoplasmic reticulum, the structures that surround

PROCEED WITH CAUTION

Adverse Reactions to Phosphodiesterase Inhibitors

Adverse reactions are uncommon, but they may include:

- arrhythmias
- nausea and vomiting
- headache
- fever
- chest pain
- hypokalemia
- thrombocytopenia (especially with inamrinone)
- mild increase in heart rate

The likelihood of adverse reactions to these drugs increases significantly over time. Prolonged use can increase the risk of complications, including death.

each muscle fiber. By directly relaxing vascular muscle, PDE inhibitors also decrease peripheral vascular resistance (called the "afterload") and the amount of blood returned to the heart (called the "preload") after each contraction.

These drugs have far fewer drug interactions than do cardiac glycosides. PDE inhibitors may react with disopyramide, causing hypertension. In addition, they reduce serum potassium levels. This means that taking them with a potassium-wasting diuretic may lead to hypokalemia.

Inamrinone

Inamrinone is available in a solution and is administered intravenously. This drug can manage heart failure in patients who have not responded adequately to treatment with cardiac glycosides, diuretics, or vasodilators. (You'll read about diuretics and vasodilators later in this chapter.) It's rarely used, however, because one possible side effect is thrombocytopenia, a severe decrease in the number of blood platelets, which can result in hemorrhaging.

Milrinone

Milrinone is another solution that is used to manage heart failure in patients who have not responded adequately to treatment with cardiac glycosides, diuretics, or vasodilators. It is administered intravenously, distributed rapidly, and excreted by the kidneys, primarily as an unchanged drug.

ANTIARRHYTHMIC DRUGS

Antiarrhythmic drugs are used to treat arrhythmias. They can be categorized into four classes:

- Class I antiarrhythmic drugs have a membrane-stabilizing or anesthetic effect on the cells of the myocardium. This class contains the largest number of antiarrhythmics and is subdivided into three groups based on slightly different mechanisms of action: IA, IB, and IC.
- Class II antiarrhythmic drugs block stimulation of the beta receptors of the heart. Adrenergic neurohormones stimulate the beta receptors of the myocardium, which increases the heart rate. Blocking the effect of the neurohormones decreases heart rate.
- Class III antiarrhythmic drugs prolong repolarization and the refractory period, the period between transmission of nerve impulses along a nerve fiber. Repolarization is the movement of the nerve cells' positive and negative ions back to their original state after an impulse passes along the nerve fiber.
- Class IV antiarrhythmic drugs are calcium channel blockers. They work by limiting the movement of calcium through channels across the myocardial cell

membranes and vascular smooth muscle. Cardiac contractions depend on this movement. Reducing this motion slows the refractory period and suppresses the arrhythmia. (You'll read more about calcium channel blockers, their other uses, and how they work later in this chapter.)

As you can see, the mechanisms of action of antiarrhythmics vary widely. A few of these drugs have properties common to more than one class; however, adenosine, a blocking agent used to treat paroxysmal supraventricular tachycardia, doesn't fall into any of them.

Class IA Antiarrhythmics

Class IA antiarrhythmics are used to treat a wide variety of atrial and ventricular arrhythmias. They do this by altering the myocardial cell membrane and interfering with autonomic nervous system control of pacemaker cells. These drugs also block parasympathetic stimulation of the SA and AV nodes.

There are risks associated with this mechanism of action, however. Because stimulation of the parasympathetic nervous system causes the heart rate to slow, drugs that block it increase the conduction rate of the AV node. This increase can produce dangerous increases in the ventricular heart rate if rapid atrial activity is present, as in a patient with atrial fib. This increased ventricular rate can offset the ability of these drugs to convert atrial arrhythmias to a regular rhythm.

When taken orally, class IA drugs are rapidly absorbed, distributed through all body tissues, and metabolized. Because they work so quickly, sustained-release forms of these drugs have been developed to help maintain therapeutic levels.

Class IA antiarrhythmics not only control arrhythmias, but they also can induce arrhythmias, especially conduction delays that may worsen existing heart blocks. Using other antiarrhythmics, such as beta-adrenergic blockers (beta blockers), with these drugs increases this risk. Drug interactions specific to class IA antiarrhythmics are discussed with each drug below.

 PROCEED WITH CAUTION

Adverse Reactions to Class IA Antiarrhythmics

Class IA antiarrhythmics—especially quinidine—may produce GI symptoms such as:

- diarrhea
- cramping
- nausea
- vomiting
- anorexia
- bitter taste

Disopyramide

Disopyramide (Norpace, Norpace CR) is used in the suppression and treatment of sustained ventricular tachycardia. It is available in capsules and extended-release capsules. When taken with macrolide antibiotics, such as clarithromycin and erythromycin, this drug increases a patient's risk of developing certain arrhythmias.

When taken with verapamil, disopyramide may increase myocardial depression. Its use should be avoided in patients with heart failure. Rifampin, phenytoin, and phenobarbital can reduce the effects of disopyramide.

Procainamide

Procainamide (Pronestyl, Pronestyl SR) is used to treat life-threatening ventricular arrhythmias. It can be taken by mouth or administered intravenously. This drug is available in tablets, extended-release tablets, and an injectable form.

Quinidine Sulfate

Quinidine sulfate is prescribed to treat several types of arrhythmias:

- premature atrial contractions
- premature ventricular contractions
- atrial tachycardia
- atrial flutter
- paroxysmal atrial fibrillation
- chronic atrial fibrillation

Quinidine sulfate is available in regular tablets and extended-release tablets. Quinidine gluconate is available in extended-release tablets and injectable solution.

Patients taking this drug may experience increased skeletal muscle relaxation if they are also taking neuromuscular blockers. Quinidine also increases the risk of digoxin toxicity. Rifampin, phenytoin, and phenobarbital can reduce quinidine's effects.

TIP Quinidine and quinine are often confused. Here's what you need to remember: Quinine is an antimalarial drug; Quinidine is an antiarrhythmic drug. Always double-check the prescription or medication order to make sure you have the correct drug. Then, check again when removing the product from the shelf to make sure you have the correct drug.

Class IB Antiarrhythmics

Class IB antiarrhythmic drugs are used to treat acute ventricular arrhythmias and ventricular ectopic (abnormal or irregular) beats. They treat only ventricular arrhythmias because they mainly affect the Purkinje fibers (fibers in the conduction system of the heart) and myocardial cells in the ventricles. They usually don't produce immediate serious adverse reactions, so they are frequently used in acute care.

Most class B antiarrhythmics are administered orally and are rapidly absorbed from the GI tract. They work by blocking the rapid influx of sodium ions during the depolarization phase of the heart's repolarization cycle. This decreases the heart's refractory period, which reduces the risk of arrhythmia.

Other antiarrhythmics such as phenytoin, propranolol, procainamide, and quinidine can either add to or inhibit the effects of this class of antiarrhythmics when they are taken together. Drug interactions specific to individual class IB antiarrhythmics are noted with each drug below.

Lidocaine

Lidocaine is perhaps best known to the general public as a local anesthetic that is used to relieve skin and rectal itching or burning, sore throat, and other topical irritations. But in its injectable form, lidocaine (Xylocaine) is a powerful antiarrhythmic drug.

Lidocaine is the only class IB antiarrhythmic that is not administered orally. In varying strengths, it may be infused as an IV solution, injected into an existing IV line (a technique called IV-push), or injected IM directly into the patient's tissues.

In addition to the other adverse reactions common to all class IB antiarrhythmics, lidocaine toxicity can cause seizures and respiratory arrest.

Mexiletine

Mexiletine is manufactured as oral capsules. When disopyramide or a beta-adrenergic blocker is used with mexiletine, the heart's ability to contract may be reduced. Rifampin may reduce mexiletine's effect. In addition, theophylline levels increase when given with mexiletine.

In addition to the adverse reactions common to drugs in this class, adverse reactions to mexiletine include:

- nausea and vomiting
- double vision
- confusion
- ataxia
- atrioventricular block

Class IC Antiarrhythmics

Like class IB antiarrhythmics, class IC antiarrhythmic drugs are used to treat life-threatening ventricular arrhythmias.

They're also used to treat supraventricular arrhythmias. They work mainly by slowing conduction of electrical impulses along the heart's conduction system.

These drugs may show additive effects with other antiarrhythmics. (As you learned in Chapter 1, an additive effect is a reaction that occurs when the combined effect of two or more drugs equals the sum of each drug given alone.) Drug interactions of specific class IC antiarrhythmics are noted in the discussion of each drug below.

Flecainide

Flecainide (Tambocor) is used to prevent paroxysmal supraventricular tachycardia, a rapid heart rate that originates above the ventricles, in patients without structural heart disease. This drug is available in tablet form. When used with digoxin, flecainide increases the risk of digoxin toxicity.

Propafenone

Propafenone (Rythmol, Rythmol SR) is available in tablets and extended-release capsules. Like flecainide, this drug is used to prevent PSVT in patients without structural heart disease. Quinidine increases propafenone's effects. When used with digoxin, propafenone increases the risk of digoxin toxicity. It also increases the serum concentration and effects of netroprolol and propranolol.

In addition to the adverse reactions common to the drugs in this class, propafenone may cause bronchospasm.

Class II Antiarrhythmics

Class II antiarrhythmic drugs consist of certain beta-adrenergic antagonists, or beta blockers. They block beta-adrenergic receptor sites in the heart's conduction system. As a result, the SA node's ability to fire is slowed. The ability of the AV node and other cells to receive and conduct electrical impulses to nearby cells is also reduced. This slows ventricular rates in patients with atrial flutter, atrial fib, and PAT.

These drugs also reduce the strength of the heart's contractions. When the heart beats less forcefully, it doesn't require as much oxygen to do its work.

Class II antiarrhythmics can cause a variety of drug interactions, however. For example, giving class II antiarrhythmics with phenothiazines and other antihypertensive

PROCEED WITH CAUTION

Adverse Reactions to Class II Antiarrhythmics

Common adverse reactions include:

- arrhythmias
- bradycardia
- heart failure
- hypotension
- bronchoconstriction
- GI reactions such as nausea, vomiting, and diarrhea

PROCEED WITH CAUTION

Adverse Reactions to Class III Antiarrhythmics

Adverse reactions to class III antiarrhythmic drugs—especially amiodarone—vary widely and commonly lead to discontinuation of the drug. A common adverse affect is aggravation of arrhythmias.

- Amiodarone may produce hypertension, nausea, and anorexia. Visual disturbances and corneal microdeposits may result. Severe pulmonary toxicity occurs in 15 percent of patients and can be fatal.
- Ibutilide may cause sustained ventricular tachycardia, prolongation of the QT interval, hypotension, nausea, and headache.
- Sotalol may cause AV block, ventricular arrhythmias, bronchospasm, and hypotension.

drugs can increase their blood pressure-lowering effect. On the other hand, giving class II antiarrhythmics with nonsteroidal anti-inflammatory drugs (NSAIDs) can cause water and fluid retention, thereby decreasing the antihypertensive affect.

Other drug interactions with class II antiarrhythmics include the following:

- The effects of sympathomimetics may be reduced when taken with class II antiarrhythmics.
- Beta blockers given with verapamil can depress the heart, causing hypotension, bradycardia, AV block, and weakened contractions.
- Beta blockers reduce the effects of sulfonylureas.
- The risk of digoxin toxicity increases when digoxin is taken with the class II antiarrhythmic drug esmolol.

Esmolol

Esmolol (Brevibloc) is usually administered in a doctor's office, clinic, or hospital setting. The drug can be injected by IV-push into an IV line or as an IV solution for infusion.

Propranolol

Propranolol (Inderal, Inderal LA, InnoPran XL) is usually administered orally as tablets or as 24-hour extended-release capsules. An oral solution and an injectable form are also available.

This drug is also used to treat angina, hypertension, migraine or vascular headache and essential tremor, and to decrease the risk of death after a myocardial infarction (MI, or "heart attack").

Acebutolol

Acebutolol (Sectral) is administered orally in capsule form and is used to treat ventricular arrhythmias and hypertension. However, this drug is rarely used.

Class III Antiarrhythmics

Class III antiarrhythmic drugs are used to treat life-threatening ventricular arrhythmias. Although their exact mechanism of action isn't known, they're thought to suppress arrhythmias by unidirectional block to a bidirectional

block. These drugs have little or no effect on depolarization. Instead, they slow repolarization, prolonging the refractory period and the duration of the heart's action potential.

Amiodarone

Amiodarone (Cordarone, Pacerone) is the first-line drug of choice for treating V-tach and V-fib. It can be taken orally in tablet form or administered intravenously.

Amiodarone increases the risk of digoxin toxicity. Too-rapid IV administration may result in hypotension. Amiodarone also increases phenytoin, procainamide, and quinidine levels when it is taken in conjunction with these three drugs.

Dofetilide

Dofetilide (Tikosyn) is available in capsule form. Because of the risk of inducing life-threatening arrhythmias, the use of this drug is contraindicated when the patient is taking:

- cimetidine
- ketoconazole
- megestrol
- prochlorperazine
- trimethoprim
- verapamil

Ibutilide

Ibutilide (Corvert) is administered by IV injection or infusion in a hospital. However, it shouldn't be given within four hours of a class I or another class III antiarrhythmic.

Sotalol

Sotalol (Betapace, Betapace AF, Sorine) is manufactured as tablets. In addition to treating life-threatening ventricular arrhythmias, it is used to maintain normal sinus rhythm or to delay the recurrence of atrial fib or atrial flutter of patients who are currently in normal sinus rhythm. Sotalol shouldn't be given with dolasetron or droperidol due to an increased risk of life-threatening arrhythmias.

Class IV Antiarrhythmics

Class IV antiarrhythmic drugs are composed of calcium channel blockers. The calcium channel blockers verapamil and diltiazem are used to treat supraventricular arrhythmias with a rapid ventricular response (a rapid heart rate in which the rhythm originates above the ventricles). You'll read more about these two drugs in the discussion of other calcium channel blockers later in the chapter.

Adenosine

Adenosine (Adenocard, Adenoscan) is an injectable IV solution that is used for acute treatment of PSVT. It works by depressing the pacemaker activity of the SA node. This reduces the heart rate and the ability of the AV node to conduct impulses from the atria to the ventricles.

Adenosine is especially effective against reentry tachycardias (when an impulse depolarizes an area of heart muscle, then returns and repolarizes it) that involve the AV node. It is typically used to treat arrhythmias associated with accessory bypass tracts (brief periods of rapid heart rate in which the rhythm originates above the ventricle).

When adenosine and the anticonvulsant carbamazepine are used together, there's an increased risk of heart block. Carbamazepine and dipyridamole increase the effects of adenosine, so smaller doses of adenosine may be necessary. On the other hand, methylxanthines block the effects of adenosine, so larger doses of adenosine may be necessary.

 T I P Caffeine blocks the effects of adenosine. If a patient is a coffee drinker, larger doses of the drug may be necessary.

ANTIANGINAL DRUGS

Although the major symptom of angina is chest pain, the drugs used to treat it typically aren't analgesics. Instead, **antianginal drugs** treat it by reducing the amount of oxygen the heart needs to do its work (myocardial oxygen

PROCEED WITH CAUTION

Adverse Reactions to Adenosine

Common adverse reactions to adenosine include:

- facial flushing
- shortness of breath
- dyspnea (labored breathing)
- chest discomfort

HOW IT WORKS

How Antianginal Drugs Work

Angina occurs when the coronary arteries—the heart's main source of oxygen—do not supply enough oxygen to the myocardium. This increases the heart's workload by increasing:

- heart rate
- preload—the volume of blood in the ventricle just before contraction
- afterload—the pressure in the arteries leading from the ventricle against which the ventricle contracts
- force of myocardial contractility—the power of the muscle fibers to execute a contraction

Antianginal drugs relieve angina by decreasing one or more of the four factors. See Figure 5-1, which summarizes how each class of antianginal drugs affects the cardiovascular system.

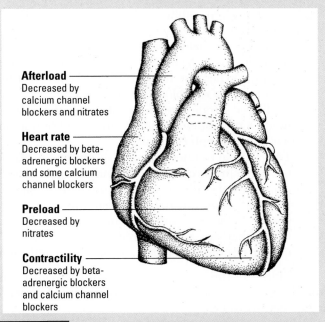

FIGURE 5-1 How antianginal drugs work. (From *Clinical Pharmacology Made Incredibly Easy.* 2nd Ed. Philadelphia, PA: Lippincott Williams & Wilkins; 2005.)

demand), by increasing the supply of oxygen to the heart, or both actions.

The three classes of antianginal drugs are:

- nitrates, which are used for treating acute angina
- beta-adrenergic blockers (beta blockers), which are used for the long-term prevention of angina
- calcium channel blockers, which are used when other drugs fail to prevent angina

Nitrates

Nitrates are the drugs of choice for relieving acute angina. They do this by causing the smooth muscles of the veins and, to a lesser extent, the arteries to relax. Here's how it happens:

1. When the veins dilate, less blood returns to the heart.
2. This reduces the amount of blood in the ventricle at the end of diastole (the heart's expansion prior to a contraction or beat).
3. By reducing preload, ventricular size and wall tension are reduced. The left ventricle doesn't have to stretch as much to pump blood.
4. The arterioles (the small branches at the end of an artery) provide the most resistance to blood pumped by the left ventricle. By dilating the arterioles, nitrates reduce this resistance and further ease the heart's workload.
5. All these actions, in turn, reduce the oxygen requirements of the heart.

Nitrates can be administered in a variety of ways:

- Nitrates given sublingually (under the tongue), buccally (in the pocket of the cheek), as chewable tablets, as lingual aerosols (sprayed onto or under the tongue), or by inhalation are absorbed almost completely because the mucous membranes of the mouth have a rich blood supply.
- Swallowed nitrate capsules are absorbed through the mucous membranes of the GI tract, and only about half the dose enters circulation.
- Transdermal nitrates—patches or ointments placed on the skin—are absorbed slowly and in varying amounts, depending on the amount of drug applied, the location on which it is applied, the surface area of skin that is used, and the skin's circulation.
- Drugs that are administered intravenously don't need to be absorbed; they go directly into circulation.

Rapidly absorbed nitrates, such as nitroglycerin (discussed below) are the drugs of choice for relief of acute angina because they:

- have a rapid onset of action
- are easy to take
- are inexpensive

Longer-acting nitrates, such as the daily nitroglycerin transdermal patch, are convenient for preventing chronic angina. Oral nitrates are also used for this purpose because they seldom produce serious adverse reactions.

There are several interactions that patients taking nitrates should be made aware of:

- Absorption of sublingual nitrates may be delayed in someone who is taking an anticholinergic drug.
- Noticeable orthostatic hypotension (drop in blood pressure when a person stands up), along with light-headedness, fainting, or blurred vision may result when nitrates and calcium channel blockers are used together.

PROCEED WITH CAUTION

Adverse Reactions to Nitrates

Most adverse reactions to nitrates result from changes in the cardiovascular system. The "three H's" may appear: *Headache* is the most common adverse reaction. *Hypotension* may also occur, accompanied by dizziness and increased *heart rate.* These reactions usually disappear when dosage is reduced.

- When alcohol interacts with nitrates, severe hypotension can result.
- Sildenafil (Viagra), vardenafil (Levitra), tadalafil (Cialis), and similar drugs used to treat erectile dysfunction should not be taken within 24 hours of taking nitrates because of potential enhanced hypotensive effects.

Isosorbide Dinitrate

Isosorbide dinitrate (Dilatrate SR, Isochron, Isordil Titradose) is swallowed or taken sublingually and is available as tablets, extended-release tablets, extended-release capsules, and as sublingual.

Isosorbide Mononitrate

Isosorbide mononitrate (Monoket, Ismo, Imdur) comes in the form of tablets and 24-hour extended-release tablets.

TIP Remember two important safety considerations regarding nitrates: (1) Nitroglycerin capsules and tablets must always be dispensed in glass containers because plastic absorbs these drugs; and (2) because the sublingual tablets are only used when needed, the patient needs to be aware of the expiration date and replace them when expired.

Nitroglycerin

Nitroglycerin (NitroDur, Minitran, Nitro-Bid, Nitrolingual Pump, Nitrostat) is administered in a wide variety of forms:

- *Extended-release capsules.* These forms are used to prevent chronic angina.
- *Sublingual tablets.* To treat acute angina attacks, patients should place one tablet under the tongue as soon as an attack begins. Another tablet can be taken in five minutes, if needed, to a maximum of three tablets. If no relief occurs after the third tablet, the patient should call 911 or go to the nearest emergency department.
- *Sublingual spray.* To prevent or treat acute angina attacks, patients should spray the medication once or twice under the tongue. Treatment can be repeated in three to five minutes, if needed, to a maximum of three doses in a 15-minute period.

- *Transdermal patch.* These patches are used to prevent chronic angina. Patches may be worn for 24 hours or for 16 hours (patient wears the patch during the day and removes it at bedtime).
- *Topical ointment.* This form of the drug is used to prevent chronic angina. A half-inch of ointment is applied initially, increasing in half-inch increments up to five inches until desired results are obtained.
- *IV solution.* This treatment, which must be administered by a medical professional, is usually limited to very acute attacks of angina. It may also be used to treat hypertension from surgery, heart failure, or myocardial infarction.

Beta-Adrenergic Antagonists

You read about beta-adrenergic antagonists, or beta blockers, and how they work earlier in this chapter, when you learned about class II antiarrhythmic drugs. While some beta blockers are used to treat arrhythmias, others are useful for the long-term prevention of angina. In addition, because their action decreases blood pressure, they are first-line therapy for treating hypertension as well. For this reason, some of the beta blockers are manufactured as combination products with a diuretic. (These combination products are included in the *Drug Classification* table at the end of this chapter.)

A number of drugs interact with beta-adrenergic blockers:

- Antacids delay the absorption of beta blockers.
- NSAIDs can decrease the hypotensive effects of beta blockers.
- Lidocaine toxicity may occur when lidocaine is taken with beta blockers.

PROCEED WITH CAUTION

Adverse Reactions to Beta-Adrenergic Antagonists

Beta-adrenergic blockers may cause:

- bradycardia
- angina
- fainting
- nausea, vomiting, and diarrhea
- fluid retention and peripheral edema
- shock
- heart failure
- arrhythmias (especially atrioventricular block)
- significant constriction of the bronchioles in the lungs

Suddenly stopping taking a beta blocker may trigger angina, hypertension, arrhythmias, or an acute MI (heart attack).

- The requirements of insulin and oral antidiabetics may be altered by beta-adrenergic blockers.
- The ability of theophylline to produce bronchodilation is impaired by nonselective beta blockers.

Atenolol and Carvedilol

Atenolol (Tenormin) is offered as tablets.

Carvedilol (Coreg, Coreg CR) is taken by mouth in tablet form. It is also manufactured as extended-release capsules. In addition to treating angina, this drug is also sometimes used in treating heart failure.

Metoprolol

Metoprolol (Lopressor, Toprol XL) is manufactured in three different formulations. It is available in tablets, 24-hour extended-release tablets, and in an injectable concentation. In acute coronary syndrome—a set of symptoms that suggest sudden and severe myocardial infarction—it is given by IV injection initially and then orally. Like carvedilol, this drug is also used in treating heart failure.

Nadolol

Nadolol (Corgard) is manufactured as oral tablets.

Propranolol

Propranolol (Inderal, Inderal LA, Innopran XL) is usually administered orally in tablet form or as 24-hour extended-release capsules. Oral solutions and injectable forms are also available.

As you learned earlier, this drug is also used in treating arrhythmias. In addition, it's used to treat hypertension. Further uses include the treatment of migraines or vascular headaches and essential tremor, and to reduce the risk of death after a heart attack.

Calcium Channel Blockers

Calcium channel blockers are commonly used to prevent angina attacks that do not respond to drugs in any of the other antianginal classes. Several of the calcium channel blockers are also used as antiarrhythmics and to treat hypertension. Like beta blockers, calcium channel blockers are often combined with other medications into a single formulation combination product. (These combination products are included in the Drug Classification table at the end of this chapter.)

The calcium channel blockers that treat angina—each of which is discussed below—are used for long-term prevention of angina only. They are not used for short-term relief of chest pain.

Like most medications, calcium channel blockers affect and are affected by the actions of other drugs. For example, calcium salts and vitamin D reduce the effectiveness of calcium channel blockers. Nondepolarizing blocking drugs may have a greater muscle-relaxing effect when taken with calcium channel blockers.

HOW IT WORKS

How Calcium Channel Blockers Work

Calcium channel blockers prevent the passage of calcium ions across the myocardial cell membrane and vascular smooth muscle cells by blocking the slow calcium channel (figure 5-2). This action causes coronary arteries—and, to a lesser extent, the peripheral arteries and arterioles—to dilate, decreasing the afterload and increasing the heart's oxygen supply. The result is less force in the heart's contractions and a reduced workload for the heart.

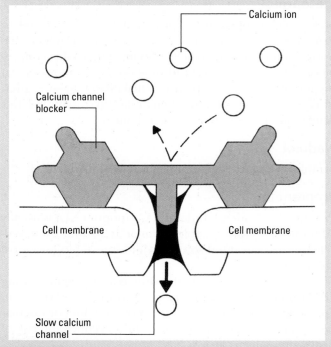

FIGURE 5-2 How calcium channel blockers work. (From *Clinical Pharmacology Made Incredibly Easy.* 2nd Ed. Philadelphia, PA: Lippincott Williams & Wilkins; 2005.)

Amlodipine and Diltiazem

Amlodipine (Norvasc) is prescribed as tablets.

Diltiazem (Cardizem, Cardizem CD, Cardizem LA, Cartia XT, Dilacor XR, Dilt-CD, Dilt-XR, Diltia XT, Taztia XT, Tiazac) is manufactured as tablets, as 24-hour extended-release tablets, and mainly as 24-hour extended-release capsules.

For hospital and clinic use, a solution is manufactured for direct injection by IV-push or for continuous infusion by mixing it with an IV solution. In this form, diltiazem is used to treat atrial fibrillation or flutter and paroxysmal supraventricular tachycardia.

There are three specific interactions and risks associated with taking this drug:

- It may increase a patient's risk of digoxin toxicity.
- It may enhance the action of carbamazepine.
- It may cause myocardial depression.

⚠ PROCEED WITH CAUTION

Adverse Reactions to Calcium Channel Blockers

As with other antianginal drugs, cardiovascular reactions are the most common adverse reactions to calcium channel blockers. These include:

- hypotension
- orthostatic hypotension
- heart failure
- arrhythmias such as bradycardia, sinus block, and AV block (with diltiazem and verapamil)

Other possible adverse reactions include:

- dizziness
- headache
- flushing
- weakness
- persistent peripheral edema

Nicardipine

Nicardipine (Cardene, Cardene SR) can be used alone or with other antianginals to treat chronic stable angina. It is available in regular and extended-release capsule form. For patients who cannot take the oral form, a solution is available for IV infusion.

Nifedipine

Nifedipine (Adalat CC, Afeditab CR, Nifediac CC, Nifedical XL, Procardia, Procardia XL) is prescribed as immediate-release capsules or as 24-hour extended-release tablets.

T I P Don't confuse *nicardipine* and *nifedipine*!

Verapamil

Verapamil (Calan, Calan SR, Covera-HS, Isoptin SR, Verelan, Verelan PM) is used in the treatment of various forms of angina as well as chronic atrial fib, supraventricular arrhythmias, and hypertension, and to prevent paroxysmal supraventricular tachycardia. It's available in immediate-release tablets, extended-release tablets, extended-release capsules, and an injectable solution.

Dosages vary greatly depending on the condition being treated and the form of verapamil being used. Like diltiazem, this drug may increase the risk of digoxin toxicity, enhance the action of carbamazepine, and cause myocardial depression.

ANTIHYPERTENSIVE DRUGS

Antihypertensive drugs are used to treat hypertension, commonly known as high blood pressure. This disorder is indicated by an elevation in systolic blood pressure, diastolic blood pressure, or both.

Treatment for hypertension usually begins with a diuretic or a calcium channel blocker. Patients may also receive beta blockers. Other drugs that are used include:

- sympatholytic drugs other than beta blockers
- vasodilators
- angiotensin-converting enzyme (ACE) inhibitors
- angiotensin II receptor blockers

At times, a combination of drugs may be used. Because of the need for combination therapy in many patients to control blood pressure effectively, many drugs come in single-dosage combination products, such as a beta blocker and a diuretic or a calcium channel blocker and a diuretic. (Combination products are included in the *Drug Classification* table at the end of this chapter.) The combination formulations give the patient the advantage of taking fewer tablets or capsules per day, making it easier for the patient to follow the physician's orders.

Sympatholytic Drugs

Sympatholytic drugs include several different types of drugs. But they all reduce blood pressure by inhibiting or blocking the **sympathetic nervous system**, the branch of the autonomic nervous system that regulates the expenditure of energy and has key effects in stressful situations.

Sympatholytic drugs are classified into four groups according to their mechanism of action. If a drug from one of these groups fails to have the desired effect, the physician may substitute one drug for another or add one from a different class.

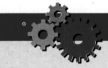

HOW IT WORKS

Blood Pressure

As you learned earlier in this chapter, oxygenated blood travels from the heart into the arteries, which carry blood to the body tissues. Blood pressure is the force of blood against the walls of the arteries.

Two variables of a person's blood pressure are measured:

- Systolic pressure, which occurs during heart muscle contraction, is less than 120 in a healthy person and is expressed in millimeters of mercury (mmHg).
- Diastolic pressure, which occurs during relaxation of the heart muscle, is less than 80 mmHg in a healthy person.

A blood pressure measurement is expressed like a fraction. The top figure is the person's systolic blood pressure; the bottom figure is her diastolic blood pressure. A normal blood pressure is less than 120/80. If the systolic figure is 140 or over, or the diastolic figure is 90 or over, the patient is considered as having high blood pressure, or hypertension.

Hypertension is serious because it causes the heart to work harder and contributes to atherosclerosis (hardening of the arteries). It increases the risk of heart disease, congestive heart failure, kidney disease, blindness, and stroke.

PROCEED WITH CAUTION

Adverse Reactions to Sympatholytics

Adverse reactions to central-acting sympatholytics include:

- depression
- drowsiness
- edema
- liver dysfunction
- numbness and tingling
- vertigo

Adverse reactions to alpha-adrenergic blockers include:

- hypotension
- orthostatic hypotension
- cardiac arrhythmias
- tachycardia

Adverse reactions to mixed alpha- and beta-adrenergic blockers include:

- fatigue
- drowsiness
- insomnia
- weakness
- hypotension
- diarrhea
- dyspnea
- skin rash

Central-Acting Sympathetic Nervous System Inhibitors

This group of drugs affects specific central nervous system centers and decreases some of the activity of the sympathetic nervous system. Although these drugs work in somewhat different ways, their results are basically the same.

Clonidine

Clonidine (Catapres, Catapres TTS, Duraclon) is used in the treatment of essential hypertension and renal hypertension. It is administered orally in tablet form, transdermally in a weekly patch, and by epidermal infusion. When taken with CNS depressants, clonidine may worsen CNS depression. When taken with antidepressants, this drug may increase blood pressure.

Methyldopa

Methyldopa is used in treating **hypertensive crisis**—a condition of impending organ damage from severely high blood pressure—as well as for ongoing treatment of hypertension.

Alpha-Adrenergic Blockers

Chemical substances called neurohormones are **neurotransmitters**. They are released at nerve endings to help transmit nerve impulses. The two neurohormones of the sympathetic nervous system are epinephrine and norepinephrine. Epinephrine is secreted by the adrenal medulla. Norepinephrine is secreted mainly at the nerve endings of sympathetic nerve fibers, which are also called adrenergic nerve fibers.

Stimulation of alpha-adrenergic fibers results in constriction of blood vessels (called vasoconstriction). If stimulation of these fibers is blocked, the result is the exact opposite effect—vasodilation, or the expansion of the blood vessels. Alpha-adrenergic blockers (commonly called alpha blockers) block the transmission of epinephrine and norepinephrine. Vasodilation and lower blood pressure result.

If diuretics and beta-andrenergic blockers fail to control hypertension, an alpha blocker or a mixed alpha- and beta-adrenergic blocker may be used.

Doxazosin

Doxazosin (Cardura, Cardura XL) is used in the treatment of essential hypertension. It is available in immediate-release tablets and 24-hour extended-release tablets.

Phentolamine

Phentolamine is an injectable drug used to prevent or control hypertension before or during certain surgical procedures. It is given intramuscularly or intravenously.

Prazosin

Prazosin (Minipress) is used to treat mild to moderate hypertension. It can be used alone, with a diuretic, or with another antihypertensive. The drug is available in capsule form.

Terazosin

Terazosin (Hytrin) is available in capsule form. It is usually taken at bedtime.

Mixed Alpha- and Beta-Adrenergic Blockers

These drugs block the stimulation of both the alpha- and beta-adrenergic receptors in the nerve fibers. As you learned earlier in this chapter, beta receptors are found mainly in the heart.

Carvedilol

Carvedilol (Coreg, Coreg CR) is available in immediate-release tablets or 24-hour extended-release capsules. Doses are individualized according to the patient's condition.

A number of drug interactions are possible when using carvedilol:

- Carvedilol taken with antidiabetics may result in increased hypoglycemic effect.
- Carvedilol taken with calcium channel blockers may result in increased conduction disturbances.
- Carvedilol taken with digoxin may result in increased digoxin levels.
- Carvedilol taken with rifampin decreases carvedilol levels.

In addition to the adverse reactions common to mixed alpha- and beta-adrenergic blockers, carvedilol may cause:

- cardiac insufficiency
- chest pain
- bradycardia

Labetalol

Labetalol (Trandate) is usually administered as tablets, but in severe hypertension or hypertensive emergencies, this drug can be given through IV-push or by infusion.

Norepinephrine Depletors

Norepinephrine depletors work by decreasing the production of norepinephrine in the brain. One of these drugs, reserpine, is available in tablet form. This group of sympatholytic drugs is rarely used.

Vasodilating Drugs

There are two types of vasodilating drugs—direct vasodilators and calcium channel blockers. Both types decrease systolic and diastolic blood pressure.

You read about calcium channel blockers earlier in this chapter. They produce arterial relaxation by preventing the entry of calcium into the cells. This prevents the contraction of vascular smooth muscle. Calcium channel blockers are sometimes used alone to treat mild to moderate hypertension.

Direct vasodilators act on arteries, veins, or both. They relax peripheral vascular smooth muscle, causing the blood vessels to dilate. The increased diameter of the blood vessels reduces total peripheral resistance, which lowers blood pressure.

Vasodilating drugs are rarely used alone to treat hypertension. They're usually combined with other drugs to treat patients with moderate to severe hypertension or

 PROCEED WITH CAUTION

Adverse Reactions to Direct Vasodilators

Direct vasodilators commonly produce adverse reactions related to reflex activation of the sympathetic nervous system. As blood pressure falls, the sympathetic nervous system is stimulated, producing compensating measures, such as vasodilation and tachycardia. Other adverse reactions to sympathetic stimulation include:

- palpitations
- angina
- edema
- breast tenderness
- fatigue
- headache
- rash
- severe pericardial effusion

hypertensive crisis. They may produce additive effects when given with nitrates such as isosorbide dinitrate, or nitroglycerin. Few other drug interactions occur. Interactions involving specific vasodilating drugs are noted with the discussion of each drug in the sections that follow.

Hydralazine

Oral hydralazine is administered in tablet form, alone or with other antihypertensives, for ongoing treatment of essential hypertension. It is generally used when the condition is resistant to other treatment or care. An injectable solution can be infused intravenously to lower severe hypertension quickly. Its antihypertensive effects are increased when it's given with methyldopa and some other antihypertensive drugs.

Minoxidil

Minoxidil is available in tablet form and is used to treat severe hypertension. Its antihypertensive effects are increased when minoxidil is administered with other antihypertensive drugs, such as methyldopa.

Nitroprusside

Nitroprusside (Nitropress) is available in an IV solution and is used to lower blood pressure quickly in hypertensive emergencies and to control hypertension during anesthesia.

Angiotensin-Converting Enzyme Inhibitors

When beta blockers or diuretics are ineffective in treating a patient's hypertension, a physician generally turns to angiotensin-converting enzyme (ACE) inhibitors next. They can be used alone or with another drug, such as a thiazide diuretic. (Combination products are included in the *Drug Classification* table at the end of this chapter.)

ACE inhibitors reduce blood pressure by interrupting the renin-angiotensin-aldosterone system. Here's how they work:

1. The kidneys maintain blood pressure in the body by releasing the hormone renin. Renin acts on the plasma protein angiotensinogen to form angiotensin I. Angiotensin I is then converted to angiotensin II.
2. A powerful vasoconstrictor, angiotensin II increases peripheral resistance and promotes the excretion of aldosterone. Aldosterone promotes the retention of sodium and water. This increases the volume of blood that the heart needs to pump.
3. ACE inhibitors prevent the conversion of angiotensin I to angiotensin II. As angiotensin II is reduced, small blood vessels dilate, reducing peripheral vascular resistance.
4. The reduced secretion of aldosterone promotes the excretion of salt and water. This reduces the volume of blood the heart needs to pump, thereby reducing blood pressure.

PROCEED WITH CAUTION

Adverse Reactions to Angiotensin-Converting Enzyme Inhibitors

ACE inhibitors can produce these adverse reactions:

- headache
- fatigue
- dry, nonproductive, persistent cough
- angioedema
- GI reactions
- increased serum potassium concentrations
- tickling in the throat
- transient elevations of blood urea nitrogen (BUN) and serum creatinine levels (indicators of kidney function)

The dry, nonproductive, persistent cough associated with ACE inhibitor use is a common reason why patients might discontinue their use of the drug.

Certain ACE inhibitors may also be used to treat patients with heart failure or following myocardial infarction. However, ACE inhibitors can cause several kinds of interactions with other cardiovascular drugs.

- All ACE inhibitors enhance the hypotensive effects of diuretics and other antihypertensives such as beta blockers.
- When ACE inhibitors are used with potassium-sparing diuretics, potassium supplements, or potassium-containing salt substitutes, hyperkalemia may occur.

ACE inhibitors also interact with other prescription and nonprescription, over-the-counter (OTC) medications. For example, patients taking ACE inhibitors should avoid NSAIDs that not only reduce the effect of ACE inhibitors, they may also alter renal function.

Benazepril

Benazepril (Lotensin) is prescribed in tablet form. For patients not also taking a diuretic, the maintenance dose is typically double the amount given to patients taking a diuretic.

Captopril

Captopril (Capoten) is taken orally in tablet form. The drug is used in treating congestive heart failure and left ventricular dysfunction after acute MI. If this drug cannot control hypertension alone, adding a diuretic can make captopril more effective.

In addition to the adverse reactions common to all drugs in this class, captopril may cause:

- protein in the urine
- reduced neutrophils and granulocytes (types of white blood cells)
- rash

- loss of taste
- hypotension
- severe allergic reaction

Enalapril

Enalapril (Vasotec) is usually taken orally in tablet form, although an IV concentration is available for injection or infusion. The injectable form of enalapril is marketed under the trade name Enalaprilat.

T I P Whenever you come across a generic drug name that ends in *-pril*, it's probably an ACE inhibitor.

Fosinopril

Fosinopril (Monopril) is available in tablet form and is used to treat hypertension and congestive heart failure.

Lisinopril

Lisinopril (Prinvil, Zestril) is taken orally in tablet form and is used to treat hypertension. If the patient is taking a diuretic, the dose of this drug is likely to be reduced. Lisinopril is also used in stable patients within 24 hours of acute MI to improve their chances for survival.

Moexipril

Moexipril (Univasc) is available in tablet form. A diuretic may be added, if needed, in which case the dose is decreased.

Quinapril

Quinapril (Accupril) is manufactured in tablet form and most often administered for hypertension, although it is occasionally prescribed for patients with congestive heart failure. Elderly patients and those taking diuretics may not need as high a dose as other patients taking this drug.

Ramipril

Ramipril (Altace) is available in tablet and capsule forms and is used in heart failure, after an MI, and to reduce the risk of MI, stroke, and death from cardiovascular causes.

Trandolapril

Trandolapril (Mavik) is produced as regular and extended-release tablets. It is most often used to treat hypertension. The extended- release tablet is combined with 180 mg or 240 mg of verapamil. It is also used in treating heart failure or ventricular dysfunction after MI.

Angiotensin II Receptor Blockers

Angiotensin II receptor blockers (ARBs) lower blood pressure by blocking the vasoconstrictive effects of angiotensin II. They are often an alternative for patients who have discontinued the use of ACE inhibitors due to the common adverse reaction of a dry, nonproductive, persistent cough. These drugs can be used alone or in combination with diuretics and other drugs. (Combination products are

HOW IT WORKS

Different Mechanisms of Action, Same Effect

ACE inhibitors and ARBs both work toward lowering blood pressure by interfering with the renin-angiotensin-aldosterone process that begins in the kidneys. But, as you've previously read, ACE inhibitors block the conversion of angiotensin I to angiotensin II. ARBs *don't* block the conversion of angiotensin I to angiotensin II. Instead, they block the binding of the angiotensin II to the AT$_1$ receptor. This prevents angiotensin II from exerting its vasoconstricting properties and from promoting the excretion of aldosterone. The result is lower blood pressure.

In short, as a treatment for hypertension, ACE inhibitors and ARBs both achieve the same result. They just do it at different stages in the process.

included in the Drug Classification table at the end of this chapter.)

There are several drug interactions associated with ARBs. For example, NSAIDs may reduce the hypertensive effects of ARBs. In addition, potassium supplements may increase the risk of hyperkalemia if they are used when taking ARBs. Specific ARBs have additional reactions with certain drugs. These are noted in the following discussions of individual ARBs.

Candesartan and Eprosartan

Candesartan (Atacand) is taken orally in tablet form and is used in treating congestive heart failure.

Eprosartan (Teveten) is available in oral tablets and is used to treat hypertension. It is taken alone or with other antihypertensives.

Irbesartan

Irbesartan (Avapro) is prescribed as oral tablets. Because irbesartan protects the renal system, it's often prescribed for patients with type 2 diabetes.

PROCEED WITH CAUTION

Adverse Reactions to Angiotensin II Receptor Blockers

Adverse reactions to ARBs include:

- headache and fatigue
- cough and tickling in the throat
- angioedema
- GI symptoms
- increased serum potassium level
- transient elevations or blood urea nitrogen (BUN) and serum creatinine levels

Losartan

Losartan (Cozaar) is taken orally in tablet form. Like irbesartan, this drug is used in patients who have type 2 diabetes. When losartan is taken with fluconazole, an increased blood level of losartan can result, leading to hypotension. On the other hand, rifampin may decrease metabolism of losartan and decrease losartan's effect.

TIP When you come across a generic drug name that ends in -*sartan*, it's most likely an ARB.

Olmesartan

Olmesartan (Benicar) is available in tablet form. In those patients with impaired renal function who are taking diuretics, a low starting dose should be considered.

Valsartan

Valsartan (Diovan) is taken orally as tablets. If the initial dose does not lower the patient's blood pressure sufficiently, the dosage can be increased, or a diuretic can be added. Valsartan is also used in treating cardiac patients. It reduces the risk of death in stable patients who have had an MI and who have left ventricular dysfunction or failure.

Aliskiren

Aliskiren (Tekturna) is a renin inhibitor used to treat hypertension. It works by relaxing blood vessels, which lowers blood pressure and helps the heart pump blood more easily. Aliskiren is available in the form of tablets.

A common adverse reaction to aliskiren is mild diarrhea. More severe adverse reactions include:

- severe allergic reactions, such as rash, difficulty breathing, or swelling of the hands, eyes, mouth, face, lips, or tongue
- symptoms of low blood pressure, including fainting, dizziness, or light-headedness
- trouble swallowing

DIURETIC DRUGS

Diuretics are used to promote the excretion of water and electrolytes by the kidneys. By doing so, they play a major role in the treatment of hypertension, as well as other cardiovascular conditions. The major types of diuretics used as cardiovascular drugs include:

- thiazide and thiazide-like diuretics
- loop diuretics
- potassium-sparing diuretics

Thiazide and Thiazide-like Diuretics

Thiazide and thiazide-like diuretics work by preventing sodium from being reabsorbed from the kidneys. As the

HOW IT WORKS

How Diuretics Work

Most diuretics act on the tubules of the kidney nephrons. The nephron is the functional unit of the kidney. Each kidney contains about a million of them. They filter the bloodstream to remove waste products such as urea and ammonia. During this process, some water, electrolytes (potassium, sodium, and chloride), and drugs may also be removed. This filtrate (the fluid removed from the blood) then passes through the proximal tubule, the loop of Henle, and the distal tubules. During this excretion process, some amino acids, glucose, electrolytes, and water are reabsorbed through tiny capillaries that surround the distal and proximal tubules and the loop of Henle, and are then returned to the bloodstream. What is not excreted goes to the bladder and is excreted as urine.

sodium is excreted, it pulls water along with it. Blood volume decreases, leading to reduced cardiac output at first. But if therapy is continued, cardiac output and blood volume stabilize.

Long-term use of these drugs also causes arteriolar vasodilation, which lowers blood pressure. This effect, combined with the decreases in blood volume that the drugs produce, makes them useful in the long-term treatment of hypertension. They're used to treat edema caused by mild or moderate heart failure, by liver or kidney disease, or by corticosteroid and estrogen therapy. In addition, because they decrease calcium levels in urine, they're used—alone or with other drugs—to prevent the development or recurrence of kidney stones.

In patients with diabetes insipidus (a disorder that causes excessive urine production and thirst), these drugs have the opposite of their usual effect. They actually *decrease* urine volume, possibly through their sodium-depleting and blood volume-reducing actions.

Thiazide diuretics include:

- bendroflumethiazide
- chlorothiazide
- hydrochlorothiazide
- methyclothiazide

Thiazide-like diuretics include:

- indapamide
- metolazone
- quinethazone

Altered fluid volume, blood pressure, and serum electrolyte levels result from interactions of other drugs with thiazide and thiazide-like diuretics. For example:

- Taking corticosteroids, corticotrophin, or amphotericin with these diuretics may cause hypokalemia.
- NSAIDS, including cyclooxygenase-2 (COX-2) inhibitors, may reduce the antihypertensive effects of these diuretics.

- These diuretics may increase blood glucose levels, requiring higher doses of insulin and oral antidiabetics.
- Hyponatremia (low levels of sodium in the blood) and thiazide resistance may also occur.
- Thiazide and thiazide-like diuretics may increase lithium levels.
- These diuretics may increase the response to skeletal muscle relaxants.

Bendroflumethiazide

Bendroflumethiazide is manufactured as an oral tablet. It may also be found in combination with other drugs. It works by decreasing the force of the heart and slowing down the heartbeat. This helps the heart beat more regularly and reduce the amount of work it has to do. The drug also increases the elimination of excess fluid, which helps decrease blood pressure.

Chlorothiazide and Hydrochlorothiazide

Chlorothiazide (Diuril) is produced as an oral suspension and tablet. It is also available as a solution for injection.

Hydrochlorothiazide (Ezide) is available as tablets or capsules. The drug is taken once daily to control hypertension or to reduce edema. When written, it is usually abbreviated as HCTZ.

Methyclothiazide and Indapamide

Methyclothiazide is available in tablet form for the treatment of hypertension and edema.

Indapamide is prescribed as oral tablets for hypertension and edema.

Chlorthalidone and Metolazone

Chlorthalidone (Thalitone) is available in tablet form for the treatment of hypertension and edema.

Metolazone (Zaroxolyn) is taken orally in tablet form to treat hypertension. This drug is also used to treat edema resulting from heart failure or renal disease.

Loop Diuretics

Loop diuretics are highly potent drugs. They are the strongest diuretics available, producing the greatest volume of urine production. They get their name because they mainly act on the loop of Henle—the part of the nephron responsible for concentrating urine—to increase the secretion of sodium, chloride, and water. These drugs may also inhibit the reabsorption of sodium, chloride, and water.

These drugs are used to treat edema associated with heart failure, liver disease, or nephritic syndrome (kidney disease). When prescribed to treat hypertension, they are usually used with a potassium-sparing diuretic or a potassium supplement to prevent hypokalemia.

Loop diuretics produce a variety of drug interactions.

- The risk of ototoxicity (damage to the hearing organs) is increased when aminoglycosides and cisplatin are taken with loop diuretics—especially with high doses of furosemide.
- When cardiac glycosides and loop diuretics are taken together, they can increase the risk of electrolyte imbalances that can trigger arrhythmias.
- Loop diuretics reduce the effect of oral antidiabetic drugs. This can result in hyperglycemia.
- Loop diuretics may increase the risk of lithium toxicity.

Bumetanide

Bumetanide is the shortest-acting diuretic. It is 40 times more powerful than even furosemide, another powerful loop diuretic that is discussed below. Bumetanide is usually taken orally in tablet form.

For patients who cannot take the drug orally, a solution is available for IM injection. It can be administered in diluted form by injection as an IV-push. The solution may also be mixed with IV fluid and infused into the patient intravenously.

 PROCEED WITH CAUTION

Adverse Reactions to Thiazide and Thiazide-like Diuretics

The most common adverse reactions to thiazide and thiazide-like diuretics include:

- reduced blood volume
- orthostatic hypertension
- hyponatremia
- hypokalemia

These drugs are contraindicated in patients who are allergic to sulfonamide drugs. A patient who's allergic to sulfas may experience an allergic reaction to thiazide and thiazide-like diuretics.

 PROCEED WITH CAUTION

Adverse Reactions to Loop Diuretics

Since loop diuretics are especially powerful drugs, adverse reactions to them may be severe. The most severe ones involve fluid and electrolyte imbalances. Common adverse reactions to loop diuretics include:

- too great a loss of fluid volume (especially in elderly patients)
- orthostatic hypertension
- hyperuricemia (excessive uric acid in the blood)
- hypochloremia
- hyponatremia
- hypocalcemia
- hypomagnesemia

TIP Patients taking diuretics, except potassium-sparing diuretics, often take a potassium supplement. When filling a prescription for a loop diuretic or a thiazide diuretic, double-check the patient's profile to see if a potassium supplement has been previously ordered. Make sure to communicate with the pharmacist if the patient is not currently taking a potassium supplement with a loop or thiazide diuretic.

Ethacrynic Acid

Ethacrynic acid (Edecrin) is administered orally in tablet form. This drug can also be administered by injection. Like other loop diuretics, ethacrynic acid is used to treat edema as well as hypertension.

Furosemide

Furosemide (Lasix) is a powerful diuretic that is available in tablet form. A solution that patients can drink is available as an alternative to tablets. An injectable form is available for treating acute pulmonary edema. Other antihypertensives are often used with this drug if it does not lower blood pressure sufficiently alone.

Torsemide

Torsemide (Demadex) is manufactured as oral tablets. The drug is also used to pull excess fluid from patients with heart failure, chronic renal failure, or liver disease. If the normal dose does not control blood pressure, another type of antihypertensive drug is often added.

Potassium-Sparing Diuretics

Potassium-sparing diuretics have weaker diuretic and antihypertensive effects than other diuretics. But they also have the advantage of conserving potassium. They're commonly used with other diuretics to increase the action of those other diuretics or to counteract their potassium-wasting

effects. In addition to hypertension, potassium-sparing diuretics are used to treat:

- edema
- heart failure
- diuretic-induced hypokalemia in patients with heart failure
- cirrhosis of the liver
- nephrotic syndrome (abnormal condition of the kidneys)

Spironolactone, one of the main potassium-sparing diuretics, is also used to treat hirsutism (excessive hair growth) and hyperaldosteronism (excessive secretion of aldosterone). You will read more about this drug below.

Potassium-sparing diuretics act on the distal tubule of the kidneys. Their action produces the following effects:

- Urinary excretion of sodium and water increases, as does excretion of chloride and calcium ions.
- The excretion of potassium and hydrogen ions decreases.
- The result is reduced blood pressure and increased serum potassium levels.

Few drug interactions are associated with potassium-sparing diuretics. Those that do occur aren't directly related to the drug, but rather are related to its potassium-sparing effects.

Spironolactone

Spironolactone (Aldactone) is manufactured as a tablet. This drug is structurally similar to aldosterone, which allows it to act as an aldosterone antagonist. Earlier in this chapter, you learned that aldosterone promotes the retention of sodium and water and the loss of potassium. Spironolactone counters these effects by competing with aldosterone for receptor sites. As a result, more sodium and water are excreted and more potassium is retained.

Amiloride and Triamterene

Amiloride (Midamor) is available in tablet form.

Triamterene (Dyrenium) is produced in capsule form. This drug is mainly used to treat edema.

 AT THE COUNTER

Furosemide

A patient receives a prescription for "furosemide 20 mg PO daily." What is the best time of day for the patient to take this medication?

Furosemide is a loop diuretic, which increases urine production. The patient should take the medication every morning so he can empty his bladder as needed. You do not want patients of advanced age to get up at night if at all possible, because this increases the chance of falls and could lead to injury. If the medication is prescribed twice a day, the second dose should be taken in the late afternoon or early evening to prevent nocturia.

 PROCEED WITH CAUTION

Adverse Reactions to Potassium-Sparing Diuretics

Few adverse reactions accompany the use of potassium-sparing diuretics. However, their potassium-sparing effects can lead to hyperkalemia, especially if they are given with a potassium supplement or a high-potassium diet.

ANTILIPEMIC DRUGS

Antilipemic drugs are used to lower abnormally high blood levels of fats such as triglycerides and cholesterol.

Triglycerides are compounds made of glycerin (a sugar alcohol) and fatty acids. They are the most common type of fat in the body and are stored in the body's fat cells for later use. In normal amounts, triglycerides are important to good health. But high levels are believed to play a role in causing heart disease. Normal triglyceride levels in the blood are below 150 mg/dL, whereas levels above 200 are considered high.

Cholesterol is one of the fat-like substances called lipids that the body needs to function. There are three types of cholesterol: high-density lipoprotein (HDL), low-density lipoprotein (LDL), and very-low-density lipoprotein (VLDL). They are described below:

- HDL consists of more protein than fat. It is sometimes called "good cholesterol" because high levels of it in the blood (45 mg/dL and above) appear to protect against heart disease.
- LDL is made up of more fat than protein. It is called "bad cholesterol" because a high level of it in the blood (above 160 mg/dL) is a risk factor for heart disease, hardening of the arteries (atherosclerosis), and stroke. An LDL level below 100 is considered healthy.
- VLDL has almost no protein. Its main purpose is to distribute the triglycerides produced by the liver. A high VLDL level can cause the buildup of cholesterol in the arteries and increase the risk of heart disease and stroke.

Total cholesterol is the sum of the blood's HDL, LDL, and VLDL levels. A total cholesterol level below 200 mg/dL is desirable, especially if LDL is below 100 and the ratio of HDL to total cholesterol is high. Total cholesterol levels above 240 are considered high and are often treated with antilipemic drugs. They are used to help lower lipid levels in combination with lifestyle changes—such as proper diet, weight loss, and exercise—and with treatment of any underlying disorder that may be causing a lipid abnormality. The classes of antilipemic drugs include:

- bile-sequestering drugs
- fibric acid derivatives
- 3-hydroxy-3-methylglutaryl coenzyme A (HMG-CoA) reductase inhibitors
- nicotinic acid
- cholesterol absorption inhibitors

Bile-Sequestering Drugs

Bile-sequestering drugs are resins that remove excess bile acids from fat deposits under the skin. They're the drugs of choice for treating familial hypercholesterolemia (type IIa hyperlipoproteinemia) when the patient can't lower his LDL levels by diet alone. Patients whose blood cholesterol levels place them at severe risk for CAD will most likely require one of these drugs in addition to dietary changes.

Bile-sequestering drugs are taken orally, but aren't absorbed in the GI tract. Instead they remain in the intestine, where they combine with bile acids for about five hours. The compound that's formed is excreted in the stool.

Meanwhile, the decreasing level of bile acids triggers the liver to produce more bile acids from cholesterol. As cholesterol leaves the bloodstream and other storage areas to replace the lost bile acids, blood cholesterol levels decrease. In addition, because the small intestine needs bile acids to break down lipids, absorption of all lipids and lipid-soluble drugs decreases until the bile acids are replaced.

Bile-sequestering drugs produce the following drug interactions:

- They may bind with acidic drugs in the GI tract and decrease the absorption and effectiveness of those drugs. Acidic drugs likely to be affected include barbiturates, phenytoin, penicillins, cephalosporins, thyroid hormones, thyroid derivatives, and digoxin.
- They may decrease absorption of propranolol, tetracycline, furosemide, penicillin G, hydrochlorothiazide, and gemfibrozil.
- They may reduce absorption of lipid-soluble vitamins such as vitamins A, D, E, and K. Poor absorption of vitamin K can affect prothrombin times significantly, increasing the risk of bleeding.

Cholestyramine

Cholestyramine (Prevalite, Questran, Questran Light) is a powder that the patient mixes with water or another liquid and drinks twice daily, usually with a meal. It comes in the form of individual packets or in bulk with a scoop in a can. Each packet or scoop of powder provides four grams of the drug.

Colestipol and Colesevelam

Colestipol (Colestid) is available as one-gram tablets and granules for oral suspension.

Colesevelam (WelChol) is prescribed in tablet form and should be taken with food and liquid.

 PROCEED WITH CAUTION

Adverse Reactions to Bile-Sequestering Drugs

Short-term reactions to these drugs are relatively mild. More severe reactions can result from long-term use. GI reactions from long-term therapy include:

- severe fecal impaction
- vomiting and diarrhea
- hemorrhoid irritation

More rarely, peptic ulcers and bleeding, gallstones, and inflammation of the gallbladder may occur.

Fibric Acid Derivatives

Fibric acid is produced by several fungi. Two derivatives of this acid are fenofibrate and gemfibrozil. These drugs are used primarily to reduce triglyceride levels, especially very-low-density triglycerides. To a lesser extent, they're also used to reduce blood cholesterol levels, especially elevated LDL levels.

The exact way in which these drugs work isn't known. But researchers believe that these fibric acid derivatives may:

- reduce cholesterol production early in its formation
- move cholesterol from body tissues
- increase cholesterol excretion
- decrease the creation and secretion of lipoproteins
- decrease the creation of triglycerides

There are several drug interactions involving fibric acid derivatives to be aware of:

- These drugs may displace acidic drugs such as barbiturates, phenytoin, thyroid derivatives, and cardiac glycosides.
- The risk of bleeding increases when these drugs are taken with oral anticoagulants.
- The use of fibric acid derivatives can have unpleasant GI effects.

Fenofibrate

Fenofibrate (Antara, Lofibra, Lipofen, Tricor, Triglide) comes in a wide variety of doses. It may be prescribed as capsules or as tablets. Daily dose varies according to the type of hyperlipidemia being treated, the brand name drug being used, and the patient's response to the drug.

Gemfibrozil

Gemfibrozil (Lopid) is manufactured only as a tablet. This drug is often used with patients who have a poor response to bile-sequestering drugs or who cannot tolerate them well.

In addition to the other affects of fibric acid derivatives, this drug also increases HDL ("good cholesterol") levels in the blood and increases the blood's ability to dissolve cholesterol.

HMG-CoA Reductase Inhibitors

HMG-CoA reductase inhibitors are commonly known as **statins**. These drugs lower lipid levels by interfering with cholesterol production. They do this by interfering with the enzyme responsible for converting HMG-CoA to mevalonate, which is an early step in the liver's production of cholesterol.

Statin drugs are used to treat primary cholesterolemia by reducing LDL ("bad cholesterol") and total blood cholesterol levels. They have the added benefit of mildly raising HDL levels. Because of their effect on LDL and total cholesterol, they're also used to reduce the risk of CAD and to prevent MI or stroke in patients with high cholesterol levels.

The use of statins can produce a number of drug interactions:

- Taking a statin drug with clarithromycin, erythromycin, fluconazole, gemfibrozil, itraconazole, ketoconazole, or niacin increases the risk of myopathy or rhabdomyolysis (a potentially fatal breakdown of skeletal muscle, causing renal failure).
- Lovastatin and simvastatin may increase the risk of bleeding when administered with warfarin (Coumadin).
- All statin drugs should be administered an hour before or four hours after the administration of any bile-sequestering drug.

Atorvastatin

Atorvastatin (Lipitor) is taken once daily in tablet form. The initial dose is adjusted upward if necessary, based on patient results. It is taken alone or as an adjunct to lipid-lowering treatments.

Fluvastatin

Fluvastatin (Lescol, Lescol XL) is produced in capsules and as 24-hour extended-release tablets.

T I P HMG-CoA reductase inhibitors are easily recognizable by their generic names. Most of the drugs in this class have generic names that end in the letters -*statin*.

Lovastatin

Lovastatin (Altoprev, Mevacor) is available as tablets and 24-hour extended-release tablets.

Pravastatin

Pravastatin (Pravachol) is manufactured in tablet form. You should be aware that the dosage of pravastatin is reduced in patients who are taking immunosuppressants.

Simvastatin

Simvastatin (Zocor) is a commonly prescribed drug used to treat hypercholesterolemia. It is available in tablet form.

 PROCEED WITH CAUTION

Adverse Reactions to HMG-CoA Reductase Inhibitors

Statin drugs may alter liver function studies, increasing aspartate aminotransferase, alkaline aminotransferase, alkaline phosphatase, and bilirubin levels. Other hepatic effects may include pancreatitis, hepatitis, and cirrhosis.

Myalgia (muscle pain) is the most common musculoskeletal effect, although joint pain and muscle cramps may also occur. Myopathy and rhabdomyolosis are rare reactions to these drugs, but they are potentially severe.

Possible adverse GI reactions include nausea, vomiting, diarrhea, abdominal pain, flatulence, and constipation.

Nicotinic Acid

Nicotinic acid, also known as niacin (Niaspan, Slo-Niacin) or vitamin B_3, is a water-soluble vitamin that decreases triglyceride and apolipoprotein B-100 levels and increases HDL levels. It can be purchased without a prescription as an OTC drug, although prescriptions are sometimes written for it. Both immediate-release tablets, and extended-release capsules and tablets are available.

Niacin is sometimes used in combination with other drugs to lower triglyceride levels in patients who are at high risk for pancreatitis. For example, niacin is available as a combination product with lovastatin. It is also useful in lowering LDL and total cholesterol, and it may be used with other antilipemics to raise HDL levels.

Even though it's an OTC drug, it must be used with care. You should keep in mind the following risks:

- Taking niacin with a statin drug may increase the risk of myopathy and rhabdomyolysis.
- Taking kava (an herbal diuretic) with niacin may increase the risk of damage to the liver.
- Niacin is contraindicated in persons who are hypersensitive to it or who have liver dysfunction, active peptic ulcer disease, or arterial bleeding.
- Bile-sequestering drugs can bind with niacin and decrease its effectiveness.

High doses of niacin may produce vasodilation and cause flushing. Extended-release forms tend to cause less vasodilation than do immediate-release forms. Taking an aspirin 30 minutes before taking niacin will help minimize flushing, as will taking the extended-release form at night.

Cholesterol Absorption Inhibitors

As the name implies, cholesterol absorption inhibitors block the absorption of cholesterol and related phytosterols from the intestine. Ezetimibe (Zetia) is the drug in this class. It reduces cholesterol levels by inhibiting absorption of cholesterol by the small intestine. This reduces the delivery of cholesterol in consumed food to the liver, which decreases the liver's stores of cholesterol and, consequently, the amount of it circulating in the blood.

 PROCEED WITH CAUTION

Adverse Reactions to Nicotinic Acid

Adverse reactions to nicotinic acid (niacin or vitamin B_3) include:

- flushing
- nausea and vomiting
- diarrhea
- epigastric or substernal pain

Nicotinic acid can also cause hepatotoxicity (toxic damage to the liver). The risk of this adverse reaction is greater with extended-release forms.

 HOW IT WORKS

How Cholesterol Absorption Inhibitors Work

Ezetimibe has a different mechanism of action than other antilipemic drugs. Instead of interfering with cholesterol production (like statins do) or increasing the liver's bile acid output (as is the case with bile-sequestering drugs), ezetimibe inhibits the absorption of cholesterol by the small intestine.

1. Ezetimibe affects the transporter Niemann-Pick C1-Like 1 (NPC1L1). This transporter is involved in the uptake of cholesterol by the small intestine.
2. The action of NPC1L1 is inhibited, which means that the intestines absorb less cholesterol.
3. As a result, less cholesterol is transported from the intestines to the liver.
4. The liver's cholesterol stores are reduced, and blood clearance of cholesterol is increased.

A 10-mg capsule of ezetimibe is taken once a day. It may be taken alone or combined with a statin drug. It can help lower LDL and total cholesterol and raise HDL when the maximum dose of statin drugs has been ineffective.

Taking cholestyramine with ezetimibe may decrease ezetimibe's effectiveness. Taking cyclosporine, fenofibrate, or gemfibrozil leads to increased levels of ezetimibe.

PROCEED WITH CAUTION

Adverse Reactions to Cholesterol Absorption Inhibitors

Adverse reactions to cholesterol absorption inhibitors include:

- fatigue
- abdominal pain and diarrhea
- pharyngitis (sore throat) and sinusitis
- arthralgia (joint pain)
- back pain
- cough

When these drugs are given with an HMG-CoA reductase inhibitor (statin drug), the most common adverse reactions are:

- chest pain
- dizziness
- headache
- pharyngitis
- sinusitis
- abdominal pain
- diarrhea
- upper respiratory tract infection
- back pain
- arthralgia
- myalgia

QUICK QUIZ

Answer the following multiple-choice questions.

1. Which statin drug is marketed under the brand name Lipitor?
   a. atorvastatin
   b. fluvastatin
   c. lovastatin
   d. pravastatin
2. Which of these antiarrhythmics is *not* a class I antiarrhythmic drug?
   a. lidocaine
   b. propranolol
   c. quinidine
   d. tocainide
3. What type of drug would most likely be taken for the same reason as an alpha-adrenergic blocker?
   a. an HMG-CoA reductase inhibitor
   b. a class IV antiarrhythmic
   c. a beta blocker
   d. an angiotensin II receptor blocker
4. In which situation would the use of digoxin be indicated?
   a. to lower blood pressure
   b. to manage chronic angina
   c. to treat heart failure
   d. to lower total cholesterol
5. Which type of diuretic drugs should be avoided if a patient is allergic to sulfa-based drugs?
   a. thiazide and thiazide-like diuretics
   b. loop diuretics
   c. potassium-sparing diuretics
   d. norepinephrine-depleting diuretics

Please answer each of the following questions in one to three sentences.

1. What is the mechanism of action of nitroglycerin?

2. How do class IA, IB, and IC antiarrhythmics differ in the ways they work?

3. How do bile-sequestering drugs and statin drugs differ in the way they reduce cholesterol?

4. How are PDE inhibitors and ACE inhibitors alike? How do they differ?

5. Why is more than one antihypertensive drug sometimes used to regulate a patient's blood pressure?

Answer the following questions as either true or false.

1. ___ The goal of antilipemic drugs is a low LDL and a high HDL.
2. ___ Diuretics are sometimes taken along with antihypertensives to help lower blood pressure.
3. ___ The popular drug Zocor is widely used to treat cardiac arrhythmias.
4. ___ Nitrates are inotropic drugs that are used to treat congestive heart failure.
5. ___ A patient who is taking a statin drug should not take over-the-counter niacin.

Match each brand name drug in the left column with its use in the right column.

1. Cardizem   a. to treat angina
2. Lanoxin   b. to treat arrhythmias
3. Lotensin   c. to treat heart failure
4. Norpace   d. to treat high cholesterol
5. Zetia   e. to treat hypertension

DRUG CLASSIFICATION TABLE

Classification	Generic Name	Trade Names(s)
Inotropic drugs	digoxin *di-jox'-in*	*tablets:* Digitek, Lanoxin *oral solution:* (no longer marketed under trade name) *injection:* Lanoxin
	inamrinone *in-am'-rih-none*	*injection:* (no longer marketed under trade name)
	milrinone *mil'-rih-none*	*injection:* (no longer marketed under trade name)
Antiarrhythmic drugs	disopyramide *die-soe-peer'-a-mide*	*capsules:* Norpace *extended-release* *capsules:* Norpace CR
	procainamide *proe-kane'-a-mide*	*tablets:* Pronestyl *extended-release* *tablets:* Pronestyl SR *injection:* (no longer marketed under trade name)
	Quinidine sulfate *kwin'-ih-deen*	*tablets:* (no longer marketed under trade name) *extended-release tablets:* (no longer marketed under trade name)
	quinidine gluconate *kwin'-ih-deen*	*extended-release tablets:* (no longer marketed under trade name) *injection:* (no longer marketed under trade name)
	lidocaine *lye'-doe-kane*	*injection:* Xylocaine
	mexiletine *max-ill'-i-teen*	*tablets:* (no longer marketed under trade name)
	flecainide *fle-kay'-nide*	*tablets:* Tambocor
	propafenone *proe-paf'-a-non*	*tablets:* Rythmol *extended-release capsules:* Rythmol SR
	esmolol *ez'-moe-lol*	*injection:* Brevibloc
	propranolol *pro-pran'-oh-lol*	*tablets:* (no longer marketed under trade name) *extended-release* *capsules:* Inderal LA, Innopran XL *injection:* Inderal *oral solution:* (no longer marketed under trade name)
	acebutolol *a-see-byoo'-toe-lol*	*capsules:* Sectral
	amiodarone *a-mee'-oh-duh-rone*	*tablets:* Cordarone, Pacerone *injection:* (no longer marketed under trade name)
	dofetilide *doe-feh'-till-ide*	*capsules:* Tikosyn
	ibutilide *eye-byoo'-tih-lide*	*injection:* Corvert
	sotalol *soe'-tah-lol*	*tablets:* Betapace, Betapace AF, Sorine
	adenosine *a-den'-oh-seen*	*injection:* Adenocard, Adenoscan
Antianginal drugs	isosorbide dinitrate *eye-soe-sor'-bide*	*tablets:* Isordil Titradose *extended release tablets:* Isochron *extended-release* *capsules:* Dilatrate SR *sublingual tablets:* (no longer marketed under trade name)

continued

DRUG CLASSIFICATION TABLE (continued)

Classification	Generic Name	Trade Names(s)
Antianginal drugs (continued)	isosorbide dinitrate and hydralazine *eye-soe-sor'-bide hye-dral'-a-zeen*	*tablets:* BiDil
	isosorbide mononitrate *eye-soe-sor'-bide*	*tablets:* Monoket, Ismo *extended-release tablets:* Imdur
	nitroglycerin *nye-troe-gli'-ser-in*	*transdermal patch:* NitroDur, Minitran *ointment:* Nitro-Bid *sublingual spray:* Nitrolingual Pump *extended-release capsules:* (no longer marketed under trade name) *sublingual tablets:* Nitrostat, Nitroquick *injection:* (no longer marketed under trade name)
	atenolol *a-ten'-oh-lol*	*tablets:* Tenormin
	atenolol and chlorthalidone *a-ten'-oh-lol klor-thal'-i-done*	*tablets:* Tenoretic
	carvedilol *kar-ve'-dil-ol*	*tablets:* Coreg *extended-release capsules:* Coreg CR
	metoprolol *me-toe'-pro-lole*	*tablets:* Lopressor *extended-release tablets:* Toprol XL *injection:* Lopressor
	metoprolol and hydrochlorothiazide *me-toe'-pro-lole hye-droe-klor-oh-thye'-a-zide*	*tablets:* Lopressor HCT
	nadolol *nay-doe'-lol*	*tablets:* Corgard
	nadolol and bendroflumethiazide *nay-doe'-lol ben-droe-floo-me-thye'a-side*	*tablets:* Corzide
	propranolol *pro-pran'-oh-lol*	*tablets:* (no longer marketed under trade name) *injection:* Inderal *extended-release capsules:* Inderal LA, Innopran XL *oral solution:* (no longer marketed under trade name)
	propranolol and hydrochlorothiazide *pro-pran'-oh-lol hye-droe-klor-oh-thye'-a-zide*	*tablets:* (no longer marketed under trade name)
	amlodipine *am-low'-dih-peen*	*tablets:* Norvasc
	amlodipine and atorvastatin *am-low'-dih-peen ah-tor'-va-stah-tin*	*tablets:* Caduet
	amlodipine and benazepril *am-low'-dih-peen ben-a'-za-pril*	*capsules:* Lotrel
	amlodipine and valsartan *am-low'-dih-peen val-sar'-tan*	*tablets:* Exforge
	amlodipine and olmesartan *am-low'-dih-peen ol-meh-sar'-tan*	*tablets:* Azor
	diltiazem *dil-tye'-a-zem*	*tablets:* Cardizem *extended-release tablets:* Cardizem LA *extended-release capsules:* Cardizem CD, Cartia XT, Dilacor XR, Dilt-CD, Dilt-XR, Diltia XT, Taztia XT, Tiazac *injection:* (no longer marketed under trade name)

continued

DRUG CLASSIFICATION TABLE *(continued)*

Classification	Generic Name	Trade Names(s)
Antianginal drugs *(continued)*	nicardipine *nye-kar'-de-peen*	*capsules:* (no longer marketed under trade name) *extended-release capsules:* Cardene SR *injection:* Cardene
	nifedipine *nye-fed'-i-peen*	*capsules:* Procardia *extended-release tablets:* Adalat CC, Afeditab CR, Nifediac CC, Nifedical XL, Procardia XL
	verapamil *ver-ap'-a-mil*	*tablets:* Calan *extended-release* *tablets:* Calan SR, Covera-HS, Isoptin SR *extended-release capsules:* Verelan, Verelan PM *injection:* (no longer marketed under trade name)
	verapamil and trandolapril *ver-ap'-a-mil tran-dole'-a-pril*	*extended-release* *tablets:* Tarka
Antihypertensive drugs	clonidine *kloe'-ni-deen*	*tablets:* Catapres *transdermal patch:* Catapres TTS *injection:* Duraclon
	clonidine and chlorthalidone *kloe'-ni-deen klor-thal'-i-done*	*tablets:* Clorpres
	methyldopa *meth'-ill-doe-pa*	*tablets:* (no longer marketed under trade name) *injection:* (no longer marketed under trade name)
	methyldopa and hydrochlorothiazide *meth'-ill-doe-pa hye-droe-klor-oh-thye'-a-zide*	*tablets:* (no longer marketed under trade name)
	doxazosin *dox-ay'-zoe-sin*	*tablets:* Cardura *extended-release tablets:* Cardura XL
	phentolamine *fen-tole'-a-meen*	*injection:* (no longer marketed under trade name)
	prazosin *praz-oh'-sin*	*capsules:* Minipress
	terazosin *ter-az'-oh-sin*	*capsules:* (no longer marketed under trade name)
	carvedilol *kar-ve'-di-lole*	*tablets:* Coreg *extended-release capsules:* Coreg CR
	labetalol *la-bet'-oh-lole*	*tablets:* Trandate *injection:* (no longer marketed under trade name)
	reserpine *re-ser'-peen*	*tablets:* (no longer marketed under trade name)
	hydralazine *hye-dral'-a-zeen*	*tablets:* (no longer marketed under trade name) *injection:* (no longer marketed under trade name)
	hydralazine and hydrochlorothiazide *hye-dral'-a-zeen hye-droe-klor-oh-thye'-a-zide*	*capsules:* Hydra-Zide
	hydralazine and isosorbide dinitrate *hye-dral'-a-zeen eye-soe-sor'-bide*	*tablets:* BiDil
	minoxidil *mi-nox'-i'-dil*	*tablets:* (no longer marketed under trade name)
	nitroprusside *nye-tro-pruss'-ide*	*injection:* Nitropress
	benazepril *ben-a'-za-pril*	*tablets:* Lotensin

continued

DRUG CLASSIFICATION TABLE *(continued)*

Classification	Generic Name	Trade Names(s)
Antihypertensive drugs *(continued)*	benazepril and hydrochlorothiazide *ben-a'-za-pril hye-droe-klor-oh-thye'-a-zide*	*tablets:* Lotensin HCT
	benazepril and amlodipine *ben-a'-za-pril am-low'-dih-peen*	*capsules:* Lotrel
	captopril *kap'-toe-pril*	*tablets:* Capoten
	captopril and hydrochlorothiazide *kap'-toe-pril hye-droe-klor-oh-thye'-a-zide*	*tablets:* Capozide
	enalapril *e-nal'-a-pril*	*tablets:* Vasotec *injection:* Enalaprilat
	enalapril and hydrochlorothiazide *e-nal'-a-pril hye-droe-klor-oh-thye'-a-zide*	*tablets:* Vaseretic
	fosinopril *foh-sin'-oh-pril*	*tablets:* Monopril
	fosinopril and hydrochlorothiazide *foh-sin'-oh-pril hye-droe-klor-oh-thye'-a-zide*	*tablets:* Monopril HCT
	lisinopril *lyse-in'-oh-pril*	*tablets:* Prinvil, Zestril
	lisinopril and hydrochlorothiazide *lyse-in'-oh-pril hye-droe-klor-oh-thye'-a-zide*	*tablets:* Prinzide, Zestoretic
	moexipril *moe-ex'-a-pril*	*tablets:* Univasc
	moexipril and hydrochlorothiazide *moe-ex'-a-pril hye-droe-klor-oh-thye'-a-zide*	*tablets:* Uniretic
	quinapril *kwin'-ah-pril*	*tablets:* Accupril
	quinapril and hydrochlorothiazide *kwin'-ah-pril hye-droe-klor-oh-thye'-a-zide*	*tablets:* Accuretic, Quinaretic
	ramipril *ra-mi'-pril*	*capsules:* Altace *tablets:* Altace
	trandolapril *tran-dole'-a-pril*	*tablets:* Mavik
	trandolapril and verapamil *tran-dole'-a-pril ver-ap'-a-mil*	*extended-release tablets:* Tarka
	candesartan *can-dah-sar'-tan*	*tablets:* Atacand
	candesartan and hydrochlorothiazide *can-dah-sar'-tan hye-droe-klor-oh-thye'-a-zide*	*tablets:* Atacand HCT
	eprosartan *ep-row-sar'-tan*	*tablets:* Teveten
	eprosartan and hydrochlorothiazide *ep-row-sar'-tan hye-droe-klor-oh-thye'-a-zide*	*tablets:* Teveten HCT
	irbesartan *er-bah-sar'-tan*	*tablets:* Avapro
	irbesartan and hydrochlorothiazide *er-bah-sar'-tan hye-droe-klor-oh-thye'-a-zide*	*tablets:* Avalide
	losartan *low-sar'-tan*	*tablets:* Cozaar
	losartan and hydrochlorothiazide *low-sar'-tan hye-droe-klor-oh-thye'-a-zide*	*tablets:* Hyzaar

continued

DRUG CLASSIFICATION TABLE (continued)

Classification	Generic Name	Trade Names(s)
Antihypertensive drugs (continued)	olmesartan *ol-meh-sar'-tan*	*tablets:* Benicar
	olmesartan and hydrochlorothiazide *ol-meh-sar'-tan hye-droe-klor-oh-thye'-a-zide*	*tablets:* Benicar HCT
	olmesartan and amlodipine *ol-meh-sar'-tan am-low'-dih-peen*	*tablets:* Azor
	valsartan *val-sar'-tan*	*tablets:* Diovan
	valsartan and hydrochlorothiazide *val-sar'-tan hye-droe-klor-oh-thye'-a-zide*	*tablets:* Diovan HCT
	valsartan and amlodipine *val-sar'-tan am-low'-dih-peen*	*tablets:* Exforge
	aliskiren *a-lis-kye'-ren*	*tablets:* Tekturna
	aliskiren and hydrochlorothiazide *a-lis-kye'-ren hye-droe-klor-oh-thye'-a-zide*	*tablets:* Tekturna HCT
Diuretic drugs	bendroflumethiazide *ben-droe-floo-me-thye'a-side*	*tablets:* Naturetin
	chlorothiazide *klor-oh-thye'-a-zide*	*oral suspension:* Diuril *tablets:* (no longer marketed under trade name) *injection:* Diuril
	hydrochlorothiazide *hye-droe-klor-oh-thye'-a-zide*	*tablets:* Ezide *capsules:* Microzide
	methyclothiazide *meth-i-kloe-thye'-a-zide*	*tablets:* (no longer marketed under trade name)
	indapamide *in-dap'-a-mide*	*tablets:* (no longer marketed under trade name)
	chlorthalidone *klor-thal'-i-done*	*tablets:* Thalitone
	metolazone *me-tole'-a-zone*	*tablets:* Zaroxolyn
	bumetanide *byoo-met'-a-nide*	*tablets:* (no longer marketed under trade name) *injection:* (no longer marketed under trade name)
	ethacrynic acid *eth-a-krin'-ik*	*tablets:* Edecrin *injection:* Edecrin
	furosemide *fur-oh'-se-mide*	*tablets:* Lasix *injection:* (no longer marketed under trade name) *oral solution:* (no longer marketed under trade name)
	torsemide *tor'-se-myde*	*tablets:* Demadex
	amiloride *a-mill'-oh-ride*	*tablets:* Midamor
	amiloride and hydrochlorothiazide *a-mill'-oh-ride hye-droe-klor-oh-thye'-a-zide*	*tablets:* (no longer marketed under trade name)
	spironolactone *speer-on-oh-lak'-tone*	*tablets:* Aldactone

continued

DRUG CLASSIFICATION TABLE *(continued)*

Classification	Generic Name	Trade Names(s)
Diuretic drugs *(continued)*	spironolactone and hydrochlorothiazide *speer-on-oh-lak'-tone hye-droe-klor-oh-thye'-a-zide*	*tablets:* Aldactazide
	triamterene *trye-am'-ter-een*	*capsules:* Dyrenium
	triamterene and hydrochlorothiazide *trye-am'-ter-een hye-droe-klor-oh-thye'-a-zide*	*capsules:* Dyazide *tablets:* Maxzide
Antilipemic drugs	cholestyramine *koe-less'-tir-a-mean*	*powder for oral suspension:* Prevalite, Questran, Questran Light
	colestipol *koe-less'-ti-pole*	*tablets:* Colestid *granules for oral suspension:* Colestid
	colesevelam *koe-leh-sev'-eh-lam*	*tablets:* WelChol
	fenofibrate *fen-oh-figh'-brate*	*tablets:* Lofibra, Tricor, Triglide *capsules:* Antara, Lofibra, Lipofen
	gemfibrozil *jem-fi'-broe-zil*	*tablets:* Lopid
	atorvastatin *ah-tor'-va-stah-tin*	*tablets:* Lipitor
	atorvastatin and amlodipine *ah-tor'-va-stah-tin am-low'-dih-peen*	*tablets:* Caduet
	fluvastatin *flue-va-sta'-tin*	*capsules:* Lescol *extended-release tablets:* Lescol XL
	lovastatin *loe-va-sta'-tin*	*tablets:* Mevacor *extended-release tablets:* Altoprev
	lovastatin and niacin *loe-va-sta'-tin nye'-uh-sin*	*extended-release tablets:* Advicor
	pravastatin *prah-va-sta'-tin*	*tablets:* Pravachol
	simvastatin *sim-va-stah'-tin*	*tablets:* Zocor
	niacin (nicotinic acid) *nye'-uh-sin*	*tablets:* (no longer marketed under trade name) *extended-release tablets:* Niaspan, Slo-Niacin *extended-release capsules:* (no longer marketed under trade name)
	ezetimibe *e-zet'-e-mibe*	*capsules:* Zetia
	ezetimibe and simvastatin *e-zet'-e-mibe sim-va-stah'-tin*	*tablets:* Vytorin

CHAPTER 6

Hematologic Drugs

CHAPTER OBJECTIVES

- Discuss the uses of iron, vitamin B$_{12}$, and folic acid
- Match brand and generic names of commonly used drugs for anticoagulation
- Describe the need for double-checking all orders and prescriptions for heparin
- Compare and contrast the two types of heparin
- Explain the monitoring parameters for patients taking anticoagulants
- Describe the complexity of dosing for warfarin, including the available strengths
- List the agents used to reverse bleeding caused by heparin and warfarin
- Match brand and generic names of commonly used thrombolytic drugs
- Compare and contrast the use of anticoagulants with thrombolytics
- Identify the time frame for initiation of thrombolytic therapy

KEY TERMS

anemia—a decrease in the number of red blood cells

anticoagulant drugs—drugs used to reduce the ability of the blood to clot

antiplatelet drugs—drugs used to prevent the formation of blood clots in arteries

darbepoetin alfa—a glycoprotein that stimulates the production of red blood cells

epoetin alfa—a glycoprotein that stimulates the production of red blood cells

erythropoietin—a hormone that stimulates bone marrow cells to produce red blood cells

folic acid—a B vitamin that is important for normal functioning of red and white blood cells

hematinic drugs—drugs used to increase the level of hemoglobin in the blood

hematologic drugs—drugs used to treat disorders of the blood and blood tissues

hemoglobin—a molecule in red blood cells that contains iron and allows the transport of oxygen

heparin—an anticlotting (antithrombolytic) agent that is used to treat and prevent clot formation

intrinsic factor—a protein produced by the gastric glands in the stomach that is needed for the metabolism of vitamin B$_{12}$

iron—a mineral needed for producing hemoglobin

megaloblastic anemia—anemia resulting from a deficiency of vitamin B$_{12}$ or folic acid

pernicious anemia—a condition characterized by decreased gastric production of hydrochloric acid and intrinsic factor deficiency

plasma—the liquid component of blood

platelets—substances in the blood that help with blood clotting

red blood cells—cells in the blood that move oxygen from the lungs to other body tissues

thrombolytic drugs—drugs that act to dissolve preexisting blood clots

vitamin B$_{12}$ deficiency pernicious anemia—a special type of anemia characterized by a deficiency of intrinsic factor

white blood cells—immune system cells in the blood that fight infection

Hematology is a branch of medicine that deals with diseases of the blood and blood tissues. The hematologic system in the body includes **plasma**, the liquid component of blood, and blood cells. There are three main types of blood cells.

- **Red blood cells (RBCs)** carry oxygen from the lungs to other cells and tissues in the body. RBCs contain **hemoglobin**, a special molecule containing **iron**. The iron in hemoglobin helps the hemoglobin pick up oxygen.
- **White blood cells (WBCs)** defend the body from infection and foreign materials. Several different types of WBCs give the body different ways to fight invading bacteria, fungi, or viruses.
- **Platelets** are substances in the blood that help in blood clotting.

Hematologic drugs are drugs used to treat disorders of the blood and blood tissues. In this chapter, you'll learn about hematologic drugs used in treating medical conditions such as:

- **anemia** (reduced blood cells or hemoglobin) caused by vitamin and mineral deficiencies
- muscle fatigue and muscle weakness
- asthma and other breathing difficulties
- abnormally high or low blood pressure
- heart conditions

The three main types of drugs used to treat disorders of the hematologic system are:

- hematinic drugs
- anticoagulant drugs
- thrombolytic drugs

HEMATINIC DRUGS

Hematinic drugs help the body produce RBCs by increasing the levels of hemoglobin in the blood to treat anemia. There are several different types of anemia:

- **Iron deficiency anemia** is a condition that results when there isn't enough stored iron to meet the body's needs. This is the most common type of anemia.
- Anemia in patients with chronic renal disease occurs when the kidneys don't produce enough of the hormone **erythropoietin**. This hormone is involved in the production of RBCs.
- **Pernicious anemia** is caused by a deficiency of **intrinsic factor**, a substance needed to absorb vitamin B_{12} in the GI tract. Untreated pernicious anemia can lead to lesions in the spinal cord.
- Anemia resulting from a folic acid deficiency is called **megaloblastic anemia**. Folic acid is a form of vitamin B that is needed to produce RBCs in the bone marrow.

Different drugs are used to treat different types of anemia. These drugs will relieve general symptoms of anemia, which include:

- fatigue
- shortness of breath
- sore tongue
- headache
- pallor

Iron

Iron preparations are used to treat iron deficiency anemia. Although iron has other roles, its most important role is in the production of hemoglobin. About 80 percent of the iron in the blood plasma goes to the bone marrow, where it's used for erythropoiesis (the production of RBCs).

Iron is transported by the blood. In the blood, iron is bound to transferrin, a protein that carries it in the blood plasma. About 66 percent of total body iron is contained in hemoglobin.

The amount of iron absorbed by the body partially depends on how much iron the body has stored. When body stores are low or RBC production is increased, iron absorption may increase by 20 to 30 percent. On the other hand, when total iron stores are large, the body absorbs only about five to ten percent of the iron available.

Iron preparations are administered orally or by parenteral administration (injection).

- Oral iron therapy is the preferred route for preventing or treating iron deficiency anemia. It's used to prevent anemia in children aged six months to two years during a period of rapid growth and development. Pregnant women may need iron supplements to replace the iron used by the developing fetus.
- Parenteral iron therapy is used for patients who can't absorb oral preparations, aren't compliant with oral therapy, or have bowel disorders (such as ulcerative colitis or Crohn disease). Patients with end-stage renal disease who are receiving hemodialysis may also receive parenteral iron therapy at the end of their dialysis session. Parenteral forms of iron may be given by IM injection or by slow, continuous IV infusion.

Iron absorption is reduced by antacids and by foods such as coffee, tea, eggs, and milk. There are also several drug interactions involving iron.

- Oral iron preparations may reduce absorption of other drugs taken with them. These drugs include tetracyclines (demeclocycline, doxycycline, minocycline, and oxytetracycline), methyldopa, quinolones (ciprofloxacin, gatifloxacin, levofloxacin, lomefloxacin, moxifloxacin, norfloxacin, ofloxacin, and sparfloxacin), levothyroxine, and penicillamine.
- Cholestyramine, cimetidine, magnesium trisilicate, and colestipol may reduce the absorption of iron in the GI tract.

Ferrous Fumarate

Ferrous fumarate (Hemocyte, Ferretts, Nephro-Fer, Ferro-Sequels, Femiron, Ircon, Tandem) is used in treating iron deficiency anemia. It's available OTC in tablets and timed-release tablets.

Ferrous Gluconate

Ferrous gluconate (Fergon, Ferate) is used as a dietary supplement and to prevent and treat iron deficiency anemia. It is available OTC as an oral tablet.

Ferrous Sulfate

Ferrous sulfate (Feosol, Feratab, Slow Fe, Fer-In-Sol, Fer-Iron, Fer-Gen-Sol) is used to treat iron deficiency anemia and is used as a dietary supplement in infants, children under the age of four years, and adults. Ferrous sulfate is available OTC in several different forms, including:

- tablets
- extended-release tablets
- extended-release capsules
- elixir
- drops
- liquid

Iron Dextran

Iron dextran (DexFerrum, Infed) is used to treat iron deficiencies in patients in whom oral administration is not possible or difficult. It is available by prescription for IM or IV injection. The maximum daily dose is 2 mL of undiluted iron dextran. Iron dextran can be used for treating adults and children over the age of four months. Rarely, anaphylactic reactions have been reported after the administration of iron dextran by injection.

Iron Sucrose

Iron sucrose (Venofer) is used to treat iron deficiency anemia in patients with chronic kidney disease. It's only administered intravenously, using slow injection or infusion techniques.

Leucovorin Calcium

Leucovorin calcium is administered by injection. It's used to treat megaloblastic anemia due to folic acid deficiency in some patients. Leucovorin is administered orally or by injection after methotrexate therapy.

Sodium Ferric Gluconate Complex

Sodium ferric gluconate complex (Ferrlecit) is used in treating iron deficiency anemia in patients undergoing long-term hemodialysis. It's not used for patients under the age of six years. Sodium ferric gluconate complex is used in patients who are receiving supplemental epoetin therapy. It's administered by IV infusion or by slow IV injection during a dialysis session.

Vitamin B_{12}

Vitamin B_{12} preparations act by restoring low levels of vitamin B_{12} in the body. Vitamin B_{12} deficiency may be seen in:

- patients who have intestinal diseases, such as ulcerative colitis
- patients who have parts of their stomach or GI tract removed, including patients who have had gastric bypass surgery
- patients with cancer of the stomach
- strict vegetarians

T I P It's rare to find a deficiency of vitamin B_{12} that is diet related. Vitamin B_{12} is found in many foods, including meats, milk, eggs, and cheese.

When vitamin B_{12} is administered, it replaces the vitamin B_{12} that the body would normally absorb from the diet. Vitamin B_{12} is needed for cell growth and replication and to maintain myelin (nerve coverings) throughout the nervous system. It may also be involved in the metabolism of lipids and carbohydrates.

Vitamin B_{12} is available in parenteral, oral, and intranasal forms.

- Oral vitamin B_{12} preparations are used to supplement nutritional deficiencies of the vitamin. To absorb oral forms of B_{12}, the body secretes a sub-

PROCEED WITH CAUTION

Adverse Reactions to Vitamin B₁₂ Therapy

There are no dose-related adverse reactions with vitamin B$_{12}$ therapy. However, some rare reactions may occur when vitamin B$_{12}$ is administered parenterally. These reactions include:

- hypersensitivity reactions
- pulmonary edema
- heart failure
- peripheral vascular thrombosis
- polycythemia vera (abnormally high levels of RBCs)
- hypokalemia
- itching, transient rash, or hives
- mild diarrhea

stance called intrinsic factor. People who have a deficiency of intrinsic factor develop a special type of anemia called **vitamin B$_{12}$ deficiency pernicious anemia.**

- Parenteral and nasal forms of vitamin B$_{12}$ are used to treat patients with pernicious anemia. Parenteral forms of vitamin B$_{12}$ are administered by IM or SubQ injection.

Common vitamin B$_{12}$ preparations include cyanocobalamin and hydroxocobalamin. The absorption of oral cyanocobalamin may be reduced when taken with alcohol, aspirin, neomycin, chloramphenicol, and colchicine.

Cyanocobalamin

Cyanocobalamin is available in several different forms. This drug may be purchased OTC in oral tablets and extended-release tablets. By prescription, cyanocobalamin is available as an intranasal spray (Nascobal, CaloMist). It's also available by prescription as cyanocobalamin crystalline for IM or SubQ injection.

Hydroxocobalamin

Hydroxocobalamin crystalline (Cyanokit) is a prescription drug used to treat several conditions related to the deficiency of vitamin B$_{12}$, including pernicious anemia, dietary deficiency of vitamin B$_{12}$, inadequate secretion of intrinsic factor, or competition for vitamin B$_{12}$ by intestinal parasites. Administration is by IM injection only and should not be given IV. Hydroxocobalamin has also been used to treat cyanide toxicity associated with sodium nitroprusside.

Folic Acid

Folic acid (also known as folate) is an essential component for the production of RBCs and growth. A deficiency in folic acid results in megaloblastic anemia and in low serum and RBC folate levels.

- This type of anemia usually occurs in patients who have tropical or nontropical sprue, a digestive disorder in which nutrients can't be absorbed properly in the GI system.
- It may also result from poor nutritional intake during pregnancy, infancy, or childhood.

Folic acid (Folacin) is available OTC and in prescription form. By prescription, folic acid and its derivatives are available as tablets and by injection. Folic acid preparations sold OTC typically contain 0.4 mg of folic acid or less. Some OTC preparations for pregnant women may contain 0.8 mg. Prescription forms of folic acid contain 1 mg of folic acid.

Who Should Take Folic Acid Supplements?

Patients may require folic acid supplementation for the following conditions or circumstances:

- pregnancy
- ongoing treatment for liver disease
- hemolytic anemia
- alcohol abuse
- skin or renal disorders

TIP It can be dangerous to give folic acid to patients with undiagnosed anemia. Folic acid may mask the symptoms of pernicious anemia without stopping its neurological effects.

Drug Interactions with Folic Acid

Folic acid may interact with other drugs:

- Methotrexate, sulfasalazine, hormonal contraceptives, aspirin, triamterene, pentamidine, and trimethoprim reduce the effectiveness of folic acid.
- In large doses, folic acid may counteract the effects of anticonvulsants, such as phenytoin, potentially leading to seizures.

PROCEED WITH CAUTION

Adverse Reactions to Folic Acid

Adverse reactions to folic acid include:

- erythema
- itching
- rash
- anorexia and nausea
- altered sleep patterns
- difficulty concentrating
- irritability
- hyperactivity

PROCEED WITH CAUTION

Adverse Reactions to Erythropoietin Agents

The most common adverse reaction to erythropoietin agents is hypertension. Other adverse reactions may include:

- headache
- joint pain
- nausea, vomiting, or diarrhea
- edema
- fatigue
- chest pain
- skin reactions at the injection site
- weakness
- dizziness

Erythropoietin Agents

Erythropoietin agents are glycoproteins that stimulate RBC production (erythropoiesis). They boost the production of erythropoietin, a hormone that stimulates bone marrow cells to produce RBCs. Normally, erythropoietin is formed in the kidneys in response to hypoxia (reduced oxygen) and anemia.

Patients with conditions that decrease the production of erythropoietin typically develop normocytic anemia. This anemia can usually be corrected after five to six weeks of treatment with an erythropoietin agent. Erythropoietin agents are used to:

- treat patients with anemia associated with chronic renal failure
- treat anemia associated with zidovudine therapy in patients with human immunodeficiency virus (HIV) infection
- treat anemia in cancer patients receiving chemotherapy
- reduce the need for allogenic blood transfusions (transfusions from genetically different individuals) in surgery patients

Erythropoietin agents have no known interactions with other drugs.

Darbepoetin Alfa

Darbepoetin alfa (Aranesp) is available in a wide range of dosage strengths for administration by SubQ injection (weekly) or IV (with dialysis). The dose is started slowly and adjusted based on the patient's levels of hemoglobin.

Epoetin Alfa

Epoetin alfa (Epogen, Procrit) is administered by SubQ injection or IV. Dosages vary depending on the patient's condition. In general, the lowest dose needed to increase hemoglobin levels is used.

ANTICOAGULANT DRUGS

Anticoagulant drugs are used to reduce the ability of the blood to clot. They stop the formation of new clots (thrombus; plural: thrombi) and stop small clots from forming larger ones. However, they don't affect clots that already exist. Anticoagulants also can't repair any damage caused by a clot. Anticoagulant therapy may be used in the following situations:

- to prevent a stroke (caused by blood clots blocking the flow of blood to the brain)
- to prevent a heart attack (caused when blood clots block the flow of blood to the heart)
- after heart valve replacement surgery
- during cardiac surgery
- for patients required to stay in bed for long periods of time after some types of surgery

Patients with a high risk of heart attack or stroke or who have deep vein thrombosis may receive anticoagulant therapy.

TIP Although they don't cause blood to thin, anticoagulants are sometimes called "blood thinners" by patients.

There are five main groups of anticoagulant drugs:

- heparin and its derivatives
- oral anticoagulants (warfarin)
- antiplatelet drugs
- direct thrombin inhibitors
- factor Xa inhibitor drugs

Heparin and Its Derivatives

Heparin is an antithrombolytic agent, which means that it works to prevent the formation of blood clots (thrombi). Heparin and its derivatives can also help prevent existing clots from growing larger. However, because heparins don't affect the synthesis of clotting factors, they can't dissolve clots that are already formed. Heparin and heparin derivatives may be used in the following situations:

- to treat disseminated intravascular coagulation, a complication of other diseases that results in faster-than-normal clotting
- to treat clotting in arteries and to prevent embolus (a blood clot that moves through the blood stream) from forming in patients with atrial fibrillation, an arrhythmia in which ineffective atrial contractions cause blood to pool in the atria
- to prevent thrombus (blood clot) formation and to promote blood circulation in the heart during MI
- to prevent clotting when the patient's blood must circulate freely outside the body through a machine, such as a cardiopulmonary bypass machine or a dialysis machine

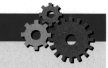

HOW IT WORKS

How Blood Clots Form

When body tissues or blood vessels are damaged, platelets stick to the injured blood vessel. These platelets release chemicals to attract other platelets to the area. This is called platelet aggregation.

The clump of platelets becomes a stable clot (thrombus) through a process called the coagulation cascade. In the coagulation cascade, several proteins work together in a systematic way to produce fibrin. Fibrin forms a network inside the clump of platelets to produce a clot.

Proteins involved in the coagulation cascade are normally inactive. They need to be converted to an active form for the next step in the coagulation process to occur. There are two different pathways in the coagulation cascade.

■ In the extrinsic pathway, coagulation begins after damaged tissues release factor VII. The active form of VII (VIIa) and tissue factor (also called thromboplastin or factor III) work to activate factor X.
■ The intrinsic pathway is activated by factor XII. Factor XII activates factors XI and IX. When activated, XIa and IXa activate factor X.

Once factor X is activated, it forms factor Xa. Factor Xa activates prothrombin (factor II) to form thrombin (factor IIa). Thrombin activates fibrinogen (factor I) to produce fibrin (factor Ia).

Different anticoagulant drugs affect different steps in the coagulation cascade.

■ Prothrombin and factors VII, IX, and X are produced in the liver and depend on vitamin K.
■ Heparin activates antithrombin III, which stops the activation of thrombin and fibrin.
■ Warfarin blocks the action of factors VII, X, and prothrombin (II).

■ to prevent clotting during blood transfusions
■ to prevent clotting during intra-abdominal or orthopedic surgery

Heparin isn't absorbed well from the GI tract. It must be administered parenterally by IV injection, IV infusion, or deep SubQ injection. Heparin is not given by IM injection because of the risk of localized bleeding. Heparin is metabolized in the liver, and its metabolites are excreted in the urine.

Heparin interacts with many other drugs, leading to either an increased risk of bleeding or a reduced effectiveness of heparin. You should be aware of the following drug interactions with heparin:

■ When heparin is taken with oral anticoagulants, there is a synergistic effect. The risk of bleeding increases. The prothrombin time (PT) and international nor-

HOW IT WORKS

How Heparin Works

Heparin's job is to prevent new clots, or thrombi, from forming. A thrombus can form in any artery or vein when blood flow is blocked. For example, a venous thrombus (blood clot in a vein) may result from decreased blood flow, an injury that damages the vein, or a change in blood coagulation (clotting). The most common type of venous thrombus is deep vein thrombosis (DVT), which occurs in the lower extremities. In arteries, clots may occur because of atherosclerosis (plaque in the arteries) or arrhythmias.

The formation of blood clots is a complex process. It requires the action of the proteins thrombin and fibrin, as well as several other chemicals in the blood called clotting factors. Each factor or component is stimulated in a specific sequence as a clot develops. Heparin prevents clots by activating antithrombin III, a protein produced by the liver. Antithrombin III stops the formation of thrombin and fibrin. Antithrombin III also inactivates factors IXa, Xa, and XII, so they can't form clots.

■ In low doses, heparin increases the activity of antithrombin III against factor Xa and thrombin and stops clots from forming.
■ Much larger doses are needed to stop fibrin formation after a clot has already been formed. This relationship between dose and effect is the reason for using low-dose heparin to prevent clotting.

malized ratio (INR), which are both used to monitor the effects of anticoagulants, may be prolonged.
■ There is an increased risk of bleeding when the patient takes heparin together with NSAIDs, iron dextran, clopidogrel, cilostazol, or an antiplatelet drug such as aspirin, ticlopidine, or dipyridamole.
■ Drugs that antagonize or inactivate heparin include antihistamines, cephalosporins, digoxin, neomycin sulfate, nicotine, nitroglycerin, penicillins, phenothiazines, quinidine, and tetracycline hydrochloride.

Nicotine may inactivate heparin, whereas nitroglycerin may inhibit the effects of heparin.

Unfractionated Heparin

Heparin is not a single drug but a mixture of drugs with low and high molecular weights. Unfractionated heparin (UFH) is typically given in a hospital or clinic, because patients require careful monitoring after administration. UFH is used to treat and prevent DVT, thrombosis, and embolism.

Heparin Sodium

Heparin sodium is used to prevent and treat venous thrombosis and peripheral arterial embolism. It's also used in

PROCEED WITH CAUTION

Adverse Reactions to Unfractionated Heparin

Heparin has relatively few adverse reactions. These reactions can usually be prevented if the patient's partial thrombo-plastin time (PTT) is kept within the therapeutic range (1.5 to 2.5 times the control).

The most common adverse reaction is bleeding. Bleeding can range from minor bruising to hemorrhaging from a major organ. Administering protamine sulfate, which binds to heparin to form a stable salt, can reverse the bleeding.

Other adverse reactions include:

- bruising
- hematoma or ulceration at injection site
- necrosis of skin or other tissue
- thrombocytopenia (low levels of platelets in the blood)

PROCEED WITH CAUTION

Adverse Reactions to Low-Molecular-Weight Heparins

LMWHs have fewer adverse reactions than heparin. Bleeding is possible, but the risk is lower than with heparin. Other adverse reactions to LMWHs include:

- bruising
- chills and fever
- erythema (redness of the skin), pain, or irritation at the injection site

Patients who are receiving LMWH therapy may be at risk for developing epidural or spinal hematomas when undergoing anesthesia that involves spinal puncture (e.g., epidural anesthesia).

low doses to prevent DVT after surgery and to prevent pulmonary embolism (blood clots moving to the lungs) in patients undergoing abdominal surgery. It may be used as an anticoagulant in blood transfusions, dialysis procedures, or other procedures in which blood circulates outside the body. Heparin sodium is administered by IV or deep SubQ injection.

Heparin sodium comes in several different strengths, including 10 units/mL, 100 units/mL, 1,000 units/mL, or 10,000 units/mL. Always double-check the order and the vial to verify that the correct medication has been pulled.

Heparin Sodium Lock Flush Solution

Heparin sodium lock flush solution is used to prevent clots in indwelling intravenous catheters (a tube that remains in-serted for IV administration of substances). Heparin lock flush solution is administered intermittently to prevent clots in several circumstances:

- after the catheter is first placed in the vein
- after each injection of a medication
- after drawing blood for laboratory tests

This solution is not appropriate for anticoagulant therapy.

Heparin sodium lock flush solution is available in a wide variety of strengths, including:

- 2 units/mL
- 10 units/mL
- 40 units/mL
- 50 units/mL
- 100 units/mL
- 1,000 units/mL
- 2,000 units/mL
- 2,500 units/mL
- 5,000 units/mL

- 10,000 units/mL
- 20,000 units/mL

Low-Molecular-Weight Heparins

Fractionated heparins or low-molecular-weight heparins (LMWHs) are used to prevent DVT after some surgical pro-cedures, including hip or knee replacement surgery. They are also used to prevent clotting associated with unstable angina or MI. When the recommended doses are adminis-tered, LMWHs produce stable responses in patients. For this reason, they don't require frequent laboratory monitoring. They may be administered at home by a home health care worker, a family member, or the patient. LMWHs are administered by SubQ injection.

Dalteparin Sodium

Dalteparin sodium (Fragmin) comes in a range of doses in prefilled syringes or as multidose vials for administration by SubQ injection. It's used to treat unstable angina/non–Q-wave MI and to prevent DVT. It may be coadministered with aspirin.

Enoxaparin Sodium

Enoxaparin sodium (Lovenox) is available in a range of single-dose, prefilled syringes or multidose vials for SubQ injection. Enoxaparin is used in several different circum-stances:

- to prevent DVT for patients undergoing hip or knee surgery
- to treat acute DVT in conjunction with warfarin
- to treat acute ST-segment elevation MI
- to prevent ischemic complications of unstable angina/non–Q-wave MI

Enoxaparin shouldn't be mixed with other injections or in-fusions.

Warfarin

Warfarin sodium (Coumadin, Jantoven) is the main oral anticoagulant used in the United States. Oral anticoagulants are prescribed in several situations:

- to treat thromboembolism (a clot that has moved through the bloodstream and blocked a blood vessel)
- to prevent DVT
- for patients with prosthetic heart valves or diseased mitral valves
- to decrease the risk of arterial clotting, in combination with an antiplatelet drug

Patients with thromboembolism typically begin taking warfarin while still receiving heparin. However, patients at high risk for thromboembolism may begin oral anticoagulant therapy without first receiving heparin.

T I P To decrease the risk of clotting in the arteries, warfarin might be combined with aspirin, clopidogrel, or dipyridamole.

Oral anticoagulants change the ability of the liver to make vitamin K-dependent clotting factors, such as prothrombin and factors VII, IX, and X. However, the anticoagulation effect doesn't begin immediately. Clotting factors already in the bloodstream continue to coagulate blood until they become depleted.

Many patients who take warfarin also receive other drugs, placing them at risk for serious drug interactions.

- Many drugs, including highly protein-bound medications, increase the effects of warfarin, resulting in an increased risk of bleeding. Examples of drugs that increase the effects of warfarin include acetaminophen, allopurinol, amiodarone, cephalosporins, cimetidine, ciprofloxacin, clofibrate, danazol, diazoxide, disulfiram, erythromycin, fluoroquinolones, glucagon, heparin, ibuprofen, isoniazid, ketoprofen, methylthiouracil, metronidazole, miconazole, neomycin, propafenone, propylthiouracil, quinidine, streptokinase, sulfonamides, tamoxifen, tetracyclines, thiazides, thyroid drugs, tricyclic antidepressants, urokinase, and vitamin E.
- Drugs metabolized by the liver may decrease or increase the effectiveness of warfarin. Examples include barbiturates, carbamazepine, corticosteroids, corticotrophin, mercaptopurine, nafcillin, oral contraceptives containing estrogen, rifampin, spironolactone, sucralfate, and trazodone.
- When phenytoin is taken with warfarin, the risk of phenytoin toxicity increases. Phenytoin may increase or decrease the effectiveness of warfarin.

Long-term alcohol abuse increases the patient's risk of clotting while taking warfarin. Short-term alcohol intoxication will increase the risk of bleeding.

Warfarin is available only by prescription. It's sold in tablets of varying strengths ranging from 1 to 10 mg. Warfarin is also available as a powder for injection. The dosage for each patient needs to be individualized based on the patient's prothrombin time and international normalized ratio (PT/INR), two measures of blood clotting. Low initial doses are recommended for elderly and disabled patients and for patients who may show a greater than expected PT/INR response. The length of treatment and time between doses also depends on the individual patient's response.

T I P Warfarin comes in many different strengths, such as 1, 2, 2.5, 3, 4, 5, 6, 7.5, and 10 mg. These tablets are color-coded to help you get it right. You also need to be aware that dosing schedules may vary for different days. For example, the patient may receive 5 mg of warfarin on even-numbered days and 7.5 mg on odd-numbered days.

Antiplatelet Drugs

Antiplatelet drugs are used to prevent arterial thromboembolism, a condition in which blood clots form in arteries and move to other parts of the body. Patients who may benefit from antiplatelet drugs include those at risk for:

- MI
- stroke
- arteriosclerosis (hardening of the arteries)

Different antiplatelet drugs work in different ways, depending on the specific medication and the dosage. In general, antiplatelet drugs act to prevent platelets from aggregating, or gathering to form clots. When artery walls are damaged or injured, platelets stick to the artery walls. They aggregate on the artery walls to form clots. Antiplatelet drugs stop the platelets from clumping together. This

AT THE COUNTER

Lab Orders with Warfarin

A medication order is received in the pharmacy for "warfarin 5 mg po qd." You notice on the same order that PT and INR labs have been requested. What are these labs, and why are they necessary? What would happen if the patient's lab values are too high or too low?

PT and INR are tests that measure how long it takes blood to clot in the extrinsic coagulation pathway. These tests involve adding a substance called a tissue factor to a patient's blood plasma and observing the clotting time. INR provides a standard measure by comparing the patient's sample to a control sample.

If the patient's lab values are too high or too low, the dose of warfarin will have to be adjusted. The labs would be repeated daily until lab values are within normal limits again.

! PROCEED WITH CAUTION

Adverse Reactions to Warfarin

The most common adverse reaction to warfarin is minor bleeding. However, severe bleeding can also occur. The most common site for severe bleeding is the GI tract. Bleeding into the brain may be fatal. Patients who have a history of stomach or bowel bleeding, high blood pressure, heart disease, cancer, or blood vessel problems in the brain may have a higher risk of bleeding when taking warfarin.

Bruises and hematomas may form at arterial puncture sites (for example, after a blood gas sample is drawn). Necrosis or gangrene of the skin and other tissues can occur in rare circumstances.

The effects of warfarin can be reversed with phytonadione (vitamin K).

reduces the chance that new clots will form. The duration of the effects of different antiplatelet drugs varies.

Antiplatelet drugs may interact with several other medications.

- Antiplatelet medications taken with NSAIDs, heparin, oral anticoagulants, or another antiplatelet medication increase the risk of bleeding.
- Aspirin and ticlopidine may reduce the effectiveness of sulfinpyrazone to relieve signs and symptoms of gout.
- Antacids may reduce the plasma levels of ticlopidine.
- Cimetidine increases the risk of ticlopidine toxicity and bleeding.

Aspirin

Aspirin (Aspergum, Bayer, Bayer Children's Aspirin, Ecotrin, Empirin, St. Joseph Adult Chewable Aspirin, Halfprin, Heartline, Bufferin, Anacin) is used in treating patients with a history of MI or who have unstable angina. It's also used in men to reduce the risk of transient ischemic attacks (TIAs), a temporary reduction in blood circulation to the brain. Aspirin is available OTC as:

- chewing gum
- tablets

! PROCEED WITH CAUTION

Adverse Reactions to Antiplatelet Drugs

Hypersensitivity reactions, particularly anaphylaxis, can occur. Bleeding is the most common adverse reaction when IV antiplatelet drugs are administered. Other adverse reactions include abdominal discomfort and nausea. Specific antiplatelet drugs may have additional adverse reactions.

- chewable tablets
- enteric-coated tablets
- extended-release tablets

By prescription, aspirin is sold in the form of controlled-release tablets (ZORprin, Easprin).

Low doses of aspirin stop clots from forming by blocking the synthesis of prostaglandin, which in turn prevents formation of the platelet-aggregating (clumping) substance thromboxane A_2. The antiplatelet effect of aspirin lasts for about ten days, or as long as platelets survive.

In addition to the drug interactions common to other antiplatelet drugs, aspirin may increase the risk of toxicity of methotrexate and valproic acid. Adverse effects specific to aspirin include:

- stomach pain
- heartburn
- constipation
- blood in stool
- slight gastric blood loss

Clopidogrel

Clopidogrel bisulfate (Plavix) is used to reduce the risk of stroke or vascular death in patients with a history of recent MI, stroke, or peripheral artery disease. It's also used to help treat coronary syndromes in the following patients:

- patients with acute ST-segment elevation MI
- patients undergoing coronary artery bypass graft
- patients being managed with percutaneous coronary intervention (PCI), a procedure in which a balloon-tipped catheter is inserted into an artery in the heart

Clopidogrel is available as oral tablets to be administered with or without food.

Clopidogrel stops platelet aggregation by preventing platelets from binding with fibrinogen, a protein involved in clotting. The effects of clopidogrel last about five days. In addition to the adverse effects noted for other antiplatelet drugs, clopidogrel increases the risk of:

- headache
- skin ulceration
- joint pain
- flulike symptoms
- upper respiratory tract infection

Dipyridamole

Dipyridamole (Persantine) is used with warfarin to prevent thromboembolism following cardiac valve replacement surgery. The combination drug dipyridamole and aspirin (Aggrenox) may be given to prevent blood clots in patients who have had coronary artery bypass grafts (bypass surgery) or prosthetic (artificial) heart valves. Dipyridamole is available in the form of tablets. It's also available as an injection.

Dipyridamole may stop platelet aggregation by increasing adenosine, a molecule that acts to stop platelet aggregation and to dilate blood vessels.

In addition to the adverse effects associated with other antiplatelet drugs, dipyridamole may lead to:

- headache
- dizziness
- flushing
- weakness
- fainting

Ticlopidine

Ticlopidine hydrochloride (Ticlid) is used to reduce the risk of thrombotic stroke in high-risk patients, such as those with a history of frequent TIAs or a previous thrombotic stroke. Ticlopidine is available in tablets of varying strengths.

Ticlopidine works by stopping platelets from binding to fibrinogen early in the coagulation cascade. Because guidelines haven't been established for administering ticlopidine with heparin, oral anticoagulants, aspirin, or fibrinolytic drugs, these drugs should be discontinued before ticlopidine therapy begins.

- When taken with aspirin, ticlopidine may reduce the effectiveness of sulfinpyrazone to relieve symptoms of gout.
- Antacids may reduce plasma levels of ticlopidine.
- Cimetidine increases the risk of ticlopidine toxicity and bleeding.

Ticlopidine can cause life-threatening adverse reactions, including:

- neutropenia/agranulocytosis (a decrease in white blood cells that fight infection)
- thrombotic thrombocytopenic purpura (a disease in which platelets and red blood cells are destroyed, resulting in excessive blood clots and kidney damage)
- aplastic anemia (a condition in which the bone marrow doesn't produce enough blood cells)

As a result, ticlopidine is recommended only for patients who can't tolerate or who have not responded to treatment with aspirin. Other adverse reactions to ticlopidine include rashes and elevated liver function test results.

Abciximab

Abciximab (ReoPro) is used to prevent blood flow complications in patients undergoing certain heart procedures, such as PCI. It may also be used for early treatment of MI. Abciximab is administered by IV injection. It's intended for use with aspirin and heparin.

Abciximab binds to receptors on platelets and blocks fibrinogen from binding. This action stops platelets from forming clots.

Eptifibatide

Eptifibatide (Integrilin) is used to treat patients with acute coronary syndrome and for patients undergoing PCI. It's administered by IV injection. Eptifibatide is a glycoprotein IIb/IIa inhibitor drug. It stops fibrinogen from binding with platelets.

HOW IT WORKS

How Intravenous Antiplatelet Drugs Work

Eptifibatide and tirofiban are antagonists of the glycoprotein IIb/IIa receptor, a major receptor involved in platelet aggregation. This receptor is found only on platelets. When this receptor is activated, fibrinogen binds with platelets, leading to platelet aggregation. Glycoprotein inhibitors stop fibrinogen from binding to the glycoprotein IIb/IIa receptor. As a result, platelets can't form clots.

Tirofiban

In combination with heparin, Tirofiban hydrochloride (Aggrastat) may be used to treat patients with acute coronary syndrome and for patients undergoing PCI. It comes as an injection or concentrate for injection by IV administration.

Like eptifibatide, tirofiban is a glycoprotein IIb/IIa inhibitor drug. It stops fibrinogen from binding with platelets.

Thrombin Inhibitors

Thrombin inhibitors help prevent the formation of blood clots. They work by blocking thrombin activity. These drugs offer several advantages over heparin.

- Direct thrombin inhibitors act against soluble and clot-bound thrombin (thrombin in clots that have already formed).
- Their anticoagulant effects are more predictable than those of heparin.
- Their actions aren't inhibited by the platelet release reaction (a process in which platelets release stored substances that promote platelet aggregation).

The binding of the drug to thrombin is reversible.

The effects of thrombin inhibitors vary depending on how they are administered.

- Direct thrombin inhibitors are typically administered by continuous IV infusion. After IV administration, levels peak in less than one hour.
- Thrombin inhibitors may also be given as an intracoronary bolus during cardiac catheterization. In this situation, the drug begins acting in two minutes, with a peak response of fifteen minutes and a duration of two hours.
- After SubQ injection, plasma levels of thrombin inhibitors peak in two hours.

Effects on PTT can be seen within four to five hours of administration. Platelet recovery is observed within three days.

Patients with liver dysfunction may require a reduced dose of direct thrombin inhibitors. Caution is also needed in administering a direct thrombin inhibitor to a patient with an increased risk of bleeding.

Drug interactions involving thrombin inhibitors involve other drugs that increase the risk of bleeding, such as thrombolytic drugs or drugs that affect platelet function.

The most common adverse reaction to direct thrombin inhibitors is bleeding.

Argatroban

Argatroban is used to prevent or treat thrombosis in patients with heparin-induced thrombocytopenia (a decrease in the number of platelets in the blood as a result of heparin therapy). It's also used for patients who are undergoing PCI and are at risk for heparin-induced thrombocytopenia. Argatroban is available in concentrated form for IV injection. It must be diluted before infusion. Doses must be adjusted based on PTT results.

Bivalirudin

Bivalirudin (Angiomax) is used as an anticoagulant for patients with unstable angina who are undergoing percutaneous transluminal coronary angioplasty. It may also be used with glycoprotein IIb/IIIa inhibitor in patients undergoing PCI. Bivalirudin should be used in conjunction with aspirin therapy. This drug is available in powder form for IV bolus injection.

Lepirudin

Lepirudin (Refludan) is used to treat patients with heparin-induced thrombocytopenia and related thromboembolic disease. It comes as a powder for IV injection.

Factor Xa Inhibitor Drugs

The only factor Xa inhibitor drug available in the United States is fondaparinux (Arixtra). It's used to prevent DVT in patients undergoing total hip and knee replacement surgery or surgery to repair a hip fracture. It is sometimes used in conjunction with warfarin.

Fondaparinux works by binding to antithrombin III. This action neutralizes the effects of factor Xa and interrupts the coagulation cascade. Because the coagulation cascade is interrupted, clots don't form.

Fondaparinux is administered by SubQ injection. Its effects peak within two hours of administration and last for about 17 to 24 hours. This drug may interact with other drugs that increase the risk of bleeding.

THROMBOLYTIC DRUGS

Thrombolytic drugs are used to dissolve a preexisting clot, or thrombus, often in an acute or emergency situation. They may be used in the following circumstances:

- to treat thromboembolic disorders such as acute MI, acute ischemic stroke, and peripheral artery occlusion
- to dissolve thrombi in arteriovenous cannulas (used in dialysis) and IV catheters

Thrombolytic drugs seem most effective when given within six hours of the onset of symptoms. After IV or intracoronary administration, thrombolytic drugs are distributed immediately throughout the bloodstream. They work by quickly converting plasminogen (a substance that occurs in blood plasma) to plasmin. Plasmin acts to dissolve thrombi, fibrinogen, and other plasma proteins.

Thrombolytic drugs interact with heparin, oral anticoagulants, antiplatelet drugs, and NSAIDs, increasing the patient's risk of bleeding.

Alteplase, tPA

Alteplase recombinant (Activase, Cathflo Activase) is used in several different situations:

- to treat acute MI, pulmonary embolism, acute ischemic stroke, and peripheral artery occlusion

PROCEED WITH CAUTION

Adverse Reactions to Fondaparinux

Adverse reactions that can occur with factor Xa inhibitor therapy include:

- bleeding
- nausea
- anemia
- fever
- rash
- constipation
- edema

PROCEED WITH CAUTION

Adverse Reactions to Thrombolytic Drugs

The main adverse reactions to thrombolytic drugs involve bleeding and allergic responses, especially with streptokinase. Bleeding may involve

- intracranial bleeding
- GI bleeding
- bleeding in the genitourinary tract
- retroperitoneal bleeding (internal bleeding that may include organs such as kidneys, bladder, and colon)

■ to restore patency (openness) to clotted grafts and IV access devices

Alteplase is available as a lyophilized powder for IV administration.

Reteplase, r-PA

Reteplase recombinant (Retavase) is used to treat acute MI. It's sold as a powder for injection in kits and half-kits, for IV administration only.

Tenecteplase, TNK-tPA

Tenecteplase (TNKase) is used to treat acute MI. This drug should be administered IV only. It's sold as a lyophilized powder.

Urokinase

Urokinase (Kinlytic) is used to treat pulmonary embolism. It is available as a lyophilized powder that is administered by IV infusion.

HOW IT WORKS

How Alteplase Helps Restore Circulation

When a thrombus forms in an artery, it blocks the blood supply. This causes ischemia (lack of blood supply) and necrosis (cell and tissue death). Alteplase can dissolve a thrombus in either the coronary or pulmonary artery (figure 6-1). This action restores the blood supply to the site beyond the blockage.

- *Obstructed artery.* A thrombus blocks blood flow through the artery, causing distal ischemia.
- *Inside the thrombus.* Alteplase enters the thrombus. The thrombus consists of plasminogen bound to fibrin. Alteplase binds to the complex of plasminogen and fibrin and begins to act on the plasminogen. Alteplase converts the plasminogen into active plasmin. The plasmin digests the fibrin, dissolving the thrombus. As the thrombus dissolves, blood flow resumes.

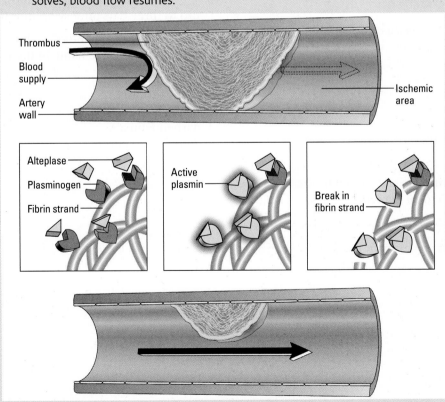

FIGURE 6-1 How alteplase works. (From *Clinical Pharmacology Made Incredibly Easy.* 2nd Ed. Philadelphia, PA: Lippincott Williams & Wilkins; 2005.)

QUICK QUIZ

Answer the following multiple-choice questions.

1. Which of the following would probably be used to treat pernicious anemia?
   a. ferrous fumarate
   b. cyanocobalamin
   c. folic acid
   d. epoetin alfa
2. What is the most common adverse reaction to erythropoietin agents?
   a. headache
   b. thrombocytopenia
   c. hypertension
   d. fever
3. Which of the following is a key difference between fractionated and unfractionated heparins?
   a. Only fractionated heparins prevent thrombi from forming.
   b. Therapy with fractionated heparins doesn't require close PTT monitoring.
   c. Only unfractionated heparins increase the risk of patient bleeding.
   d. none of the above
4. Which of the following would probably *not* require treatment with antiplatelet drugs?
   a. MI
   b. arteriosclerosis
   c. megaloblastic anemia
   d. stroke
5. Which of the following is *not* a direct inhibitor of thrombin?
   a. argatroban
   b. bivalirudin
   c. lepirudin
   d. dipyridamole

Please answer each of the following questions in one to three sentences.

1. Why does the amount of iron absorbed by the body vary (for example, from 5 to 30 percent)?

   _____

   _____

2. Why are folic acid supplements recommended for pregnant women?

   _____

   _____

3. Identify three situations when warfarin may be used.

   _____

   _____

4. Explain why it may be complicated to decide on the appropriate dose of warfarin for a patient.

   _____

   _____

5. In what way does the action of thrombolytic drugs differ from the action of anticoagulant drugs?

   _____

   _____

Answer the following questions as either true or false.

1. ___ Oral iron therapy is the preferred route for preventing or treating iron deficiency anemia.
2. ___ Heparin sodium lock flush solution is often used for anticoagulant therapy.
3. ___ The effects of warfarin can be reversed with phytonadione (vitamin K).
4. ___ Ticlopidine is often used in conjunction with aspirin.
5. ___ Thrombolytic drugs are most effective when given two to three days after symptoms first appear.

Match the generic name of each drug in the left column with the correct trade name in the right column.

1. clopidogrel   a. Plavix
2. fondaparinux   b. Aggrastat
3. tirofiban   c. Aranesp
4. darbepoetin alfa   d. Arixtra
5. dalteparin sodium   e. Fragmin

DRUG CLASSIFICATION TABLE

Classification	Generic Name	Trade Name(s)
Hematinic drugs	ferrous furmarate *fair'-us fyoo'-ma-rare*	*tablets:* Hemocyte, Ferretts, Nephro-Fer, Femiron, Ircon *capsules (polysaccharide-iron complex):* Tandem *tablets (timed release):* Ferro-Sequels *capsules (liquid filled):* (no longer marketed under trade name)
	ferrous gluconate *fair'-us gloo'-koe-nate*	*tablets:* Fergon, Ferate
	ferrous sulfate *fair'-us sull'-fate*	*tablets:* Feosol, Fe-Max, Feratab *elixir:* (no longer marketed under trade name) *drops:* Fer-In-Sol, Fer-Iron, Fer-Gen-Sol, Fer-iron *liquid:* Fer-Gen-Sol *extended-release capsules:* (no longer marketed under trade name) *extended-release tablets:* Slow Fe oral solution: (no longer marketed under trade name)
	iron dextran *eye'-run dex'-tran*	*injection:* PriDextra, DexFerrum
	iron sucrose *eye'-run soo'-krose*	*injection:* Venofer
	leucovorin calcium *loo-koe-vor'-in*	*tablets, injection:* (no longer marketed under trade name)
	sodium ferric gluconate complex *sow'-dee-um fer'-ik gloo'-koe-nate*	*injection:* Ferrlecit
	polysaccharide-iron complex *pah'-lee-saa'-kah-ride-eye'-run*	*capsules:* EZFE, FerUS 150, Ferrex-150, iFerex 150, Nu-Iron *elixir:* Niferex
	carbonyl iron *car'-bah-nill eye'-run*	*suspension:* ICAR Pediatric *chewable tablets:* Iron Chews Pediatric, ICAR Pediatric
	cyanocobalamin *sye-an-oh-koe-bal'-a-min*	*tablets (OTC):* (no longer marketed under trade name) *tablets (extended release) (OTC):* (no longer marketed under trade name) *nasal spray (Rx):* Nascobal, CaloMist *injection (Rx):* Nutri-Twelve,
	hydroxocobalamin *hye-drox-oh-koe-bal'-a-min*	*injection:* Cyanokit
	folic acid *foe'-lik*	*tablets (OTC):* Folacin *tablets (Rx):* (no longer marketed under trade name) *injection (Rx):* (no longer marketed under trade name)
	darbepoetin alfa *dar-bah-poe-e'-tin*	*injection:* Aranesp
	epoetin alfa *e-po'-e-tin*	*injection:* Epogen, Procrit

continued

DRUG CLASSIFICATION TABLE (continued)

Classification	Generic Name	Trade Name(s)
Anticoagulant drugs	heparin sodium *hep'-ah-rin*	*injection:* (no longer marketed under trade name)
	dalteparin sodium *dal-tep'-a-rin*	*injection:* Fragmin
	enoxaparin sodium *en-ocks'-a-par-in*	*injection:* Lovenox
	warfarin sodium *war'-far-in*	*injection:* Coumadin *tablets:* Jantoven, Coumadin
	aspirin *ass'-purr-in*	*chewing gum (OTC):* Aspergum *tablets (OTC):* Bayer, Empirin, Bufferin, Anacin *chewable tablets (OTC):* Bayer Children's Aspirin, St. Joseph Adult Chewable Aspirin *extended-release tablets (OTC):* Ecotrin, Empirin, Halfprin *enteric-coated tablets (OTC):* Ecotrin, Halfprin, Heartline *tablets (Rx):* ZORprin, Easprin
	clopidogrel bisulfate *kloe-pid'-oh-grel*	*tablets:* Plavix
	dipyridamole *dye-peer-id'-a-mole*	*tablets:* Persantine *injection:* (no longer marketed under trade name)
	dipyridamole and aspirin *dye-peer-id'-a-mole*	*tablets:* Aggrenox
	ticlopidine *tye-kloe'-pi-deen*	*tablets:* Ticlid
	abciximab *ab-siks'-ih-mab*	*injection:* ReoPro
	eptifibatide *ep-ti-fib'-ih-tide*	*injection:* Integrilin
	tirofiban *tye-roe-fye'-ban*	*injection:* Aggrastat
	argatroban *ar-ga'-troh-ban*	*injection:* (no longer marketed under trade name)
	bivalirudin *bye-val'-ih-ruh-din*	*injection:* Angiomax
	lepirudin *le-peer'-u-din*	*injection:* Refludan
	fondaparinux *fon-da-pare'-i-nux*	*injection:* Arixtra
Thrombolytic drugs	alteplase recombinant, tPA *al'-te-plaze*	*injection:* Activase, Cathflo Activase
	reteplase recombinant, r-PA *ret'-ah-plaze*	*injection:* Retavase
	tenecteplase, TNK-tPA *teh-nek'-ti-plaze*	*injection:* TNKase
	urokinase *yoor-oh'-kye-nase*	*injection:* Kinlytic

Respiratory Drugs

CHAPTER OBJECTIVES

- Match brand and generic names of commonly used respiratory drugs
- Identify the classification of commonly used respiratory drugs
- List the uses of commonly used respiratory drugs
- Identify commonly used respiratory drugs with a significant number of drug interactions
- Compare and contrast the use of short-acting beta$_2$-adrenergic agonists with long-acting beta$_2$-adrenergic agonists
- Identify special populations that may require special care when taking corticosteroids
- Explain the mechanism of action for a leukotriene modifier and a mast cell stabilizer
- Discuss dosing complications of methylxanthines
- Compare and contrast the uses of expectorants with antitussives
- Identify medications that are available over the counter and medications that require a prescription

KEY TERMS

anticholinergic drug—a drug that acts as a bronchodilator by blocking the parasympathetic nervous system and is used in treating asthma, COPD, and other respiratory disorders

antitussives—drugs used to relieve coughing

asthma—an obstructive pulmonary disease of the lower airway; characterized by difficulty breathing and wheezing that results from spasming of the bronchial tubes or by swelling of their mucous membrane

beta2-adrenergic agonists—drugs that act as bronchodilators by stimulating the sympathetic nervous system and are used to treat symptoms associated with asthma and COPD

bronchoconstriction—the narrowing of airway passages in the bronchi as muscles in the walls tighten and the walls swell

bronchodilator—a drug used to relieve the bronchial spasms and constriction that are often associated with respiratory disorders

chronic obstructive pulmonary disease (COPD)—a permanent, destructive pulmonary disorder that is a combination of chronic bronchitis and emphysema

corticosteroids—anti-inflammatory drugs available in inhaled and systemic forms for short- and long-term control of asthma symptoms

decongestants—drugs that reduce the swelling of nasal passages

dyspnea—difficulty breathing

emphysema—a lung disorder in which the terminal bronchioles or alveoli become enlarged and plugged with mucus

expectorants—drugs that aid in removing thick, sticky mucus from respiratory passages by coughing

histamines—substances in various body tissues, such as the heart, lungs, gastric mucosa, and skin, that are produced in response to injury

leukotriene modifiers—a class of drugs mainly used to prevent and control asthma attacks in persons with mild to moderate levels of the disease

leukotrienes—substances that are released by the body during the inflammatory process and constrict the bronchi

mast cell stabilizers—drugs that prevent and control asthma symptoms by preventing the release of histamines from mast cells that would swell and tighten airways

methylxanthines—a class of drugs that stimulates the central nervous system and results in bronchodilation; also called *xanthines*

mucolytics—drugs that loosen respiratory secretions

nebulizer—a therapeutic device that disperses liquid medication in a mist of extremely fine particles that can be inhaled into the deeper parts of the respiratory tract

nonproductive cough—a dry, hacking cough that produces no secretions

productive cough—a cough that expels secretions from the lower respiratory tract

sympathomimetic drugs—drugs that imitate the activities or actions of the central nervous system

xanthines—see *methylxanthines*

The respiratory system performs the vital function of gas exchange between the body and the environment. In other words, it takes in oxygen and expels carbon dioxide. In this chapter, you'll learn about drugs used to treat disorders of the respiratory system, the uses and varying actions of these drugs, and interactions and adverse reactions to them.

THE RESPIRATORY SYSTEM AND DISORDERS

We take a breath about 12 to 20 times each minute. Although breathing seems like a simple, automatic process that we usually don't even notice, it involves some complicated body structures.

The Respiratory System Close Up

Air enters the body through the nose and mouth. The pharynx (throat) then directs the air into the trachea (windpipe). As you can see in figure 7-1, the trachea divides into two main tubes. These tubes, known as bronchi, subdivide into smaller and smaller "branches" that deliver air throughout the lung tissue.

The smallest of these conducting tubes are called bronchioles. At the end of the bronchioles there are clusters of tiny air sacs called alveoli. The alveoli are covered in millions of tiny capillaries (blood vessels). In the lungs, blood passes through the capillaries around the alveoli, where gas exchange takes place.

The air we inhale normally contains about 21% oxygen and 0.04% carbon dioxide. The alveoli are responsible for taking in the oxygen from inhaled air and diffusing it into the blood. The oxygenated blood then travels to the heart, which delivers it to the tissues throughout the body. As the body's cells take in oxygen from the blood, they release carbon dioxide.

The blood, now relatively low in oxygen and high in carbon dioxide, returns from the tissues and enters the lung capillaries. There, carbon dioxide is removed from the body through air that is exhaled from the lungs.

Other parts of the respiratory system help ensure that the air reaching the lungs is as clean and pure as possible. For example, the walls of the nasal cavity are covered with mucous membrane. The cells of this membrane secrete a large amount of fluid—up to one quart each day. As air comes in contact with the lining of the nose, impurities, such as dust and pathogens (germs), are filtered out by the hairs of the nostrils or caught in the surface mucus. In addition, the trachea, bronchi, and other conducting passageways of the respiratory tract are lined with cells that have cilia (small, hairlike projections). The cilia also work to keep impurities from entering the lungs. The cilia function by driving impurities toward the throat, where they can be swallowed or eliminated by coughing, sneezing, or blowing the nose.

Respiratory Disorders

Breathing disorders such as asthma and emphysema can keep the respiratory system from functioning properly. As a result, the lungs are unable to do their work effectively.

Asthma is an obstructive pulmonary disease of the lower airway. It is characterized by **dyspnea** (difficulty breathing) and wheezing that results from spasming of the bronchial tubes or by swelling of their mucous membrane. The body's response is a massive release of histamines from the mast cells of the respiratory tract.

Histamines are substances in the beta cells within various tissues that are produced in response to injury. $Beta_1$ cells are located in the heart and $beta_2$ cells are located in the lungs, stomach, and skin. When histamines are released, symptoms such as increased mucus production, inflammation, and edema (swelling) of the lining of the bronchi and bronchioles appear.

The extra mucus can worsen the situation by plugging the smaller airways. Gas exchange is impaired. Carbon dioxide becomes trapped in the alveoli, and oxygen cannot enter.

Other disorders of the lower respiratory tract include:

- **emphysema**—a lung disorder in which the terminal bronchioles or alveoli become enlarged and plugged with mucus
- **bronchitis**—inflammation and possible infection of the bronchi
- **chronic obstructive pulmonary disease (COPD)**—a permanent, destructive pulmonary disorder that is a combination of chronic bronchitis and emphysema

Asthma that is persistent and present most of the time may also be referred to as COPD.

DRUGS AND THE RESPIRATORY SYSTEM

The drugs used to improve the functioning of an impaired respiratory system are mainly available in three forms:

- mists that are inhaled through the nose or mouth
- ointments or creams that are applied topically to the skin
- pills or capsules that are swallowed and absorbed through the digestive tract

In addition, some inhaled or topical medications act locally, whereas others are systemic drugs. That is, these medications eventually reach the bloodstream, which circulates them throughout the body.

Ten different classes of drugs are used to treat a variety of respiratory disorders. These classes of drugs are:

- $beta_2$-adrenergic agonists
- anticholinergics
- corticosteroids
- leukotriene modifiers
- mast cell stabilizers

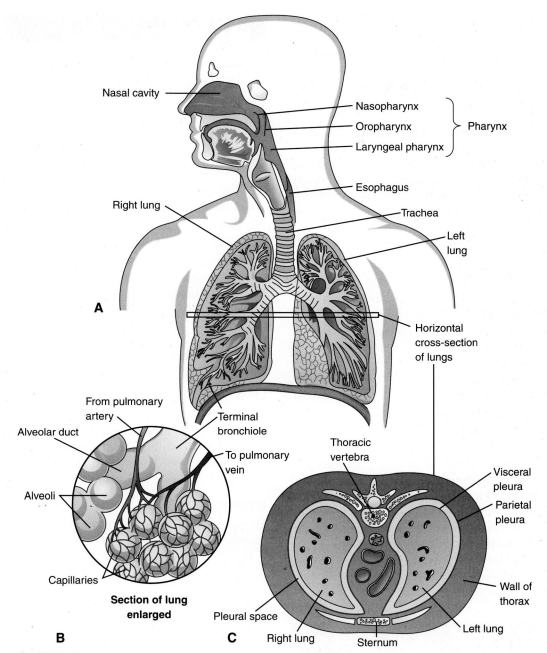

Nasal cavity

Nasopharynx
Oropharynx
Laryngeal pharynx

} Pharynx

Esophagus

Right lung

Trachea

Left lung

A

Horizontal cross-section of lungs

From pulmonary artery

Alveolar duct

Terminal bronchiole

To pulmonary vein

Thoracic vertebra

Alveoli

Visceral pleura

Parietal pleura

Capillaries

Wall of thorax

Section of lung enlarged

Pleural space

Left lung

B

C

Right lung

Sternum

FIGURE 7-1 (A) The respiratory system is a complex arrangement of spaces and passageways that conduct air into the lungs. (B) In lung tissue, the bronchioles end in clusters of tiny air sacs called alveoli, which is where gas exchange takes place. (C) Transverse view of the lungs. (From *Memmler's Structure and Function of the Human Body.* 9th Ed. Baltimore, MD: Lippincott Williams & Wilkins; 2009.)

- methylxanthines
- mucolytics
- expectorants
- antitussives
- decongestants

BETA₂-ADRENERGIC AGONISTS

Beta₂-adrenergic agonists are **bronchodilators**—drugs used to relieve the bronchial spasms and constriction that are often associated with respiratory disorders. **Beta₂-**adrenergic agonists** are used to treat symptoms associated with asthma and COPD. The inhaled forms of these drugs are preferred because they act locally. They seem to be absorbed over several hours from the respiratory tract. Because they act locally, there are fewer adverse reactions than with systemically absorbed beta₂-adrenergic agonists.

Interactions with the inhaled forms of these drugs are also uncommon. However, beta-adrenergic blockers (beta blockers) decrease the bronchodilating effects of beta₂-adrenergic agonists. Therefore, they should be used together cautiously. Beta₂-adrenergic agonists also may lose their selectivity at higher doses. This can increase the risk of toxicity.

The drugs in this class can be either short acting or long acting.

Short-Acting Beta₂-Adrenergic Agonists

Short-acting beta₂-adrenergic agonists are the drugs of choice for fast relief from asthma and COPD. A patient with COPD may use them around the clock on a scheduled basis. However, excessive use of a short-acting beta₂-adrenergic agonist may be a sign of poor asthma control and indicates that the patient's treatment regimen should be reassessed.

Albuterol

Albuterol may be administered:

- by inhalation using an inhaler (Proair HFA, Proventil HFA, Ventolin HFA) or a **nebulizer (Accuneb)** (a therapeutic device that disperses liquid medication in a mist that can be inhaled into the deeper parts of the respiratory tract)
- by mouth in extended-release tablet (Vospire ER), single-dose tablet, or syrup form

For administration by inhalation, albuterol is available in an aerosol container or as a solution in a vial. The aerosol container delivers a premeasured spray when placed in an inhaler. When the medication is needed, the inhaler is first shaken and then placed into the mouth and pumped once, releasing a dose of the drug to be inhaled. To administer the solution by nebulizer, the vial is opened and poured into the reservoir of the nebulizer. As the patient breathes, the medication is delivered through a tube and mouthpiece or face mask into the mouth or the nose and mouth. The concentrated form of the solution must

HOW IT WORKS

Beta₂-Adrenergic Agonists

Beta₂-adrenergic agonists stimulate the beta₂-adrenergic receptors in smooth muscle, which causes bronchodilation.

The patient would have trouble moving air through the lung on the right—that is, breathing—because of **bronchoconstriction**. In asthma, the bronchi become narrow as muscles in their walls tighten and the airway walls become swollen. In addition, the swollen walls give off extra mucus, which clogs the airways and makes breathing even more difficult.

The lung on the left is functioning normally. Air breathed in through the trachea is passing through bronchi that have been opened by a bronchodilator to reach the air sacs deep in the lungs, where gas exchange takes place.

PROCEED WITH CAUTION

Adverse Reactions to Beta₂-Adrenergic Agonists

Adverse reactions to short-acting beta₂-adrenergic agonists include:

- paradoxical bronchospasm
- tachycardia
- palpitations
- tremors
- dry mouth

Adverse reactions to long-acting beta₂-adrenergic agonists include:

- bronchospasm
- tachycardia
- palpitations
- hypertension
- tremors

be mixed with normal saline in the nebulizer before administration.

Levalbuterol

Levalbuterol (Xopenex, Xopenex HFA) is available as a solution for use in nebulizers in 3-mL vials. It also comes in a concentrated solution that must be mixed with normal saline before use. The drug is also available as an aerosol container for use in an inhaler.

Metaproterenol

Metaproterenol (Alupent) is available in the following forms:

- aerosol inhalant
- oral solution
- single-dose tablets
- solution vials for use in nebulizers

Pirbuterol and Terbutaline

Pirbuterol (Maxair) is produced as an aerosol inhalant. A 14-g canister provides 400 metered doses.

Terbutaline can be administered by injection or as a single-dose oral tablet. The injectable form comes in small, single-use vials.

Long-Acting Beta₂-Adrenergic Agonists

Long-acting beta₂-adrenergic agonists tend to be used with anti-inflammatory agents—specifically inhaled corticosteroids (which you'll read about later in this chapter)—to help control asthma. These drugs must be administered on a set schedule. These drugs aren't useful for relieving acute asthma attacks because they don't act fast enough. They also don't affect the chronic inflammation associated with asthma.

TIP Long-acting beta$_2$-adrenergic agonists should be used daily as prescribed and should never be used as a "rescue" inhaler. If you notice that a prescription for a long-acting beta$_2$ agonist is being refilled early, alert the pharmacist so she can question the patient about how he is using the medication.

Formoterol

Formoterol (Foradil, Perforomist) is available as a solution for inhalation and in blister packs of 12 or 60 capsules of formoterol powder. The powder form of the drug is administered by placing a capsule in a special inhaler that breaks the capsule and delivers the fine powder into the patient's mouth. The powder is to be inhaled, not swallowed.

Aformoterol and Salmeterol

Aformoterol (Brovana) is available as a solution for inhalation using a nebulizer.

Salmeterol (Serevent Diskus) is manufactured as a ready-to-use inhaler that contains either 28 doses or 60 doses of the drug. Each dose consists of a very fine powder that is inhaled into the mouth.

TIP Long-acting beta$_2$-adrenergic agonists are especially useful for people who have nocturnal asthmatic symptoms.

ANTICHOLINERGICS

Ipratropium is the most commonly used **anticholinergic drug** (a drug that acts as a bronchodilator by blocking the parasympathetic nervous system) for treating respiratory disorders. It is used to treat COPD and sometimes, on a scheduled basis, in combination with short-acting beta$_2$-adrenergic agonists to relieve the symptoms of asthma. Ipratropium is less effective in long-term management of asthma, however.

The drug is administered by inhalation:

- into the mouth from a handheld aerosol inhaler (Atrovent HFA)
- into the nose via a nasal spray (Atrovent)
- through the nose and/or mouth via a nebulizer and mask

Unlike beta$_2$-adrenergic agonists, which stimulate the sympathetic nervous system, this drug works by blocking the parasympathetic nervous system. Specifically, it inhibits muscarinic receptors on bronchial smooth muscle, resulting in bronchodilation.

Drug interactions are uncommon when using the inhaled forms of ipratropium. However, this drug should be used cautiously when administered with other anticholinergics and with antimuscarinic drugs.

PROCEED WITH CAUTION

Adverse Reactions to Anticholinergics

The most common adverse reactions to anticholinergics include:

- nervousness
- tachycardia
- nausea and vomiting
- paradoxical bronchospasm (with excessive use)

Ipratropium is also found in combination with albuterol as both an aerosol for inhalation (Combivent) and a solution for inhalation (Duoneb) via a nebulizer.

CORTICOSTEROIDS

Corticosteroids are anti-inflammatory drugs available in inhaled and systemic forms for short- and long-term control of asthma symptoms. They are the most effective drugs for the long-term treatment and prevention of acute asthma attacks. They work by inhibiting:

- the production of cytokines (substances involved in responses by the body's immune system), leukotrienes (substances that take part in allergic responses), and prostaglandins (substances that control smooth muscle contractions)
- the recruitment of eosinophils (a type of white blood cell involved in immune system responses)
- the release of other inflammatory agents

Corticosteroids also affect other body systems and can have adverse effects with long-term use. Some patient populations require special attention when taking corticosteroids:

- *Children.* Growth should be monitored, especially when children are taking systemic corticosteroids or high doses of inhaled corticosteroids.
- *Older adults.* This population may benefit from receiving drugs that prevent osteoporosis during corticosteroid therapy, especially if they're taking high doses of systemic or inhaled steroids.
- *Diabetics.* This population may require closer monitoring of blood glucose levels while taking steroids.
- *Breastfeeding women.* Corticosteroid levels are negligible in the breast milk of mothers who take less than 20 mg of prednisone a day. Amounts in breast milk may be minimized if the mother waits four hours after taking the drug to nurse her child.

Drug interactions are uncommon when using inhaled forms of corticosteroids. However, hormonal contraceptives, ketoconazole, and macrolide antibiotics may increase the activity of corticosteroids in general. As a result, steroid dosage may need to be reduced. In addition, barbiturates, cholestyramine, and phenytoin may decrease the effectiveness of corticosteroids, resulting in the need to increase steroid dosage.

T I P Corticosteroids have a variety of uses aside from treating asthma. They are available in a number of other dosage forms, including topical sprays, ointments, creams, and lotions. Because these drugs reduce inflammation, topical forms may be used to treat conditions such as skin rashes and joint injuries.

Inhaled Corticosteroids

Inhaled corticosteroids are the preferred drugs for preventing attacks in patients with mild to severe asthma. The use of inhaled forms reduces the need for systemic steroids in many cases. This in turn reduces the patient's risk of developing serious long-term adverse reactions.

Beclomethasone Dipropionate

Beclomethasone dipropionate is available as a nasal spray (Beconase AQ). An aerosol solution (QVAR) that is administered by an inhaler is also available.

T I P The generic names of corticosteroids typically end in the letters -sone.

Budesonide

Budesonide is available in a variety of forms and strengths:

- Pulmicort Respules is a suspension that is used by squeezing the contents of premeasured ampules into a nebulizer.
- Pulmicort Flexhaler contains a fine powder that the patient receives by placing the inhaler between his lips and breathing in deeply and forcefully though the mouth. Inhalers deliver a premeasured dose of the drug.
- Rhinocort Aqua is a liquid nasal spray that contains the drug in suspension. A metered-dose spray pump delivers the required dose in each spray.

 PROCEED WITH CAUTION

Adverse Reactions to Inhaled Corticosteroids

Adverse reactions to inhaled corticosteroids include:

- mouth irritation
- oral candidiasis (a type of fungal infection)
- upper respiratory tract infection

To reduce the risk of adverse reactions, patients should:

- use the lowest possible dose to maintain control
- administer oral doses using a spacer
- rinse out the mouth after administration

In addition, budesonide is marketed as Entocort EC, an oral sustained-release capsule that delivers the drug over a 24-hour period. It is also available in a combination powder for inhalation with formoterol (Symbicort).

T I P A patient with asthma or COPD may be using multiple inhalers. Always make sure that the dose is correct and that the patient is receiving medications from different classifications. Patients are not usually prescribed two oral corticosteroids or two short-acting beta$_2$-adrenergic agonists simultaneously. However, a patient might be prescribed one of each.

Flunisolide

Flunisolide is manufactured as the aerosol inhalants AeroBid and AeroBid-M. Another trade name, Nasarel, is available in the form of a nasal spray.

Fluticasone

For respiratory use, fluticasone (Flovent HFA, Flovent Diskus, Flonase, Veramyst) is produced in several types of inhalers and as a nasal spray. Flovent HFA is an aerosol inhalant. Flovent Diskus is an aerosol inhaler that delivers the drug in fine powder from premeasured blister packs. Flonase and Veramyst are manufactured as nasal sprays. Fluticasone is also available as a topical cream, ointment and lotion under the trade name Cutivate for the treatment of a wide variety of skin conditions.

T I P Over the past few years, HFA inhalers have replaced traditional inhalers that used CFCs as the propellant. The FDA ruled that CFC inhalers could no longer be produced or marketed as of December 31, 2008, because of the damage CFCs cause to the ozone layer.

Triamcinolone

Triamcinolone is marketed as a nasal spray under the trade name Nasacort AQ. An aerosol inhalant is manufactured under the name Azmacort. In addition to its inhaled forms, triamcinolone acetonide is available as an injection. The injectable form of the drug is manufactured under various trade names, including Aristospan and Kenalog.

Like other corticosteroids, triamcinolone has a variety of nonrespiratory uses. For example, topical forms of the drug (lotions, creams, ointments, and sprays) are used to treat skin diseases such as psoriasis. It also comes in oral tablets and a dental paste. The injectable form of triamcinolone is also useful in treating arthritis, gout, and other inflammatory problems.

Oral Corticosteroids

Systemic corticosteroids include those that are taken orally and those that are administered intravenously. The systemic forms are usually reserved for moderate to severe attacks. But they're also used for persons with milder asthma who don't respond well to other measures.

AT THE COUNTER

Oral Inhalers

A patient is prescribed albuterol and fluticasone oral inhalations for asthma. In what order should the patient use the inhalers and why?

The patient would use the albuterol (bronchodilator) first to open the airways. The fluticasone (corticosteroid) would be used second and would have better penetration because the airways would then be open.

Why would a patient need a spacer for these inhalers?

A spacer is a chamber that receives a dose of medication from the oral inhaler prior to inhalation by the patient. Spacers are often used to make administration of the product easier. The spacer does not require the coordination that using the inhaler alone requires. If a spacer is not used, the patient must depress the canister, keep the tongue down, and inhale all at the same time. The spacer gives the patient a moment after depressing the canister to move the tongue down and inhale. In addition, the spacer moves the inhaler farther from the face and prevents the apprehension that some patients feel when things are right in front of their eyes. Spacers are especially helpful for pediatric and geriatric patients.

Prednisolone

Prednisolone is manufactured in several oral forms. A conventional tablet (Prednoral) is available, as well as tablets of varying strengths that dissolve in the mouth (Orapred ODT). Physicians also may prescribe it as an oral solution (Orapred, Pediapred, Millipred) or syrup (Prelone). In addition, prednisolone eye drops are also available under a variety of trade names.

T I P The names sound similar, but be sure not to confuse prednisolone and prednisone.

Prednisone

Prednisone is available in the form of tablets and an oral solution. The tablets are also available in 6- and 12-day unit dose blister packs (Sterapred DS) for short-term taper dosing.

Intravenous Corticosteroids

Like all systemic corticosteroids, intravenous use of this class of drugs should be at the lowest effective dosage and over the shortest possible period of time to minimize the risk of adverse reactions.

Hydrocortisone

Hydrocortisone (A-Hydrocort, Solu-Cortef, Cortef, Hydrocortone) is manufactured as an injectable solution and tablets. Injections are usually given in a physician's office or clinic, but patients sometimes self-administer this drug.

Like several other corticosteroids, hydrocortisone is produced in several other forms—such as ointments, creams, eye and ear solutions, suppositories, and even enemas—for treating a variety of other nonrespiratory conditions. For example, topical hydrocortisone is used as an anti-inflammatory drug. (You'll read more about hydrocortisone in Chapter 10.)

Methylprednisolone

Methylprednisolone (A-Methapred, Depo-Medrol, Solu-Medrol) is a powder. It is put in suspension in liquids for injection. It is also available as oral tablets (Medrol).

LEUKOTRIENE MODIFIERS

Leukotriene modifiers are mainly used to prevent and control asthma attacks in patients with mild to moderate asthma. These drugs also may be prescribed instead of steroids, if possible, so that patients may be spared the adverse effects of long-term steroid use.

However, leukotriene modifiers are metabolized, induced, or inhibited by the cytochrome P450 system. This can result in a number of drug interactions. For example, the risk of toxicity may be increased if leukotriene modifiers are used with the following drugs:

- amiodarone
- cimetidine
- fluconazole
- fluoxetine
- fluvoxamine
- itraconazole
- isoniazid
- ketoconazole
- metronidazole
- voriconazole

In addition, the effectiveness of these leukotriene modifiers may be reduced if they are used with the following drugs:

- carbamazepine
- phenobarbital

PROCEED WITH CAUTION

Adverse Reactions to Leukotriene Modifiers

Adverse reactions that may occur with leukotriene modifiers include:

- headache
- dizziness
- nausea and vomiting
- myalgia (muscle pain)

- phenytoin
- primidone
- rifampin

You'll read about drug interactions that are specific to certain leukotriene modifiers in the sections that follow.

Leukotriene Receptor Antagonists

As their name suggests, these drugs block leukotriene receptor sites in the respiratory tract. Although they prevent airway swelling, they're not bronchodilators and should not be used in place of rescue inhalers during an acute asthma attack.

TIP A generic drug name ending in *-lukast* indicates that the drug is most likely a leukotriene receptor antagonist.

Montelukast

Montelukast (Singulair) is available as conventional tablets and chewable tablets. It is also available in oral granules that can be taken by mouth or sprinkled on soft food. This drug is appropriate for use in adults and in children older than two years old.

Unlike the other leukotriene modifiers, montelukast is not contraindicated in patients with liver impairments. Therefore, it isn't necessary to monitor liver function in patients who are taking this drug.

In addition to the drug interactions associated with all leukotriene modifiers, the risk of toxicity may be increased if the following are used with montelukast:

- clarithromycin
- cyclosporine
- erythromycin
- grapefruit juice

The following drugs and supplements can decrease the effectiveness of montelukast:

- efavirenz
- garlic supplements
- modafinil
- nevirapine
- oxcarbazepine
- rifabutin
- St. John's wort

Zafirlukast

Zafirlukast (Accolate) is used in the prevention and treatment of chronic and severe asthma in patients aged 12 years or older. It is manufactured as oral tablets. Dosages may need to be adjusted for patients with liver impairments, and these patients must be closely monitored.

The risk of toxicity may be increased when zafirlukast is used with the following drugs:

- amlodipine
- atorvastatin

- carbamazepine
- clarithromycin
- cyclosporine
- erythromycin
- hormonal contraceptives
- lovastatin
- nelfinavir
- nifedipine
- phenytoin
- ritonavir
- sertraline
- simvastatin
- warfarin

These interactions are in addition to the drug interactions associated with other leukotrienes.

Leukotriene Formation Inhibitors

Leukotriene formation inhibitors reduce the body's formation of leukotrienes. The main drug in this class is zileuton (Zyflo CR), which comes in an extended-release tablet form.

In addition to the drug interactions that may occur with other leukotriene modifiers, the risk for toxicity may be increased if zileuton is taken with the following:

- amlodipine
- atorvastatin
- carbamazepine
- amitriptyline
- clarithromycin
- clozapine
- cyclosporine
- desipramine
- erythromycin
- grapefruit juice
- hormonal contraceptives
- imipramine
- lovastatin
- nelfinavir
- nifedipine
- ritonavir
- sertraline
- simvastatin
- theophylline
- warfarin

The effectiveness of zileuton may be decreased if it is taken with any of the following substances:

- efavirenz
- garlic supplements
- modafinil
- nevirapine
- oxcarbazepine
- rifabutin
- ritonavir
- St. John's wort
- tobacco

HOW IT WORKS

Leukotriene Modifiers and Mast Cell Stabilizers: How Do They Work?

Leukotrienes are substances that are released by the body during inflammation. They can cause smooth muscle contraction in the body's airways, as well as increased secretions and the activation of other inflammatory agents. As a drug class, leukotriene modifiers work either to inhibit the body's formation of leukotriene or to inhibit its receptor sites. The results are the same—edema (swelling) is prevented, and bronchodilation is facilitated.

Mast cell stabilizers also control the inflammatory process. Here's how they work:

1. The antigen enters.
2. The mast cell releases histamine immediately to respond.
3. The mast cell also produces arachidonic acid and facilitates the conversion into leukotrienes.

MAST CELL STABILIZERS

Mast cell stabilizers are mainly used to prevent asthma attacks in:

- children (the drug of choice)
- adults and children with mild disease
- adults and children with mild to moderate persistent asthma
- patients with exercise-induced asthma (the drug of choice)

Like leukotriene modifiers, mast cell stabilizers are used for the prevention and long-term control of asthma symptoms. They're minimally absorbed from the GI tract and are available in inhaled forms that have only local effects. As a result, drug interactions are uncommon when using the inhaled forms of these drugs. However, their use by pregnant or nursing women or by patients with impaired renal or liver function should be closely monitored.

Like leukotriene modifiers, mast cell stabilizers are not rescue inhalers for use in acute asthma attacks. In fact, they

! PROCEED WITH CAUTION

Adverse Reactions to Mast Cell Stabilizers

Inhaled mast cell stabilizers may cause these adverse reactions:

- pharyngeal and tracheal irritation
- cough
- wheezing
- bronchospasm
- headache

can worsen bronchospasm if they're used during an attack. Instead, these drugs are intended for regular, long-term use to prevent such attacks. However, they must be taken for two to four weeks before they reach their maximum therapeutic effect.

Cromolyn Sodium

Cromolyn sodium is available in several different dosage forms. For prevention of asthma symptoms, an aerosol inhaler (Intal) and an aerosol nasal spray (Nasalcrom) deliver premeasured doses of the drug. A solution is also available for nebulizer use (Intal).

In concentrated oral solution form (Gastrocrom), cromolyn sodium is used to treat inflammatory bowel disease. This drug is also manufactured as an ophthalmic solution for the treatment of conjunctivitis (pinkeye).

Nedocromil

Nedocromil (Tilade) is marketed as an aerosol inhalant. Like cromolyn sodium, it is also available as an ophthalmic solution (Alocril) for pinkeye.

METHYLXANTHINES

Methylxanthines, which are also called **xanthines**, are another class of drug used to treat respiratory disorders. These drugs are used to relieve or prevent bronchospasm associated with chronic bronchitis and emphysema and to treat bronchial asthma. Methylxanthines work in several ways, depending on which drug is used, its dosage form, and its route of administration.

- These drugs relieve bronchospasm and create bronchodilation by relaxing the smooth muscles of the bronchi.
- In treating apnea and other nonreversible obstructive airway diseases (such as chronic bronchitis and emphysema), methylxanthines cause the brain to stimulate the respiratory drive.
- In patients with chronic bronchitis and emphysema, these drugs reduce fatigue of the diaphragm (the respiratory muscle that separates the abdomen from the thoracic cavity). Methylxanthines also improve ventricular function and, therefore, the heart's pumping action.

Theophylline

Theophylline is the most commonly prescribed oral methylxanthine. This drug is used as second- or third-line therapy for the longer-term control and prevention of the symptoms of asthma, chronic bronchitis, and emphysema. It's also been used to treat neonatal apnea (periods of not breathing in newborn infants) and to reduce bronchospasm in infants with cystic fibrosis.

! PROCEED WITH CAUTION

Adverse Reactions to Methylxanthines

Adverse reactions to methylxanthines may be temporary, or they can be signs of toxicity.

Adverse GI system reactions include:

- nausea and vomiting
- abdominal cramping
- epigastric pain
- anorexia
- diarrhea

Adverse central nervous system reactions include:

- headache
- irritability
- restlessness
- anxiety
- insomnia
- dizziness

Adverse cardiovascular reactions include:

- tachycardia
- palpitations
- arrhythmias

Theophylline is available in several forms:

- as extended-release tablets (Theochron, Uniphyl)
- as extended-release capsules (Theo-24)
- as an oral elixir (Elixophylline)
- as a solution for IV injection

High-fat meals can increase the concentration of theophylline in the body and the risk for toxicity. Food and gastric pH also can alter absorption of some of theophylline's slow-release forms.

A number of drugs and other substances can interact with theophylline to affect its action and benefits:

- Inhibitors of the CYP1A2 enzyme—such as cimetidine, ciprofloxacin, clarithromycin, erythromycin, fluvoxamine, hormonal contraceptives, isoniazid, ketoconazole, ticlopidine, and zileuton—decrease the metabolism of theophylline, which can increase its serum level and the risk of adverse reactions and toxicity.
- Inducers of the CYP1A2 enzyme—such as carbamazepine, phenobarbital, phenytoin, rifampin, St. John's wort, and charbroiled meats—increase the metabolism of theophylline, which can reduce its serum level and make it less effective.
- Smoking cigarettes or marijuana increases theophylline elimination, thus decreasing its serum level and effectiveness.
- Taking adrenergic stimulants or drinking beverages that contain caffeine result in additive adverse reactions to theophylline or symptoms of theophylline toxicity.
- The use of enflurane, halothane, isoflurane, or methoxyflurane with theophylline increases the risk of cardiac toxicity.
- Theophylline may reduce the effects of lithium.
- Thyroid hormones may reduce theophylline levels. Antithyroid drugs may increase theophylline levels.

Theophylline levels must be measured to evaluate the drug's effect and to avoid toxicity. The therapeutic serum level is 10 to 20 mcg/mL. Theophylline levels must be measured when treatment begins, when the dosage is changed, and when other drugs are added or removed from the patient's drug regimen.

Aminophylline

Aminophylline is a derivative of theophylline. Therefore, the drug interactions and other warnings that apply to theophylline apply to this drug, too. It is available as a tablet and as a solution for intravenous injection. Aminophylline is preferred when an intravenous methylxanthine drug is required.

MUCOLYTIC AND EXPECTORANT DRUGS

A **mucolytic** is a drug that breaks down and loosens mucus in the respiratory system. Mucus is a thick, sticky secretion from the body's mucous membranes. An **expectorant** is a drug that aids in raising thick mucus from the respiratory passages so that it can be expelled by coughing.

Mucolytics

Mucolytics are used with other therapies to treat patients with abnormal or thick mucous secretions, as in patients with:

- atelectasis caused by mucus obstruction, such as may occur in pneumonia, bronchiectasis, or chronic bronchitis
- bronchitis, chronic emphysema, or emphysema with bronchitis
- pulmonary complications related to cystic fibrosis

These drugs may also be used to prepare a patient for certain bronchial tests and studies.

Acetylcysteine is the only mucolytic drug used clinically in the United States for patients with abnormal or thick mucus. It decreases the thickness of respiratory tract secretions by altering the molecular composition of mucus. It also irritates the mucosa to bring about a "runny nose" to clear out the mucus.

Acetylcysteine is manufactured as a solution that is inhaled as a mist through a nebulizer and mask. This drug is also available in the form of a solution for IV injection

(Acetadote). The injectable form of acetylcysteine may be mixed with diet soda and used as an oral antidote for an overdose of acetaminophen. Although acetylcysteine won't fully protect against liver damage caused by acetaminophen overdose, its action in the liver does somewhat reduce acetaminophen toxicity.

During administration, acetylcysteine has a "rotten egg" odor that may cause nausea. With long-term or frequent use, this drug may produce:

- bronchospasm
- drowsiness
- nausea and vomiting
- severe runny nose
- stomatitis (inflammatory disease of the mouth)

Because it can cause bronchospasm, acetylcysteine isn't recommended for use by persons with asthma.

Expectorants

Coughing expels air from the lungs forcefully. A **productive cough** is one that expels secretions from the lower respiratory tract. A **nonproductive cough** is a dry hacking one that produces no secretions. Antitussive drugs are used to relieve coughing. (You'll read more about antitussives shortly.) For a patient with a productive cough, however, a physician may prescribe an expectorant as well. Expectorants are used to help the patient rid the lungs of secretions. If these secretions become pooled in the lungs, they can lead to more serious health problems, such as pneumonia.

Expectorants provide a soothing effect on the mucous membranes of the respiratory tract. These drugs also thin mucus so it may be cleared out of the airways more easily. Expectorants do this by increasing production of respiratory tract fluids, which reduces the thickness, adhesiveness, and surface tension of mucus, making it easier to clear from the airways. The result is a more productive cough.

The most commonly used expectorant is guaifenesin, which is available in both prescription and over-the-counter products. This drug is available in a number of forms, including tablets (Liquibid, Organidin NR, XPECT), extended-release tablets (Humibid, Mucinex), dissolving granules (Mucinex Mini-Melts), and oral solutions (Diabetic Tussin EX Expectorant, Mucinex Children's, Scot-Tussin Expectorant, Naldecon Senior EX, Organidin NR) and syrups (Q-Tussin, Robitussin) in a variety of strengths and concentrations. Some formulations combine guaifenesin with an antitussive or a decongestant to reduce coughing or relieve congestion and to thin secretions.

Guaifenesin is used to relieve symptoms due to ineffective productive coughs from many disorders, including:

- bronchial asthma
- bronchitis
- colds
- emphysema
- influenza

- minor bronchial irritation
- sinusitis

By itself, this drug is not known to have any specific drug interactions. However, it does cause some adverse reactions, including:

- nausea
- vomiting (if taken in large doses)
- diarrhea
- abdominal pain
- drowsiness
- headache
- hives
- rash

ANTITUSSIVES

Antitussives are typically used to treat dry, nonproductive coughs. Many brands are available in prescription strength and in OTC formulations. The opioid antitussives (typically codeine and hydrocodone) are **controlled substances**—substances that have been identified by the federal government as potentially addictive. These drugs are more strictly regulated in their use than other antitussives and are therefore available by prescription only or through a pharmacist, depending on state law. The use of opioid antitussives is mainly reserved for treating intractable coughs, such as those associated with lung cancer. In recent years, however, some OTC antitussives that do not contain controlled substances have been abused by some users who take them for nontherapeutic reasons.

The uses of different antitussives vary slightly, as does the way in which each drug works. However, each antitussive treats a serious nonproductive cough that interferes with the user's ability to rest or to carry out the activities of daily living.

Dextromethorphan

Dextromethorphan suppresses the cough reflex by acting on the cough center in the medulla of the brain, thus lowering the cough threshold. It is the most widely used cough suppressant in the United States and may provide better antitussive effects than codeine. Its popularity may stem from the fact that it isn't associated with sedation, respiratory depression, or addiction when taken as directed.

Dextromethorphan is available in a variety of dosage forms, including:

- lozenges (Sucrets DM Cough Formula)
- gel caps that contain an extended-release liquid (Robitussin CoughGels)
- oral liquid (Robitussin Maximum Strength Cough, Simply Cough, Vicks 44 Cough Relief)
- syrup (Robitussin Pediatric Cough, Triaminic Long Acting Cough)
- strips (Triaminic Thin Strips Long Acting Cough)
- extended-release oral suspension (Delsym 12-Hour)

This is a commonly sold OTC drug. Note that when it is taken by patients who are also taking monoamine oxidase inhibitors (MAOIs), excitation, elevated body temperature, hypotension, and coma can result.

Adverse Reactions to Dextromethorphan

At usual doses, adverse reactions to dextromethorphan may include:

- dizziness
- drowsiness
- GI disturbances

Dextromethorphan Abuse

Because dextromethorphan is available over the counter, it has become a drug of choice for abuse (called DXM abuse), mainly by teenagers, because of the "high" it can produce when taken in large amounts.

Overdosage from products containing dextromethorphan can cause dangerous side effects, including:

- mental confusion
- respiratory depression
- toxic psychosis (hyperactivity and visual and auditory hallucinations)

DXM abuse is sometimes combined with other medications, alcohol, and illegal drugs. The risk of harmful side effects increases when dextromethorphan is taken with these substances.

Codeine

Like dextromethorphan, codeine works through the brain and CNS to suppress the cough reflex. As an antitussive alone, codeine is available as a solution for injection and in tablet form as a Schedule II controlled substance. Codeine is also available in combination with expectorants. For example, the combination drug codeine and guaifenesin comes in a variety of dosage forms, including:

- syrup (Cheracol with Codeine, Mytussin AC)
- tablets (Brontex)
- liquid (Tussi-Organidin NR, Dex-Tuss, TussidenC)
- oral solution (Gani-Tuss NR, GuaiCo, Iophen C NR, Robafen C NR, Romilar AC)

Taking codeine with other CNS depressants—including alcohol, barbiturates, phenothiazines, and sedative-hypnotics—may increase CNS depression, resulting in drowsiness, lethargy, stupor, respiratory depression, coma, and even death. When taken with MAOIs, codeine may cause excitation, an extremely elevated temperature, hypertension or hypotension, and coma.

Hydrocodone

Hydrocodone, like dextromethorphan and codeine, works by suppressing the brain's cough reflex. This drug is not used alone as an antitussive, although it is available in combination with various expectorants.

The combination drug hydrocodone bitartrate and guaifenesin is available in several forms, including:

- caplets (Ztuss ZT)
- extended-release caplets (Tusso-HC)
- extended-release capsules (Atuss HX)

AT THE COUNTER

Selecting an Antitussive

A customer comes to the pharmacy window and asks the pharmacist for an over-the-counter product to treat her cough. You hear the pharmacist's recommendation of Delsym and know that this product contains dextromethorphan as the only active ingredient. A few minutes later, the customer returns with a bottle of your "house" brand of Robitussin DM. She wants to know if this is the same because it is used to relieve coughing and is much cheaper than what the pharmacist recommended. What do you tell her?

You can show her the box for Delsym and the box of the product that she has in their hand. Point out that the active ingredients are different between the two products. The product the pharmacist recommended contains dextromethorphan only, a cough suppressant. The product the customer has selected contains dextromethorphan and guaifenesin, a cough suppressant and an expectorant. If she wants further explanation, refer her to the pharmacist.

PROCEED WITH CAUTION

Adverse Reactions to Opioid Antitussives

The most common adverse reactions to opioid antitussives are:

- nausea
- vomiting
- sedation
- dizziness
- constipation

Other adverse reactions include:

- pupil constriction
- bradycardia
- tachycardia
- hypotension
- stupor
- seizures
- circulatory collapse
- respiratory arrest

Opioid antitussives should be used with caution in patients with past or current opioid addiction or with respiratory disorders such as asthma or COPD.

- tablets (EndaCof-Tab, Pneumotussin, Touro HC)
- extended-release tablets (Extendryl HC, XPECT-HC)
- oral syrup (Codiclear DH, Vi-Q-Tuss, Vitussin Expectorant)
- oral liquid (FluTuss XP, Kwelcof, Maxi-Tuss HCG, Relasin-HCX, Z-Cof HCX)
- oral solution (Canges-XP)

In combination with the expectorant potassium guaiacolsulfonate, hydrocodone (Pro-Clear, Marcof Expectorant, Prolex DH) is manufactured in oral liquid and syrup forms.

TIP There are many combination products available over the counter, including combinations of antihistamines, decongestants, expectorants, and/or cough suppressants. Because these medications often contain multiple ingredients, patients may not always be aware of which drugs they're actually taking. This can cause unintentional duplication in therapy. As a pharmacy technician, it's important that you read product labeling and stay up-to-date on product reformulations. Combination products can change rapidly, especially in the OTC market.

Benzonatate

Benzonatate (Tessalon Perles) is a capsule that is taken orally to relieve coughs caused by pneumonia, bronchitis, the common cold, and chronic pulmonary diseases such as emphysema. It can also be used during bronchial diagnostic tests, such as bronchoscopy, when the patient must avoid coughing. It acts by anesthetizing stretch receptors throughout the bronchi, alveoli, and pleurae (the membranes around the lungs).

Adverse reactions to benzonatate include:

- dizziness
- sedation
- headache
- nasal congestion
- burning in the eyes
- nausea or GI upset
- constipation
- rash, eruptions, or itching
- chills
- chest numbness

Benzonatate capsules should be swallowed whole. Chewing or crushing the capsules can produce a local anesthetic effect in the mouth and throat, which can compromise the airway.

DECONGESTANTS

Decongestants may be classified as systemic or topical, depending on how they're administered. Some decongestants are available as both systemic and topical drugs. Both types are powerful vasoconstrictors that reduce swelling in the respiratory tract's vascular network, although they do so in a slightly different manner. Both are used to relieve the symptoms of swollen nasal membranes resulting from:

- acute coryza (large amounts of discharge from the nose)
- allergic rhinitis (hay fever)
- the common cold
- sinusitis
- vasomotor rhinitis (swelling of nasal membranes from factors other than allergies, such as air pollution or sudden temperature change)

TIP Decongestants do more than simply clear up nasal congestion. They're used in rectal suppositories and creams for treating hemorrhoids, in ophthalmic solutions for treating red, irritated eyes, and in dental implants and solutions to shrink blood vessels and reduce swelling.

Systemic Decongestants

Systemic decongestants stimulate the sympathetic nervous system to reduce swelling in the respiratory tract. They do

PROCEED WITH CAUTION

Adverse Reactions to Decongestants

Most adverse reactions to decongestants result from CNS stimulation. These reactions include:

- nervousness
- restlessness
- insomnia
- nausea
- palpitations
- tachycardia
- difficulty urinating
- elevated blood pressure

Systemic decongestants are excreted in the milk of breast-feeding women. They also can exacerbate the following conditions:

- hypertension
- hyperthyroidism
- diabetes
- benign prostatic hypertrophy
- glaucoma
- heart disease

The most common adverse reaction associated with topical decongestants is rebound nasal decongestion after more than five days' use. Other adverse reactions include:

- burning and stinging of the nasal mucosa
- sneezing
- mucosal dryness or ulceration

Patients who are hypersensitive to other sympathomimetic amines may also be hypersensitive to decongestants.

this by stimulating alpha-adrenergic receptors in the body's blood vessels. This reduces the blood supply to the nose, which decreases swelling of the nasal mucosa.

These drugs may also act indirectly by causing the release of norepinephrine from storage sites in the body, resulting in peripheral vasoconstriction. Systemic decongestants cause contraction of urinary and GI sphincters, dilated pupils, and decreased insulin secretion. They are commonly given with other drugs such as antihistamines, antimuscarinics, antipyretic analgesics, and antitussives.

Systemic decongestants may interact with other drugs.

- Using systemic decongestants with MAOIs may cause severe hypertension or a hypertensive crisis, which can be life threatening. These drugs should never be used together.
- Increased CNS stimulation may occur when systemic decongestants are taken with other drugs that act on the sympathetic nervous system, such as epinephrine, norepinephrine, dopamine, dobutamine, isoproterenol, metaproterenol, terbutaline, phenylephrine, and tyramine.

Ephedrine

As a systemic decongestant, ephedrine is available as capsules and in a solution for injection. As an injection, it may be injected subcutaneously or directly into a large vein. This is in contrast to many other injectable drugs that are given only by infusion with a bag of IV solution or IV push through a port in a patient's IV line.

In addition to relief of nasal congestion, the oral forms are usually prescribed for shortness of breath, tightness in the chest, and wheezing caused by bronchial asthma. Injection or IV infusion is usually reserved for treatment of acute asthma attacks and allergy-related asthma disorders. Ephedrine is also a component in several combination respiratory medicines.

Phenylephrine

As a systemic decongestant, phenylephrine is used in combination with acetaminophen, codeine, dextromethorphan, guaifenesin, and several other drugs.

- Orally dissolving tablets (Nasop)
- Orally dissolving film (Sudafed PE Quick Dissolve, Triaminic Thin Strips)
- Oral tablets (Sudafed PE)
- Oral suspension (Nasop)
- Chewable tablets (Nasop 12)
- Oral solution (PediaCare Children's Decongestant)

Pseudoephedrine

Pseudoephedrine is manufactured as:

- single-dose tablets (Sudafed)
- extended-release tablets (Dimetapp Maximum Strength Decongestant for Adults, Sudafed 12-Hour, Sudafed 24-Hour)

- oral solution (ElixSure Cold, Sudafed Children's Nasal Decongestant)
- suspension (Entex, Nasofed)
- syrup

This powerful vasoconstrictive decongests nasal passages as well as the eustachian tubes that run between the ear and mouth. It is available by prescription and in a large number of medications sold over the counter. Patients should be made aware, however, that taking alkalinizing drugs can increase pseudoephedrine's effects by reducing its excretion in urine.

Federal law restricts over-the-counter sales of cold medicines that contain pseudoephedrine. The law was enacted to curb the use of these medicines in making methamphetamine, a powerful, highly addictive stimulant that is produced in secret, illegal labs. Although these medicines are available without a prescription, products that contain pseudoephedrine must now be kept behind the counter. Customers must produce photo identification to purchase these products, and the amount they can buy is limited. Pharmacies are required to record and keep information about purchasers for two years.

Topical Decongestants

Topical decongestants are also powerful vasoconstrictors. When applied directly to the swollen mucous membranes of the nose, they provide immediate relief from nasal congestion.

Like systemic decongestants, these drugs stimulate alpha-adrenergic receptors in the smooth muscle of nasal blood vessels. The result is vasoconstriction, which limits blood flow to the mucous membranes and thereby reduces swelling. This action improves breathing by helping to drain sinuses, clear nasal passages, and open eustachian tubes. Because these effects are local, absorption of the drug is limited, and few adverse reactions and drug interactions result.

Topical decongestant drugs include:

- sympathomimetic amines
- derivatives of sympathomimetic amines
- propylhexedrine

Sympathomimetic Amines

Sympathomimetic drugs are drugs that imitate the activities or actions of the central nervous system. Amines are compounds that are created from the chemical element ammonia.

Epinephrine

Epinephrine is produced as an aerosol inhaler (Primatene Mist), solutions for injection (Adrenalin) and nebulizer (Micronefrin, Nephron, S2) use, and self-contained devices for intramuscular or subcutaneous injections (EpiPen,

EpiPen Jr, Twinject). The nebulizer solution and aerosol inhaler are bronchodilators used in acute asthma attacks. Epinephrine injections are also used to treat bronchospasm and anaphylaxis—a severe and sometimes life-threatening allergic reaction to some foreign antigen, such as peanuts or bee venom. Only the nasal solution form (Adrenalin) of epinephrine serves as a topical decongestant.

Phenylephrine

You read about the systemic forms of phenylephrine above. As a topical decongestant, phenylephrine (4-Way, Neo-Synephrine, Nostril, Rhinall, Sinex, Little Noses Decongestant, Afrin Children's, Neo-Synephrine, Vicks) is available as nasal spray and nasal drops. A stronger solution of this drug is used in eye drops to dilate pupils during eye exams or as a topical anesthetic to treat itching or burning in the eyes.

Derivatives of Sympathomimetic Amines

Derivatives of sympathomimetic amines include:

- naphazoline
- oxymetazoline
- tetrahydrozoline

Naphazoline

Naphazoline is manufactured as a nasal solution (Privine) and as an ophthalmic solution both prescription (AK-Con, Albalon) and over-the-counter (All ClearAR, All Clear, Naphcon, Clear Eyes) that is used as an ocular decongestant and to treat eye irritation and itching. The nasal solution is dispensed as drops that the user places into her nose, with her head back, using the dropper that comes with the bottle.

Oxymetazoline

Oxymetazoline (Afrin, Duramist Plus, Four-Way, Mucinex Full Force, Mucinex Moisture Smart, Nasal 12 Hour, Nasal LA, Neo-Synephrine 12-Hour, Sinex Long-Acting, Visine Long Lasting, Zicam Congestion Relief, Zicam Sinus Relief) is a nasal solution that is produced as a conventional nasal spray and as a 12-hour formulation. Both are available in OTC formulations. Another type of solution is dispensed as eye drops (Tyzine) and serves as an ocular decongestant to treat redness caused by minor eye irritation. The drops work by constricting blood vessels in the eye that are swollen by irritation. This reduces redness in the whites of the eyes. This medicine is also available in an prescription form.

Tetrahydrozoline

Tetrahydrozoline is a nasal decongestant available by prescription as a nasal solution (Tyzine). It is also available OTC as an opthalmic solution (Murine Tears Plus, Visine).

QUICK QUIZ

Answer the following multiple-choice questions.

1. Which type of respiratory drug has the largest number of potential drug interactions?
   a. leukotriene modifiers
   b. inhaled corticosteroids
   c. inhaled beta$_2$-adrenergic agonists
   d. mucolytics
2. Which of the following drugs would be *most likely* to be taken during an acute asthma attack?
   a. ipratropium bromide
   b. albuterol
   c. montelukast
   d. cromolyn sodium
3. Which of the following is *not* a special population that requires extra attention when taking corticosteroids?
   a. older adults
   b. children
   c. people with diabetes
   d. people with asthma
4. What type of drug is *most likely* to assist the action of an expectorant?
   a. a corticosteroid
   b. a mucolytic
   c. a nasal spray
   d. an antitussive
5. Which of the following is likely to be found in an OTC medication?
   a. codeine
   b. hydrocodone
   c. oxymetazoline
   d. none of the above

Please answer each of the following questions in one to three sentences.

1. How do short-acting beta$_2$-adrenergic agonists differ in use from long-acting beta$_2$-adrenergic agonists?

_____

_____

2. How do leukotriene modifiers and mast cell stabilizers differ in their mechanism of action?

_____

_____

3. What lifestyle behaviors can affect treatment outcomes for patients taking theophylline?

_____

_____

4. Why might using an antitussive be contraindicated when a patient is already taking an expectorant?

_____

_____

5. Why are sprays and other topical forms of respiratory drugs generally safer to take than systemic forms of such drugs?

_____

_____

Answer the following questions as either true or false.

1. ___ Mast cell stabilizers are often prescribed as rescue inhalers.

2. ___ Corticosteroids are the most effective drugs for long-term treatment and prevention of asthma attacks.

3. ___ Decongestants should be used with care by persons with high blood pressure because the drugs work by constricting blood vessels to limit blood supply to swollen tissues.

4. ___ Some drugs used as nasal decongestants also have therapeutic uses as eye drops.

5. ___ Corticosteroids are popular drugs for treating respiratory disorders because they are relatively safe for long-term use.

Match each generic drug in the left column with its classification in the right column.

1. albuterol   a. antitussive
2. dextromethorphan   b. beta$_2$-adrenergic agonist
3. epinephrine   c. corticosteroid
4. guaifenesin   d. decongestant
5. prednisone   e. expectorant

DRUG CLASSIFICATION TABLE

Classification	Generic Name	Trade Names(s)
Beta$_2$-adrenergic agonists	albuterol *al-byoo'-ter-ole*	*tablets:* (no longer marketed under trade name) *extended-release tablets:* Vospire ER *aerosol inhalant:* Proair HFA, Proventil HFA, Ventolin HFA *solution for inhalation:* Accuneb *syrup:* (no longer marketed under trade name)
	levalbuterol *lev-al-byoo'-ter-ole*	*aerosol inhalant:* Xopenex HFA *solution for inhalation:* Xopenex
	metaproterenol *met-a-proe-ter'-e-nole*	*aerosol inhalation:* Alupent *solution for inhalation:* (no longer marketed under trade name) *oral solution:* (no longer marketed under trade name) *tablets:* (no longer marketed under trade name)
	pirbuterol *peer-byoo'-ter-ole*	*aerosol inhalant:* Maxair
	terbutaline *ter-byoo'-ta-leen*	*tablets:* (no longer marketed under trade name) *injection:* (no longer marketed under trade name)
	formoterol *for-moh'-te-rol*	*powder for inhalation:* Foradil *solution for inhalation:* Perforomist
	aformoterol *eh-for-moh'-te-rol*	*solution for inhalation:* Brovana
	salmeterol *sal-mee'-ter-ol*	*powder for inhalation:* Serevent
Anticholinergics	ipratropium *ih-prah-trow'-pea-um*	*aerosol inhalant:* Atrovent HFA *nasal spray:* Atrovent *solution for inhalation:* (no longer marketed under trade name)
Corticosteroids	beclomethasone dipropionate *be-kloe-meth'-a-sone*	*aerosol inhalant:* QVAR *nasal spray:* Beconase AQ

continued

DRUG CLASSIFICATION TABLE (continued)

Classification	Generic Name	Trade Names(s)
Corticosteroids (continued)	budesonide *bue-des'-oh-nide*	*sustained-release capsules:* Entocort EC *nasal spray:* Rhinocort Aqua *powder inhalant:* Pulmicort Flexhaler *suspension for inhalation:* Pulmicort Respules *powder for inhalation:* Symbicort
	flunisolide *floo-niss'-oh-lide*	*aerosol inhalant:* AeroBid, AeroBid-M *nasal spray:* Nasarel
	fluticasone *flew-tick'-ah-sone*	*aerosol inhalant:* Flovent HFA *nasal spray:* Flonase, Veramyst *powder inhalant:* Flovent Diskus *topical cream:* cutivate
	triamcinolone *trye-am-sin'-oh-lone*	*injection:* various trade names including Aristospan and Kenalog *aerosol inhalant:* Azmacort *nasal spray:* Nasacort AQ
	prednisolone *pred-niss'-oh-lone*	*tablets:* Prednoral *orally disintegrating tablets:* Orapred ODT *oral solution:* Orapred, Pediapred, Millipred *syrup:* Prelone
	prednisone *pred'-ni-sone*	*tablets:* (no longer marketed under trade name) *tablets:* (unit-dose blister pack) Sterapred DS *oral solution:* (no longer marketed under trade name)
	hydrocortisone *hye-droe-kor'-ti-zone*	*powder for injection:* A-Hydrocort, Solu-Cortef *tablets:* Cortef, Hydrocortone
	methylprednisolone *meth-il-pred-niss'-oh-lone*	*injection:* variety of trade names including Depo-Medrol, A-Methapred and Solu-Medrol *tablets:* Medrol
Combination Respiratory Products	budesonide and formoterol *bue-des'-oh-nide for-moh'-te-rol*	*aerosol inhalant:* Symbicort
	fluticasone and salmeterol *flew-tick'-ah-sone sal-mee'-ter-ol*	*powder for inhalation:* Advair Diskus *inhalation aerosol:* Advair HFA
	ipratropium and albuterol *ih-prah-trow'-pea-um al-byoo'-ter-ole*	*solution for inhalation:* DuoNeb *inhalation aerosol:* Combivent
Leukotriene modifiers	montelukast *mon-tell-oo'-kast*	*tablets:* Singulair *chewable tablets:* Singulair *oral granules:* Singulair
	zafirlukast *zah-fir'-luh-kast*	*tablets:* Accolate
	zileuton *zye-loot'-on*	*extended-release tablets:* Zyflo CR
Mast cell stabilizers	cromolyn sodium *kroe'-moe-lin*	*aerosol inhalant (Rx):* Intal *nebulizer solution (Rx):* Intal *aerosol nasal spray (OTC):* Nasalcrom *concentrated oral solution (Rx):* Gastrocrom
	nedocromil *nee-doc'-ro-mill*	*inhalation aerosol:* Tilade

continued

DRUG CLASSIFICATION TABLE (continued)

Classification	Generic Name	Trade Names(s)
Methylxanthines	theophylline *thee-off'-i-lin*	*extended-release tablets:* Theochron, Uniphyl *extended-release capsules:* Theo-24 *elixir:* Elixophylline *injection:* (no longer marketed under trade name)
	aminophylline *am-in-off'-i-lin*	*tablets:* (no longer marketed under trade name) *injection:* (no longer marketed under trade name)
Mucolytics	acetylcysteine *a-se-teel-sis'-tay-een*	*solution for inhalation:* (no longer marketed under trade name) *injection:* Acetadote
Expectorants	guaifenesin *gwye-fen'-e-sin*	*tablets (Rx):* variety of trade names including Liquibid, Organidin NR, XPECT
		extended-release tablets (OTC): Humibid, Mucinex *liquid/oral solution (OTC):* variety of trade names including Diabetic Tussin EX, Mucinex Children's, Naldecon Senior EX, Scot-Tussin Expectorant, *liquid/oral solution (Rx):* Organidin NR *syrup (OTC):* variety of trade names including Q-Tussin and Robitussin *dissolving granules (OTC):* Mucinex Mini-Melts
Antitussives	dextromethorphan *dex-troe-meth-or'-fan*	*capsules:* Robitussin CoughGels *lozenges:* Hold DM, Sucrets Cough Control Formula *oral liquid:* variety of trade names including Robitussin Maximum Strength Cough, Simply Cough, Vicks 44 Cough Relief *syrup:* variety of trade names including Robitussin Pediatric Cough, Triaminic Long Acting Cough *extended-release syrup:* Delsym *orally dissolving strips:* Triaminic Thin Strips Long Acting Cough
	codeine *koe'-deen*	*tablet:* (no longer marketed under trade name)
	codeine and guaifenesin *koe'-deen gwye-fen'-e-sin*	*syrup:* Cheracol with Codeine, Mytussin AC *tablets:* Brontex *liquid:* Tussi-Organidin NR, Dex-Tuss, Tussiden C *oral solution:* Gani-Tuss NR, GuaiCo, Iophen C NR, Robafen C NR, Romilar AC
	hydrocodone and guaifenesin *hye-droe-koe'-done gwye-fen'-e-sin*	*caplets:* Ztuss ZT *extended-release caplets:* Tusso-HC *extended-release capsules:* Atuss HX *liquid:* FluTuss XP, Kwelcof, Maxi-Tuss HCG, Relasin-HCX, Z-Cof HCX *tablets:* EndaCof-Tab, Pneumotussin, Touro HC *extended-release tablets:* Extendryl HC, XPECT-HC *solution:* Canges-XP *syrup:* variety of trade names including Codiclear DH, Vi-Q-Tuss, Vitussin Expectorant

continued

DRUG CLASSIFICATION TABLE *(continued)*

Classification	Generic Name	Trade Names(s)
Antitussives *(continued)*	hydrocodone bitartrate and potassium guaiacolsulfonate *hye-droe-koe'-done*	*syrup:* variety of trade names including Pro-Clear *oral liquid:* variety of trade names including Marcof Expectorant, Prolex DH
	benzonatate *ben-zoe'-naa-tate*	*capsules:* Tessalon Perles
Decongestants	ephedrine *e-fed'-rin*	*injection:* (no longer marketed under trade name) *capsules:* (no longer marketed under trade name)
	phenylephrine *fen-ill-ef'-rin*	*orally dissolving tablets:* Nasop *orally dissolving film:* Sudafed PE Quick Dissolve, Triaminic Thin Strips *oral tablets:* Sudafed PE *oral suspension:* Nasop *chewable tablets:* Nasop 12 *oral solution:* PediaCare Children's Decongestant *nasal spray:* 4-Way, Synephrine, Nostril, Rhinall, Sinex *nasal drops:* Little Noses Decongestant, Neo-Synephrine *nasal solution:* Rhinall, Little Noses, Afrin Children's, Neo-Synephreine, Vicks, 4-Way
	pseudoephedrine *soo-dow-e-fed'-rin*	*tablets:* variety of trade names including Sudafed *extended-release tablets:* Dimetapp Maximum Strength Decongestant for Adults, Sudafed 12-Hour, Sudafed 24-Hour *oral solution:* ElixSure Cold, Sudafed Children's Nasal Decongestant *oral syrup:* (no longer marketed under trade name) *oral suspension:* Entex, Nasofed
	epinephrine *ep-i-nef'-rin*	*nasal solution (Rx):* Adrenalin *aerosol inhalant (OTC):* Primatene Mist *solution for inhalation (OTC):* Micronefrin, Nephron, S2 *injection (Rx):* Adrenalin, EpiPen, EpiPen Jr, Twinject *topical solution (Rx):* Adrenalin
	naphazoline *na-faz'-o-line*	*nasal solution (OTC):* Privine *ophthalmic solution (OTC):* variety of trade names including All Clear AR, All Clear, Naphcon, Clear Eyes *ophthalmic solution (Rx):* AK-Con, Albalon

continued

DRUG CLASSIFICATION TABLE (continued)

Classification	Generic Name	Trade Names(s)
Decongestants (continued)	oxymetazoline oxy-met-az'-oh-leen	nasal solution (OTC): variety of trade names including Afrin, Duramist Plus, Four-Way, Mucinex Full Force, Mucinex Moisture Smart, Nasal 12 Hour, Nasal LA, Neo-Synephrine 12-Hour, Sinex Long-Acting, Visine Long Lasting, Zicam Congestion Relief, Zicam Sinus Relief ophthalmic solution (OTC): Visine Long Lasting opthalmic solution (Rx): Tyzine
	tetrahydrozoline tet-rah-hi-draz'-oh-leen	nasal solution (Rx): Tyzine ophthalmic solution (OTC): Murine Tears Plus, Visine

CHAPTER 8

Gastrointestinal Drugs

CHAPTER OBJECTIVES

- Match brand and generic names of commonly used gastrointestinal drugs
- Identify the classification of commonly used gastrointestinal drugs
- Identify the uses of commonly used gastrointestinal drugs
- Organize commonly used gastrointestinal drugs into the correct category of scheduled (II-V), prescription, or over-the-counter drugs
- List drugs used to treat *Helicobacter pylori* and construct a successful treatment plan
- Compare and contrast the uses of antacids, H$_2$ receptor antagonists, proton pump inhibitors, and other antiulcer drugs
- Compare and contrast the different types of laxatives based on the mechanism of action and how long they take to work
- Compare and contrast the uses and mechanisms of action of activated charcoal and ipecac syrup in treating poisoning
- List the national poison control number

KEY TERMS

adsorbents—drugs that are used as antidotes for ingested toxins

antacids—drugs that neutralize or reduce the acidity of stomach and duodenal contents

antidiarrheals—drugs that act systemically or locally to control diarrhea

antiemetics—drugs that are used to treat or prevent nausea

antiflatulents—drugs that work against flatus (gas)

bulk-forming laxatives—drugs that contain natural and synthetic substances that act similarly to dietary fiber

dietary fiber—the part of plants not digested in the small intestine

digestive drugs—drugs that help digestion in patients who are missing enzymes or other substances needed to digest food

emetics—drugs that induce vomiting

emollients—drugs that soften stool and make bowel movements easier; also known as *stool softeners*

H$_2$ receptor antagonists—commonly prescribed antiulcer drugs that reduce acid secretion

Helicobacter pylori—bacteria that cause a type of chronic gastritis and peptic and duodenal ulcers; often abbreviated to *H. pylori*

hyperosmolar laxatives—drugs that stimulate bowel movements by drawing water into the intestine

ipecac syrup— emetic; substance used to induce vomiting

irritant cathartics—see *stimulant laxatives*

laxatives—drugs used to stimulate bowel movements and relieve constipation

lubricant laxatives—substances that smooth the lining of the gastrointestinal tract and moisten the stool

peptic ulcer—an open sore in the mucous membrane lining of the lower esophagus, stomach, duodenum, or jejunum

peptic ulcer drugs—drugs used to treat sores in the lining of the esophagus, stomach, or small intestine

proton pump inhibitors (PPIs)—drugs with antisecretory properties

stimulant laxatives—drugs that promote peristalsis by irritating the lining of the gastrointestinal tract; also known as *irritant cathartics*

stool softeners—see *emollients*

systemic antibiotics—drugs that affect the entire body as they work to kill or inhibit the growth of bacteria

The gastrointestinal (GI) tract is basically a hollow, muscular tube that begins at the mouth and ends at the anus (figure 8-1). It includes several different structures:

- pharynx (throat)
- esophagus
- stomach
- small intestine, which has three parts called the duodenum, the jejunum, and the ileum
- large intestine or colon

The main functions of the GI tract are to digest food, absorb nutrients, and excrete waste. Food passes through the esophagus to the stomach. The stomach produces gastric acid, which mixes with food in the process of digestion.

As the food travels through the three parts of the small intestine, nutrients from the food are absorbed. Digestive enzymes break the food into key elements for the body. The colon stores waste products of digestion before they are excreted.

In this chapter, you'll learn about digestive system drugs that are used to treat conditions such as:

- **peptic ulcers**—an open sore in the mucous membrane lining of the lower esophagus, stomach, duodenum, or jejunum.
- heartburn and indigestion
- spastic or irritable colon
- diarrhea and constipation
- nausea and vomiting

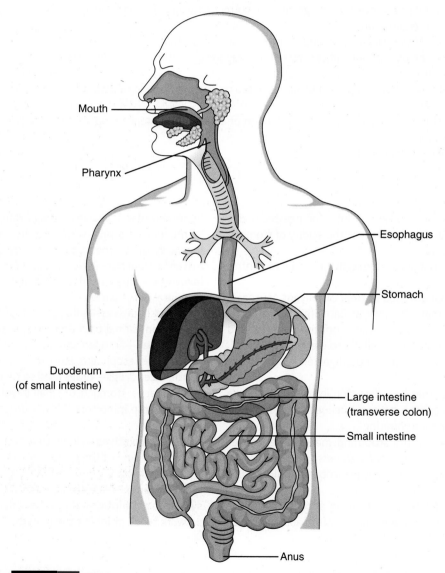

Mouth

Pharynx

Esophagus

Stomach

Duodenum
(of small intestine)

Large intestine
(transverse colon)

Small intestine

Anus

FIGURE 8-1 The GI tract is a continuous passageway beginning at the mouth, where food is taken in, and ending at the anus, where the solid waste products of digestion are expelled from the body. (From *Memmler's Structure and Function of the Human Body*. 9th Ed. Baltimore, MD: Lippincott Williams & Wilkins; 2009.)

ANTIULCER DRUGS

There are five major causes of peptic ulcers:

- bacterial infection with *Helicobacter pylori (H. pylori)* —a bacterium that's believed to cause peptic ulcers and gastritis (inflammation of the stomach lining)
- the use of nonsteroidal anti-inflammatory drugs (NSAIDs)
- hypersecretory states such as Zollinger-Ellison syndrome (a condition in which excessive secretion of gastric acid leads to peptic ulcers)
- cigarette smoking, which can cause hypersecretion of digestive enzymes and impair healing of ulcers
- a genetic predisposition, which accounts for 20 to 50 percent of peptic ulcers

Peptic ulcer drugs act in different ways. Some drugs work to get rid of *H. pylori*. Others act to restore the balance between acid and pepsin secretions and the GI mucosal defense. These drugs include:

- **systemic antibiotics**—drugs that affect the entire body as they work to kill or inhibit the growth of bacteria
- histamine-2 (H_2) receptor antagonists
- proton pump inhibitors (PPIs)—drugs with antisecretory properties
- antacids—drugs that neutralize or reduce the acidity of stomach and duodenal contents
- other peptic ulcer drugs, such as misoprostol and sucralfate

Systemic Antibiotics

Eliminating *H. pylori* helps heal ulcers and decrease their recurrence. Treatment of peptic ulcers usually involves the use of two or more antibiotics in combination with other drugs such as acid suppressants (drugs that reduce stomach acid). Systemic antibiotics act by treating the *H. pylori* infection. This reduces the risk of a duodenal ulcer. The antibiotics are used in conjunction with an H_2 receptor antagonist or a proton pump inhibitor because these drugs decrease stomach acid and further promote healing. Antibiotics commonly used in combinations for ulcer treatment are:

- amoxicillin
- clarithromycin
- metronidazole
- tetracycline

Because combination therapies may involve three or more different drugs, there are many potential drug interactions. These interactions vary depending on which drugs are included in the combination. Some interactions for combinations to treat *H. pylori* are as follows:

- Combination therapies for *H. pylori* may increase the risk of heart arrhythmias if taken with HIV protease oral solutions, such as amprenavir.

- Using combination therapies for *H. pylori* with certain other drugs may increase the risk of adverse effects for the other drugs. These drugs include anticoagulants, digoxin, ergot alkaloids, and ranolazine.

Triple Therapy

In triple therapy, two antibiotics are combined with a proton pump inhibitor. Triple therapy is effective for 80 to 90 percent of patients.

One common triple therapy includes the following combination of drugs:

- amoxicillin
- clarithromycin
- lansoprazole

This combination (Prevpac Daily Administration Pack) is used to treat patients with *H. pylori* infection and duodenal ulcer disease.

Each drug has a different effect that acts to promote ulcer healing.

- Amoxicillin stops the growth of *H. pylori* by blocking the building of new bacterial cells.
- Clarithromycin stops the growth of *H. pylori* by stopping the bacteria from making proteins.
- Lansoprazole reduces gastric acid secretion.

Quadruple Therapy

In quadruple therapy, two antibiotics are combined with bismuth subsalicylate and a proton pump inhibitor or an H_2 receptor antagonist. Quadruple therapy is effective for more than 90 percent of patients.

A common combination of drugs for quadruple therapy is:

- metronidazole
- tetracycline
- bismuth
- H_2 receptor antagonist

The combination of metronidazole, tetracycline, and bismuth subcitrate potassium is available by prescription in

PROCEED WITH CAUTION

Adverse Reactions to Antibiotics

Adverse reactions to combination therapies containing systemic antibiotics to treat *H. pylori* depend on which drugs are used in the treatment combination.

- Metronidazole, clarithromycin, and tetracycline commonly cause GI disturbances.
- Clarithromycin and metronidazole may produce abnormal tastes.
- Amoxicillin may cause diarrhea.

capsule form (Pylera). The combination of metronidazole, tetracycline, and bismuth subsalicylate is also available by prescription. In this combination, tablets and capsules for each drug are packaged together (Helidac Therapy Kit). However, individual tablets or capsules for each drug can also be purchased separately. To treat duodenal ulcers, one of these three-drug combinations is taken with a prescribed H_2 receptor antagonist, such as ranitidine.

Each drug has a different effect that acts to promote ulcer healing.

- Metronidazole kills *H. pylori* by blocking the transport of proteins.
- Tetracycline halts the growth of *H. pylori* by stopping the bacteria from making proteins.
- Bismuth protects the stomach lining.
- The H_2 receptor antagonist blocks the action of histamine, reducing gastric acid.

In addition to the drug interactions already noted, the following drug interactions may occur with tetracycline and metronidazole:

- Tetracycline increases digoxin levels and, when combined with methoxyflurane, increases the risk of kidney toxicity.
- Metronidazole and tetracycline increase the risk of bleeding when taken with oral anticoagulants.
- Metronidazole can cause a severe reaction when combined with alcohol.

H_2 Receptor Antagonists

H2 receptor antagonists prevent a body substance called histamine from producing acid in the stomach. They are used therapeutically to:

- promote healing of duodenal and gastric ulcers
- provide long-term treatment of pathological GI hypersecretory conditions such as Zollinger-Ellison syndrome
- reduce gastric acid production and prevent stress ulcers in severely ill patients and in patients with upper GI bleeding or reflux esophagitis (an inflammation of the esophagus caused by acid from the stomach)

H_2 receptor antagonists work by blocking the action of histamine in the stomach. Histamine controls the production of stomach acid and is involved in immune system responses in allergic reactions. When the action of histamine is blocked, less gastric acid is produced. This decrease in gastric acid allows peptic ulcers to heal.

Food and **antacids**, or drugs that neutralize or reduce the acidity of stomach and duodenal contents, may reduce the absorption of H_2 receptor antagonists.

T I P It's important to note that H_2 receptor antagonists affect the histamine-2 receptor only. These drugs are not used to treat allergic reactions.

PROCEED WITH CAUTION

Adverse Reactions to H_2 Receptor Antagonists

The use of H_2 receptor antagonists may lead to adverse reactions, especially in older adult patients and patients with altered liver or kidney function.

Adverse reactions to cimetidine and ranitidine may include:

- dizziness
- headache
- malaise (discomfort, uneasiness)
- muscle pain
- nausea
- diarrhea or constipation
- rash
- itching
- loss of sexual desire
- impotence

Famotidine and nizatidine, on the other hand, produce few adverse reactions:

- headache
- constipation or diarrhea
- rash

Cimetidine

Cimetidine is sold OTC (Tagamet HB) in tablet and oral solution form to relieve heartburn. It is also available by prescription in vials or premixed containers for injection and in oral solution.

Cimetidine by prescription is used to treat several conditions:

- uncomplicated gastric ulcers
- active duodenal ulcers
- gastroesophageal reflux disease (GERD), a condition in which the contents of the stomach and duodenum flow back into the esophagus
- hypersecretory conditions such as Zollinger-Ellison syndrome

For ulcer treatment, the oral form of the drug is typically given four times a day with meals and at bedtime or as a single dose at bedtime. The parenteral form is administered by IM or IV injection and through continuous IV infusion. For heartburn relief, one oral dose is taken as needed, up to twice a day.

Cimetidine causes more drug interactions than other H_2 receptor antagonists, including the following:

- Cimetidine may increase the blood levels of anticoagulants, propranolol (and possibly other beta-adrenergic blockers), benzodiazepines, tricyclic antidepressants, theophylline, procainamide, quinidine, lidocaine, phenytoin, calcium channel blockers, cyclosporine, carbamazepine, and opioid analgesics. Cimetidine inhibits the metabolism of these drugs in the liver, which reduces their subsequent excretion from the body.

■ When taken with carmustine, cimetidine increases the risk of bone marrow toxicity.

■ Cimetidine inhibits metabolism of ethyl alcohol in the stomach, resulting in higher blood alcohol levels.

In addition to the adverse reactions associated with other H_2 receptor antagonists, cimetidine may also cause gynecomastia (breast enlargement in male patients).

Famotidine

Famotidine is available by prescription to treat:

- benign gastric ulcers
- duodenal ulcers
- GERD
- pathological hypersecretory conditions

Forms of famotidine available by prescription (Pepcid) include tablets, powder for oral suspension, single and multidose vials for injection, and premixed injections in single-dose containers. Famotidine is also sold OTC (Pepcid AC) for heartburn relief as tablets, and chewable tablets.

For ulcer treatment, it is taken once a day at bedtime. Doses may be more frequent for GERD or hypersecretory conditions. Parenteral forms are administered intravenously. For heartburn relief, patients may take it once or twice a day.

Famotidine is also available OTC in combination with calcium carbonate and magnesium hydroxide, which are both antacids, in chewable tablets (Pepcid Complete).

T I P Patients shouldn't take the maximum daily dose of OTC famotidine for more than two weeks at a time unless directed to do so by their health care provider.

Nizatidine

Nizatidine is available by prescription to treat:

- benign gastric ulcers
- duodenal ulcers
- GERD

In prescription form, nizatidine is manufactured as capsules or as oral solution (Axid). Nizatidine therapy for treating ulcers is typically dosed twice a day or once a day at bedtime.

Nizatidine is also sold over the counter in a lower-strength oral tablet (Axid AR) for the treatment of heartburn. The OTC drug may be taken up to twice per day.

Ranitidine

Ranitidine is prescribed to treat:

- benign gastric ulcers
- duodenal ulcers

- erosive esophagitis
- GERD
- pathological hypersecretory conditions

Prescription forms of ranitidine include oral tablets, capsules, and oral solution under the trade name Zantac, and effervescent tablets (Zantac Efferdose). Oral dosage forms are typically given twice a day. It is also available in vials or premixed containers for IM injection or IV infusion. Injectable forms of the drug are used to treat pathological hypersecretory conditions or duodenal ulcers that are difficult to manage. Ranitidine is also sold OTC in lower strengths tablets (Zantac) to treat heartburn, acid indigestion, and sour stomach. OTC ranitidine may be taken up to twice a day.

Proton Pump Inhibitors

Proton pump inhibitors (PPIs) are used therapeutically in a variety of situations:

- short-term treatment of active gastric ulcers
- active duodenal ulcers
- erosive esophagitis
- symptomatic GERD that doesn't respond to other therapies
- active peptic ulcers associated with *H. pylori* infection, in combination with antibiotics
- long-term treatment of hypersecretory conditions such as Zollinger-Ellison syndrome

Proton pump inhibitors act to disrupt chemical binding in stomach cells, reducing acid production. The reduced acid production lessens irritation and allows peptic ulcers to heal. Proton pump inhibitors work by blocking

HOW IT WORKS

How H_2 Receptor Antagonists and Proton Pump Inhibitors Work

Acid secretion in the stomach depends on the binding of gastrin, acetylcholine, and histamine to receptors on the parietal cells within the stomach lining. If the binding of one of these substances is blocked, acid secretion is reduced.

H_2 receptor antagonists work by binding with H_2 receptors. This blocks the action of histamine in the stomach, reducing the secretion of gastric acid. The total amount of pepsin is also reduced.

Proton pump inhibitors don't act on the H_2 receptors. Instead, they combine with hydrogen, potassium, and adenosine triphosphate in the parietal cells of the stomach. An enzyme system in the parietal cells is the "acid pump" of the gastric mucosa. By blocking this system, proton pump inhibitors block the final step in acid production. This reduces the secretion of gastric acid.

the last step in the secretion of gastric acid. They combine with hydrogen, potassium, and adenosine triphosphate in the parietal cells of the stomach.

Because proton pump inhibitors are highly unstable in acid, they are administered orally in enteric-coated formulas. These formulas allow the drug to bypass the stomach. In the small intestine, they dissolve and are absorbed rapidly.

Proton pump inhibitors can interfere with the absorption of several other drugs.

- Proton pump inhibitors may increase plasma levels and absorption time of diazepam, phenytoin, and warfarin.
- Proton pump inhibitors may also interfere with absorption of drugs that depend on gastric pH for absorption. These include ketoconazole, digoxin, ampicillin, and iron salts.

Esomeprazole

Esomeprazole (Nexium) is available by prescription only. It is used in the treatment of:

- erosive esophagitis
- duodenal ulcers (as part of triple therapy)
- pathological hypersecretory conditions
- GERD

In addition, esomeprazole may be prescribed for patients undergoing continuous NSAID therapy to reduce the risk of gastric ulcers.

This drug is manufactured as delayed-release oral capsules and powder for oral suspension. It's also available in the form of a powder that must be reconstituted before being administered by IV injection or IV infusion.

Lansoprazole

Like esomeprazole, lansoprazole is available in prescription form only. This drug is used for:

- short-term treatment of duodenal or gastric ulcers
- reducing the risk of duodenal ulcers (in dual or triple therapy)
- maintaining healed duodenal or gastric ulcers
- short-term treatment of gastric ulcers
- healing gastric ulcers related to NSAID use
- reducing the risk of gastric ulcers due to NSAID use

PROCEED WITH CAUTION

Adverse Reactions to Proton Pump Inhibitors

Adverse reactions to proton pump inhibitors include:

- abdominal pain
- diarrhea
- nausea and vomiting

- short-term treatment of GERD or erosive esophagitis
- maintaining healing for erosive esophagitis
- treating pathological hypersecretory conditions

T I P After ulcers are healed, the patient may receive a reduced dose of ulcer medication for a long period of time to prevent new ulcers from forming.

Lansoprazole is manufactured as orally disintegrating delayed-release tablets (Prevacid Solutab), delayed-release capsules (Prevacid), granules for oral suspension (Prevacid), and powder to be reconstituted for injection (Prevacid IV). Injectable forms are used in short-term treatment of erosive esophagitis when patients are not able to take oral forms.

This drug is also available in combination with naproxen (Prevacid NapraPAC) for the treatment of gastric ulcers related to NSAID use. Prevacid NapraPAC is manufactured in a therapy kit that contains naproxen tablets and lansoprazole delayed-release capsules.

Omeprazole

Omeprazole is manufactured as a prescription drug and in OTC form. Prescription-strength omeprazole is used for:

- short-term treatment of duodenal and gastric ulcers
- treatment of duodenal ulcers associated with *H. pylori* (in triple therapy)
- short-term treatment of erosive esophagitis
- treatment of symptoms associated with GERD

Omeprazole is chemically very closely related to esomeprazole. By prescription, omeprazole is available in the form of delayed-release capsules (Prilosec). Omeprazole is sold OTC to relieve frequent heartburn (more often than two days per week). The OTC form of the drug comes as delayed-release tablets (Prilosec OTC).

Omeprazole is also manufactured in combination forms, capsules and powder for oral suspension, with sodium bicarbonate (Zegerid). In addition to the other uses for omeprazole, it is also used as stress ulcer prophylactic therapy in critically ill patients.

T I P Prilosec OTC should be used for no longer than 14 days at a time. However, this OTC drug can be purchased in boxes of 42, which is a three-month supply. Because the prescription and OTC strengths are the same (20 mg), a patient could substitute Prilosec OTC for a prescription form of the drug and take the OTC form continually without being monitored by a physician. If you think this might be occurring, be sure to alert the pharmacist.

Pantoprazole

Pantoprazole (Protonix) is available as a prescription drug only. This medication is used in several situations:

- to maintain healing of erosive esophagitis
- to reduce heartburn symptoms in patients with GERD

- long-term treatment of pathological hypersecretory conditions
- short-term treatment (eight weeks or less) of erosive esophagitis related to GERD

Pantoprazole is manufactured as delayed-release tablets, granules for oral suspension and as powder to be reconstituted for injection. This drug may be administered orally or by IV infusion. Other parenteral routes of administration shouldn't be used.

Rabeprazole

Rabeprazole (Aciphex) is available by prescription only. It's used therapeutically in the following situations:

- for short-term healing of erosive or ulcerative GERD
- to maintain healing of erosive or ulcerative GERD
- to treat heartburn and other symptoms of GERD
- for short-term treatment (4 weeks or less) in the healing of duodenal ulcers
- for long-term treatment of pathological hypersecretory conditions, including Zollinger-Ellison syndrome

Rabeprazole is manufactured in the form of delayed-release oral tablets.

Antacids

Antacids are OTC medications used as adjunct therapy in treating peptic ulcers. They are mainly prescribed to relieve pain and to relieve symptoms of GI disorders, including:

- acid indigestion
- heartburn
- dyspepsia (burning or indigestion)
- GERD

Antacids work locally in the stomach by neutralizing gastric acid. They don't need to be absorbed by the body to treat peptic ulcers. The acid-neutralizing action reduces the total amount of acid in the GI tract. This reduction in acid gives peptic ulcers time to heal.

Although some people think antacids work by coating the lining of the stomach, this isn't true. Antacids affect one of the stomach secretions called pepsin. Pepsin acts more effectively when the stomach is highly acidic. As antacids lower the acidity in the stomach, the action of pepsin is also reduced.

Along with reducing acid and slowing the action of pepsin, antacids also increase the muscle tone of the esophageal sphincter (the opening between the esophagus and the stomach). This helps in treating GERD.

All antacids can interfere with the absorption of certain oral drugs given at the same time. Absorption of the following drugs may be reduced if taken within two hours of antacids:

- digoxin
- phenytoin

PROCEED WITH CAUTION

Adverse Reactions to Antacids

All adverse reactions to antacids are dose related. They vary for different antacids. Common adverse reactions to antacids include:

- diarrhea (typically caused by magnesium salts)
- constipation (typically caused by aluminum salts)

- ketoconazole
- iron salts
- isoniazid
- quinolones
- tetracyclines

Antacids may also affect the absorption of enteric-coated drugs. Antacid doses should be separated from doses of enteric-coated drugs and from doses of the drugs in the list above by at least an hour.

Aluminum Salts

Aluminum hydroxide (Alternagel) is used in treating peptic ulcers and stomach acidity. This drug releases aluminum ions in the GI tract. These ions stop smooth muscle contractions and reduce gastric emptying. They also bind with phosphate ions, reducing phosphate levels.

Aluminum hydroxide is administered orally in the form of a suspension. One dose of the oral suspension may be taken as needed between meals and at bedtime.

AT THE COUNTER

Aluminum and Magnesium as Comrades

A customer comes to the counter with your store brand of a popular antacid that contains aluminum hydroxide, magnesium hydroxide, and simethicone. The customer asks you why there are three ingredients in the product. What should you tell him?

Aluminum hydroxide and magnesium hydroxide are both antacids. Some antacid products contain only one ingredient, but others contain two. Usually, a combination of two products will help minimize the adverse reactions seen with each one individually. Simethicone is included because it's often used to treat gas.

Why do products often contain both aluminum and magnesium?

Aluminum causes constipation. Magnesium causes diarrhea. By combining the two in a single product, the result is generally no change in bowel function.

TIP Antacids may also be added to aspirin, such as in the products Ascriptin and Bufferin. The antacids in these medications decrease GI irritation caused by aspirin.

Calcium Carbonate

Calcium carbonate (Tums, Maalox Children's, Maalox Quick Dissolve, Maalox Antacid Barrier Maximum Strength, Mylanta Children's, Pepto-Bismol Children's, Titralac, Alka-Mints, Rolaids Extra Strength) is used to treat symptoms such as:

- heartburn
- acid indigestion
- sour stomach

It may also be used to treat calcium deficiencies and related conditions (for example, osteoporosis, rickets).

This drug is sold as tablets, chewable tablets, soft chews, and oral suspension. For use as an antacid, the dosing schedule may vary according to the product being used. With many products, one dose may be taken after each meal as needed. As with all antacids, patients should read the package insert or drug label carefully so as not to exceed the maximum daily dosage.

Magnesium Salts

Magnesium hydroxide (Phillips' Milk of Magnesia, Phillips' Laxative, Ex-Lax Milk of Magnesia) is sold OTC to relieve heartburn, acid indigestion, and sour stomach. It may also be used to relieve occasional constipation.

Magnesium hydroxide comes in chewable tablets and as a liquid. For use as an antacid, one dose may be taken up to four times a day.

Combination Products

Many antacid products contain combinations of antacids with or without simethicone, an **antiflatulen**t. Some common combination products include:

- Aluminum hydroxide and magnesium carbonate/trisilicate (Gaviscon)
- Aluminum hydroxide and magnesium hydroxide (Mylanta Ultimate Strength)
- Aluminum hydroxide, magnesium hydroxide, simethicone (Gelusil)
- Calcium carbonate, magnesium hydroxide (Mylanta, Rolaids)
- Calcium carbonate, magnesium hydroxide, simethicone (Rolaids Multi-Symptom)

Other Antiulcer Drugs

Scientists continue to research the usefulness of other drugs to treat peptic ulcer disease. The specific actions of these drugs vary. However, each drug works to protect the GI tract from the effects of gastric acid.

 PROCEED WITH CAUTION

Adverse Reactions to Other Antiulcer Drugs

Although adverse reactions differ for specific peptic ulcer drugs, some common reactions include:

- nausea
- vomiting

Misoprostol

Misoprostol (Cytotec) is used to prevent gastric ulcers for:

- patients who may have ulcers as a result of long-term NSAID therapy
- patients with a history of ulcers

This drug works by blocking the secretion of acids in the stomach. It also may increase the production of mucus and bicarbonate. NSAIDs stop the body from making prostaglandins, which in turn may lead to reduced mucus secretion. By increasing mucus production, misoprostol may counteract these effects.

Misoprostol is available by prescription only. It's manufactured as tablets. The recommended dosing schedule for the prevention of NSAID-induced ulcers is one dose four times daily. Misoprostol should be taken with food, and the last dose of the day should be at bedtime.

Misoprostol has no known interactions with other drugs. However, in addition to nausea and vomiting, this drug may cause the following adverse reactions:

- abdominal pain
- diarrhea
- gas
- indigestion
- spontaneous abortion (in pregnant women)

Misoprostol shouldn't be given to women who are or who may become pregnant because of the high risk of abortion, premature birth, or birth defects.

Misoprostol is also manufactured in tablet form in combination with NSAIDs, such as diclofenac (Arthrotec), for the treatment of arthritis.

Sucralfate

Sucralfate (Carafate) is used for:

- short-term treatment of active duodenal ulcers
- maintenance therapy after healing of duodenal ulcers

Sucralfate has a local effect. Although the way it works is not fully known, part of its effect comes through blocking the activity of pepsin. It may also cover the ulcer site and protect it from acid, pepsin, and bile salts.

Like misoprostol, sucralfate is available by prescription only. It comes in the form of tablets or oral suspension and is taken on an empty stomach.

Sucralfate may interact with other medications:

■ Antacids may reduce the binding of sucralfate to the gastric and duodenal mucosa, reducing its effectiveness.
■ Certain drugs may decrease the body's absorption of sucralfate, including cimetidine, digoxin, fluoroquinolones, ranitidine, tetracycline, and theophylline.

Adverse reactions to sucralfate are rare. The most common adverse reaction is constipation.

ADSORBENT, ANTIFLATULENT, AND DIGESTIVE DRUGS

Adsorbent, antiflatulent, and digestive drugs are used to fight unwanted toxins, acids, and gases in the GI tract. They increase healthy GI function.

■ **Adsorbents** are prescribed as antidotes for ingested toxins, or substances that can lead to poisoning or overdose.
■ **Antiflatulents** are drugs that work against flatus (gas).
■ **Digestive drugs** aid digestion in patients who are missing enzymes or other substances needed to digest food.

Adsorbent Drugs

Drugs that act to counteract toxins may be natural or synthetic. The most commonly used clinical adsorbent is activated charcoal (Actidose-Aqua, EZ Char Pellets, Actidose with Sorbitol, Charcoal Plus DS, CharcoCaps). This substance is a black powder residue that is produced by distilling organic materials. It's a general purpose antidote used for many types of poisoning by mouth.

Activated charcoal works by attracting and binding to toxins in the intestine. When the adsorbent binds with the toxin, it stops the toxin from being absorbed by the GI tract. Because the adsorbent can bind only to a toxin that has not already been absorbed from the GI tract, it should be administered soon after the drug or poison is taken.

After initial absorption, some poisons move back into the intestines, where they're reabsorbed. Activated charcoal may be administered repeatedly to break this cycle.

Activated charcoal is not absorbed or metabolized by the body. It's excreted unchanged in stool.

Although activated charcoal is used to treat many types of oral poisoning, there are several cases where it should not be used:

■ Activated charcoal is not used for acute poisoning from mineral acids, alkalines, cyanide, ethanol, methanol, iron, sodium chloride alkali, inorganic acids, or organic solvents.

■ It shouldn't be administered to a child younger than one year old.
■ It shouldn't be administered to a patient who has a risk of GI obstruction, perforation, or hemorrhage. It is also not advised for patients with decreased or absent bowel sounds or who have had recent GI surgery.

Activated charcoal is available OTC in several oral forms:

■ liquid
■ granules
■ powder
■ suspension

Activated charcoal can decrease the absorption of oral medications. Patients should not take medications other than those used to treat the ingested toxin within two hours of taking the activated charcoal. The effectiveness of activated charcoal may be reduced by vomiting that is induced by **ipecac syrup**—a substance used to induce vomiting in the early management of poisoning or drug overdose. If both drugs are used to treat oral poisoning, activated charcoal should be used after vomiting has ceased.

Antiflatulent Drugs

Antiflatulents break up gas pockets in the GI tract, relieving symptoms of bloating or pain. These drugs are available alone or in combination with antacids. Antiflatulents are used therapeutically in many situations where excess gas may be a problem, including the following:

■ functional gastric bloating
■ gaseous bloating after surgery
■ diverticular disease (characterized by abnormal side pockets in the GI tract usually related to a lack of **dietary fiber**)
■ spastic or irritable colon
■ air swallowing

Antiflatulents work by providing defoaming action in the digestive tract. They stop mucus-enclosed gas pockets from forming in the GI tract. Antiflatulents also cause gas bubbles to combine into larger bubbles that can be passed more easily.

 PROCEED WITH CAUTION

Adverse Reactions to Activated Charcoal

Activated charcoal may cause the following adverse reactions:

■ black stool
■ constipation

A laxative, such as sorbitol, is usually given with activated charcoal to prevent constipation and improve taste.

The main antiflatulent available in the United States is simethicone (Gas-X, Mylanta Gas, Phazyme, Mylicon). It's available OTC in several oral forms:

- chewable tablets
- capsules
- drops (in solution and suspension forms)
- orally disintegrating strips

Simethicone doesn't interact significantly with other drugs and doesn't cause any known adverse reactions.

Digestive Drugs

Digestive drugs are designed to improve digestion in patients who are missing enzymes or other substances needed to digest food. These drugs act in the GI tract, liver, and pancreas in much the same way as the body substances they replace.

In the body, the pancreas produces enzymes that act to break down and digest fats, starches, and proteins in foods. Pancreatic enzyme drugs are prescribed for patients who don't produce enough of these enzymes naturally. Pancreatic enzyme drugs may contain several different substances:

- protease to digest proteins
- amylase to digest carbohydrates
- lipase to digest fats

Different amounts of each enzyme may be included in different formulations.

These drugs work in the duodenum and upper jejunum of the GI tract. The actions of these drugs vary, depending on the enzymes the drug is intended to replace.

One pancreatic enzyme drug, pancrelipase (Pancrease, Creon, Lipram, Ultrase, Dygase, Plaretase, Viokase, Palcaps, Pangestyme, Panocaps, Pancrecarb, Panokase, is used to treat cystic fibrosis in adults and children. It's also used to treat steatorrhea (a disorder related to fat metabolism that is characterized by fatty, foul-smelling stool) and other disorders caused by pancreatic enzyme deficiency. Pancrelipase is available as delayed-release capsules, tablets, and oral powder. Pancreatic enzyme drugs can interact with other substances.

- Antacids reduce the effectiveness of pancreatic enzymes.
- Pancreatic enzymes may decrease the absorption of folic acid and iron.

! PROCEED WITH CAUTION

Adverse Reactions to Pancrelipase

Adverse reactions to pancrelipase are dose related. They may include the following:

- abdominal cramping
- diarrhea
- nausea

ANTIDIARRHEAL DRUGS

Antidiarrheals act systemically or locally to control diarrhea. Diarrhea is one of the main symptoms related to disturbances of the large intestine. Antidiarrheals work by decreasing intestinal peristalsis, the wave-like muscle contractions that push fecal matter through the GI tract.

Opioid-Related Drugs

Opioid-related drugs are used to treat diarrhea. They slow the movement of fecal matter through the intestines and colon by decreasing peristalsis. Peristalsis is usually increased in patients with diarrhea. Opioid-related drugs also decrease expulsive contractions (muscle movements to push out fecal matter) in the colon.

Opioid-related drugs may interact with other substances. They may enhance the depressive effects of the following:

- barbiturates
- alcohol
- opioids
- tranquilizers
- sedatives

Diphenoxylate with Atropine

Diphenoxylate with atropine (Lomotil, Lonox) is used as adjunctive therapy to treat diarrhea. This drug is a Schedule V controlled substance and is available by prescription only in oral tablets and as a liquid.

Loperamide

Loperamide is available OTC and by prescription. OTC loperamide (Imodium A-D) is sold to control diarrhea, including traveler's diarrhea. By prescription, this drug is used:

- to relieve acute nonspecific diarrhea
- to treat chronic diarrhea associated with inflammatory bowel disease

! PROCEED WITH CAUTION

Adverse Reactions to Opioid-Related Drugs

There are several potential adverse reactions for opioid-related antidiarrheals:

- nausea and vomiting
- abdominal discomfort or distention
- drowsiness
- fatigue
- central nervous system depression
- tachycardia (rapid heart rate)
- paralytic ileus (reduced or absent peristalsis in the intestines)

■ to reduce the volume of discharge from an ileostomy (an opening in the ileum for stool to leave the body following surgical removal of the colon)

The prescription form of loperamide is available in 2-mg capsules. Loperamide is available OTC as 2-mg tablets or as an oral suspension, or fast dissolving tablet. Loperamide is also available OTC in a combination product with Simethicone (Imodium Advanced).

 The dosing for loperamide is the same for both prescription and OTC forms of the drug. Loperamide is not recommended for children under two years of age.

5-HT$_3$ Receptor Antagonists

Alosetron (Lotronex) is a selective 5-HT$_3$ receptor antagonist used for short-term treatment of diarrhea-predominant irritable bowel syndrome (IBS) in women. This drug is thought to work by blocking serotonin (a body substance that regulates mood and stimulates smooth muscles in the intestines) in the GI tract. By blocking the action of serotonin, alosetron reduces symptoms of IBS including abdominal cramping, urgency, and diarrhea.

 Alosetron shouldn't be taken if the patient is constipated and should be stopped if constipation develops.

Alosetron may interact with other drugs.

■ Alosetron blocks about 30 percent of the action of *N*-acetyltransferase and CYP1A2 (a cytochrome P-450 enzyme), substances that are important in metabolism.
■ Alosetron could cause constipation when given with other drugs that decrease GI motility.

This drug is available by prescription only through a restricted marketing program because of reported serious GI adverse effects. (See *Adverse Reactions to Alosetron.*) Only prescribers enrolled in the prescribing program may write

! PROCEED WITH CAUTION

Adverse Reactions to Alosetron

Alosetron can cause serious and sometimes fatal adverse reactions. These reactions may include:

■ ischemic colitis (a disease caused by decreased blood flow to the colon)
■ complications of constipation, such as obstruction, perforation, and toxic megacolon (a condition in which the colon becomes abnormally enlarged due to inflammation)

Older adult patients may have increased sensitivity to the effects of alosetron. This increases their risk of developing serious constipation.

! PROCEED WITH CAUTION

Adverse Reactions to Bismuth Subsalicylate

The main adverse reactions to bismuth subsalicylate are darkened stool and black tongue. Bismuth subsalicylate may also increase the risk of Reye syndrome in children who are recovering from chickenpox or the flu.

a prescription for it. Alosetron is manufactured in the form of oral tablets.

Bismuth Subsalicylate

Bismuth subsalicylate (Kaopectate, Pepto-Bismol, Maalox Total Stomach Relief) is used to control diarrhea. It's also used to treat the following symptoms:

■ gas
■ upset stomach
■ indigestion
■ heartburn
■ nausea

This drug is available over the counter in the form of tablets, chewable tablets, and oral suspension.

Bismuth subsalicylate may interact with other drugs.

■ When taken with aspirin or other salicylates, bismuth subsalicylate may result in salicylate toxicity.
■ High doses of bismuth subsalicylate may increase the effects of oral anticoagulants or oral antidiabetic drugs.
■ Bismuth subsalicylate may decrease absorption of the antibiotic tetracycline.

LAXATIVE DRUGS

Laxatives are commonly prescribed to prevent or relieve constipation. They work by stimulating bowel movements. There are several different types of laxatives, which act differently to relieve constipation.

 Constipation is an adverse reaction to certain drugs. Laxatives or stool softeners may be prescribed to prevent constipation when patients are taking anticholinergics, antihistamines, phenothiazines, opiates, iron preparations, or other drugs.

Hyperosmolar Laxatives

Hyperosmolar laxatives act to draw more water into the colon from surrounding body tissues. This softens stool and makes it easier to pass. The enlargement of the colon leads to increased peristalsis, resulting in a bowel movement. Some hyperosmolar laxatives work quickly and are used to empty the colon before rectal or bowel examinations or

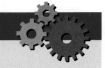

HOW IT WORKS

Laxatives in Action

Different types of laxatives have different ways of acting on the body.

- **Hyperosmolar laxatives** are drugs that stimulate bowel movements by drawing water into the intestine from body tissues. Most of these drugs take effect within 15 minutes to 3 hours. Lactulose, however, takes 24 to 48 hours.
- **Bulk-forming laxatives** add bulk and moisture to stool, encouraging peristalsis. Bacteria in the intestines break down the polysaccharides in the laxatives into metabolites that draw water into the intestine. The onset of action for bulk-forming laxatives ranges from 12 to 72 hours.
- **Emollient laxatives** soften stool in the large intestine. These drugs take effect within 12 to 72 hours.
- **Stimulant laxatives** irritate the intestinal mucosa, promoting peristalsis. The onset of action for this type of laxative varies. For example, cascara sagrada, senna, and bisacodyl tablets take effect within 6 to 10 hours. Bisacodyl suppositories, however, have a more rapid onset of action—15 minutes to an hour. Castor oil takes effect within 2 to 6 hours.
- **Lubricant laxatives** moisten and coat the intestinal walls and stool. This helps the stool hold water and eases movement. It takes between 6 and 8 hours for these drugs to take effect.

surgery. Others are more suitable for long-term treatment of constipation.

Glycerin

Glycerin (Colace, Fleet Babylax) is an OTC drug that is helpful in bowel retraining (a process of developing strategies or skills for bowel control in patients who are unable to

PROCEED WITH CAUTION

Adverse Reactions to Hyperosmolar Laxatives

Adverse reactions vary depending on the type of hyperosmolar laxative used. Hyperosmolar laxatives commonly cause the following reactions:

- abdominal cramping
- diarrhea
- gas
- increased thirst
- nausea

High doses or use for long periods of time can result in fluid and electrolyte imbalances. With prolonged use, patients can develop dependency on the laxative to have a bowel movement.

control bowel movements). Glycerin has a local effect. It's placed directly into the colon by rectal suppository. A liquid suppository form of the drug is available for pediatric use. An oral solution is also available. Adverse reactions to glycerin may include weakness and fatigue.

Lactulose

Lactulose (Acilac, Constulose, Cephulac, Enulose) is used to treat constipation. It's also used to reduce ammonia production and absorption from the intestines in patients with elevated ammonia levels. (This occurs in patients with cirrhosis and liver failure.)

Lactulose is available by prescription only and is administered orally. It is manufactured as a solution that may be taken by itself or mixed with juice, water, or milk.

The effectiveness of lactulose may be reduced when taken with antacids, antibiotics, or oral neomycin. In addition to the adverse reactions associated with other hyperosmotic laxatives, lactulose may cause:

- belching
- gaseous distention
- flatulence

Saline Compounds

Saline compounds are used when prompt and complete emptying of the bowel is needed. They may be used to empty the bowel before surgery or to relieve constipation.

Saline compounds are administered orally or as an enema. They work by attracting water into the colon. This increases the pressure in the colon, promoting peristalsis. Some of the ions from saline compounds are absorbed by the GI tract. Absorbed ions are excreted in urine. The unabsorbed drug is eliminated in stool.

These drugs may cause the following adverse reactions:

- weakness
- lethargy
- dehydration
- hypernatremia (high blood sodium level)
- hypermagnesemia (high blood magnesium level)
- hyperphosphatemia (high blood phosphate level)
- hypocalcemia (low blood calcium level)
- cardiac arrhythmias
- shock

Magnesium Salts

Magnesium salts are used to empty the bowel before examinations or surgery. They are not for long-term or repeated use. These drugs may also be used in small amounts to relieve acid indigestion. There are various types of magnesium salts, including the following:

- Magnesium citrate is available OTC as an oral solution. It's typically used to empty the bowel before medical procedures.
- Magnesium hydroxide (Phillips' Milk of Magnesia, Phillips' Laxative, Ex-Lax Milk of Magnesia) is avail-

able OTC in the form of chewable tablets, soft chews, and oral suspension. It's used to relieve acid indigestion and upset stomach as well as for a laxative effect. Doses vary depending on the product.

Sodium Phosphates

The combination drug sodium phosphate and sodium biphosphate (Osmo Prep, Visicol) is used in treating constipation. This drug works by drawing water into the small intestine. It is sold OTC as oral tablets, oral solution, or an enema. Sodium phosphates should not be used by patients who are following sodium-restricted diets.

Polyethylene Glycol

Polyethylene glycol (PEG) is used in treating occasional constipation. PEG solution is not absorbed by the body, so it doesn't change the electrolyte balance.

This drug is available OTC (MiraLax) and by prescription (GlycoLax) in the form of a powder to be dissolved in water. A typical daily dose is 17 g (or one heaping tablespoonful) dissolved in eight ounces of water. Laxatives that are sold as powders must be mixed by the patient. It's important to read package labels to see how long the mixed solution can be stored before use.

Polyethylene Glycol and Electrolytes

PEG and electrolyte solution (MoviPrep, GolYTELY, NuLYTELY, TriLyte, Colyte) is used to cleanse the bowel before GI examinations. It is available by prescription only in the form of a powder to be reconstituted as an oral solution.

Patients should fast for three to four hours before taking this solution. A typical dose is 4 L of oral solution. This large dose is consumed on a schedule provided by the physician to ensure that the bowel is emptied prior to the examination. The electrolytes in the solution reduce the absorption of ions.

Dietary Fiber and Related Bulk-Forming Laxatives

The most natural way to prevent and treat constipation is through a high-fiber diet. Dietary fiber is the part of plants that is not digested in the small intestine. Like dietary fiber, bulk-forming laxatives are not absorbed by the body. They contain natural and partially synthetic polysaccharides (sugars) and cellulose (a fiber found in plant cells). Dietary fiber and bulk-forming laxatives are used to:

- treat simple cases of constipation, especially constipation resulting from a low-fiber or low-fluid diet
- help patients recovering from MI or cerebral aneurysms who need to avoid Valsalva maneuver (forced breathing against a closed airway) and maintain soft stool
- manage patients with IBS and diverticulosis (a disorder in which small fluid-filled pouches develop in the intestinal wall)

Bulk-forming laxatives work because the polysaccharides and cellulose absorb water and expand to increase the bulk and the moisture in stool. Bacteria in the intestine break down the polysaccharides into metabolites that draw water into the intestine. The added bulk and water content in the stool encourages peristalsis.

Fiber and bulk-forming laxatives may affect the absorption of some other drugs. Decreased absorption of digoxin, warfarin, and salicylates occurs if these drugs are taken within two hours of taking fiber or bulk-forming laxatives.

Methylcellulose

Methylcellulose (Citrucel) is used to relieve constipation and to maintain bowel regularity. It's sold OTC as a powder for mixing with liquid or as tablets. This medication is taken orally.

Polycarbophil

As a bulk-forming laxative, polycarbophil (FiberCon, Equalactin) is used to maintain normal bowel function and to relieve constipation. This drug may also be used for its antidiarrheal effects. It's available OTC as tablets and chewable tablets.

Polycarbophil may interact with tetracycline. It should be taken at least one hour before or two hours after medications that contain tetracycline.

Psyllium

Psyllium (Reguloid, GenFiber, Hydrocil, Metamucil) is an OTC drug used to treat:

- occasional constipation
- constipation associated with GI disorders
- IBS
- diverticulosis

It comes in several dosage forms, including capsules, chewable bars, oral suspension, and a powder to be reconstituted as an oral suspension. All forms are administered orally.

Psyllium may interact with other medications. It should be taken two hours before or two hours after other oral

PROCEED WITH CAUTION

Adverse Reactions to Bulk-Forming Laxatives

Adverse reactions may include:

- gas
- abdominal fullness
- intestinal obstruction
- fecal impaction (hard stool that can't be removed from the rectum)
- esophageal obstruction (if sufficient liquid hasn't been taken with the drug)
- severe diarrhea

medications. Along with the adverse reactions common to other bulk-producing laxatives, psyllium may cause allergic reactions.

TIP Psyllium is a dietary fiber that comes from the seed coat of a plant. It is also found in some cereals because it may lower blood cholesterol levels.

Emollient Laxatives

Emollients are also known as stool softeners. These drugs soften stool and make bowel movements easier. Emollients are often used for softening stools in patients who should avoid straining during a bowel movement. This includes patients with:

- recent MI or surgery
- disease of the anus or rectum
- increased intracranial pressure
- hernias
- postpartum constipation (constipation following childbirth)

Emollients act in the small and large intestines. They work by emulsifying, or blending, the fat and water components of stool. This detergent action allows water to enter the stool, making it softer and easier to pass.

Emollients may interact with other drugs.

- Drugs with low margins of safety (narrow therapeutic index) must be administered with caution with emollients. Emollients may increase the body's absorption of these drugs.
- Emollients may increase the systemic absorption of mineral oil, leading to tissue deposits of the oil.

Docusate Calcium

Docusate calcium (Sur-Q-Lax, Kaopectate) is sold OTC in capsules to be taken by mouth. It's used to relieve occasional constipation and to prevent dry, hard stools. It's also used for patients who should not strain during bowel movements.

Docusate Sodium

Docusate sodium (Colace, Correctol, Dulcolax, Phillips' Stool Softener, DocuLace, Doc-Q-Lace, Diocto, Silace) is an

! PROCEED WITH CAUTION

Adverse Reactions to Emollients

Adverse reactions to emollients are rare. When adverse reactions do occur, they may include:

- bitter taste
- diarrhea
- throat irritation
- mild abdominal cramping

AT THE COUNTER

Softening Stool After Surgery

In the pharmacy, you receive a medication order for a new mother whose baby was delivered by Caesarean section. What GI product would you most likely expect to see prescribed for this patient?

A stool softener, such as docusate calcium or docusate sodium, is often ordered for patients who have undergone surgery where the strain of pushing out a bowel movement might cause further injury, such as popping stitches. Stool softeners are commonly prescribed after a Caesarean section, an episiotomy, or after open heart surgery. Stool softeners are also recommended or prescribed with opioid/opiate pain management therapy because constipation is a common adverse reaction to those drugs.

OTC medication that is taken orally as capsules to relieve occasional constipation. It's also sold in oral solution, suspension and syrup forms for patients who need to avoid the strain of bowel movements.

Stimulant Laxatives

Stimulant laxatives, also known as **irritant cathartics**, act directly on the intestine to stimulate peristalsis. They are the preferred drugs to empty the bowels before:

- general surgery
- sigmoidoscopic procedures, in which an instrument is used to examine the lower part of the bowel
- proctoscopic procedures, in which an instrument is used to examine the rectum
- radiologic procedures, such as barium studies of the GI tract

Stimulant laxatives are also used to treat constipation caused by:

- prolonged bed rest
- neurological dysfunction of the colon
- constipating drugs such as opioids

Stimulant laxatives work by irritating the mucosa, or lining, of the large intestine. They stimulate nerve endings of the smooth muscle in the intestine. These effects increase peristalsis and produce a bowel movement.

There are no significant drug interactions with stimulant laxatives. However, because these drugs increase the movement of material inside the intestine, they reduce the absorption of other oral drugs. Other drugs, especially sustained-release drugs, shouldn't be administered at the same time as a stimulant laxative.

Bisacodyl

Bisacodyl (Dulcolax, Ex-Lax Ultra, Doxidan) is used to treat occasional constipation. In addition to acting as a stimulant in the large intestine, bisacodyl draws in water to soften stool. It's sold OTC as capsules, tablets, and enteric-coated tablets for oral use, and as suppositories for rectal use.

Bisacodyl may be affected by substances that reduce stomach acid.

- When taken with antacids, bisacodyl may cause stomach irritation. Bisacodyl should be taken one hour after antacids or other medications that reduce stomach acid.
- Bisacodyl shouldn't be taken with milk or dairy products because they may reduce stomach acid.

Cascara Sagrada

Cascara sagrada is a natural laxative derived from tree bark. It's used to relieve occasional constipation. Cascara sagrada is sold OTC as an oral liquid. In addition to the adverse effects noted for other stimulant laxatives, cascara sagrada may discolor urine.

Castor Oil

Castor oil is most often used to empty the small and large intestines before medical procedures. It may also be used to treat occasional constipation. Castor oil is sold OTC as an oral liquid.

Castor oil not only acts as an irritant in the large intestine, it also increases peristalsis in the small intestine. One hour after taking castor oil, the patient needs to drink water to flush out the colon and prevent cramping.

Senna

Senna (Black Draught, Ex-Lax, Perdiem, Senokot, Fletcher's Laxative) is sold OTC for relief of occasional constipation. It comes in several different forms to be taken orally, including:

- tablets
- chewable tablets
- syrup
- oral solution

Senna should be taken with a full glass of water or juice.

In addition to the adverse reactions common to other drugs in this group, senna may cause:

- bloating
- discoloration of urine

- flatulence
- vomiting

Senna also comes in a combination tablet product with docusate sodium (Doc-Q-Lax, Peri-Colace, Senokot-S).

Lubricant Laxatives

The main lubricant laxative currently in use is mineral oil. Mineral oil lubricates the intestinal walls so stool passes more easily. It's used therapeutically for the following reasons:

- to treat constipation
- to maintain soft stool for patients who need to avoid straining
- to treat fecal impaction

Mineral oil may be administered orally or by enema. It works by making the intestinal mucosa slippery. This prevents water from being reabsorbed from the material in the bowel. The increased fluid in the stool increases peristalsis. Administering mineral oil by enema produces bowel distention.

Mineral oil can affect the absorption of other drugs.

- Mineral oil may block the absorption of fat-soluble vitamins, hormonal contraceptives, and anticoagulants.
- Mineral oil may interfere with the antibacterial activity of nonabsorbable sulfonamides.

To reduce drug interactions, mineral oil should be taken at least two hours before these medications.

Mineral oil shouldn't be given to anyone with a cough, since it can be aspirated, or breathed into the lungs. This could cause lipid pneumonia, a type of lung inflammation that occurs when fats (lipids) enter the bronchial passages.

ANTIEMETIC AND EMETIC DRUGS

Antiemetics and **emetics** are two groups of drugs with opposing actions. Antiemetic drugs decrease nausea, reducing the urge to vomit. In contrast, emetic drugs induce vomiting.

Antiemetic Drugs

Antiemetics are used to treat nausea and vomiting in:

- patients who are undergoing chemotherapy or radiotherapy
- individuals with motion sickness
- patients who are experiencing nausea and vomiting as a side effect of other medications, such as opioid analgesics or general anesthetics

There are several different types of antiemetics. The action varies depending on the drug.

Antihistamines

Antihistamines are used to treat nausea and vomiting caused by inner ear stimulation. They are often used to prevent or treat motion sickness. These drugs are most effective when taken before activities that produce motion sickness. They are less effective when nausea or vomiting has already started.

Drug interactions associated with antihistamines include the following:

- Antihistamines can produce additive CNS depression and sedation when taken with barbiturates, tranquilizers, antidepressants, alcohol, or opioids.
- Antihistamines shouldn't be used with morphine or other respiratory depressants.
- When taken with anticholinergic drugs (including tricyclic antidepressants, phenothiazines, and antiparkinsonian drugs), antihistamines can cause additive anticholinergic effects, such as constipation, dry mouth, vision problems, and urine retention.

Cyclizine Hydrochloride

Cyclizine hydrochloride (Marezine) is used to prevent and treat motion sickness, including symptoms of dizziness, nausea, and vomiting. It's sold OTC in oral tablet form.

 PROCEED WITH CAUTION

Adverse Reactions to Antihistamines

Adverse reactions to antihistamines used as antiemetics include:

- drowsiness
- hypotension (decreased blood pressure)
- urinary frequency, difficulty urinating, or urinary retention

Overdosage of antihistamines can have serious consequences, such as:

- drowsiness with hyperexcitability
- convulsions
- hallucinations
- respiratory paralysis

Dimenhydrinate

Dimenhydrinate (Dramamine) is used to prevent and treat nausea, vomiting, and dizziness related to motion sickness. It's sold OTC as tablets, and chewable tablets. It's also available by prescription in the form of vials for injection.

In addition to the adverse effects common to other antihistamines, dimenhydrinate taken with some antibiotics may cause ototoxicity (damage to the ear leading to hearing and balance problems). This drug shouldn't be given to children younger than two years old.

Diphenhydramine Hydrochloride

Diphenhydramine hydrochloride (Simply Sleep, Sominex, Nytol, Unisom Sleepgels) is used to treat motion sickness and insomnia. It may also be used to treat or ease nausea and vomiting resulting from chemotherapy. Diphenhydramine is available OTC in the form of tablets, chewable tablets, dissolving tablets, capsules, orally disintegrating film, oral suspension, oral solution, syrup, and elixir. It is also available by prescription as an injection.

Along with the drug interactions noted for other antihistamines, the drying effects of diphenhydramine may be intensified when taken with MAO inhibitors.

In addition to the adverse effects common to antihistamine drugs, diphenhydramine may cause thickening of bronchial secretions and abdominal pain.

Hydroxyzine

Hydroxyzine (Vistaril) is administered with other medications either before or after surgery to control nausea and vomiting. It's available by prescription only. Hydroxyzine is manufactured as tablets, capsules, and oral suspension. It also comes in injection form for deep IM administration.

Hydroxyzine is believed to work by blocking activity in key regions of the CNS. It may interact with opioid drugs such as meperidine, resulting in severe hypotension. Adverse reactions of hydroxyzine are mild. The most common adverse reaction is drowsiness.

Meclizine

Meclizine is used to treat symptoms of motion sickness, including dizziness, nausea, and vomiting. This drug is available in both prescription and OTC forms. By prescription, meclizine is manufactured as tablets (Antivert). It's sold OTC in the form of tablets and chewable tablets (Dramamine Less Drowsy Formula, Bonine).

Meclizine tablets may contain a yellow dye (tartrazine) that can cause allergic-type reactions in some individuals, especially those with a sensitivity to aspirin.

Trimethobenzamide

Trimethobenzamide (Tigan) is used to treat nausea and vomiting after surgery. It's also used in treating nausea associated with gastroenteritis (irritation of the stomach and intestines). Trimethobenzamide is a prescription-only drug. It's administered by mouth in the form of capsules or by injection.

Phenothiazines

Phenothiazines are used to treat severe nausea and vomiting in a variety of situations, including:

- postsurgical patients
- patients with viral nausea and vomiting
- patients with nausea and vomiting resulting from chemotherapy or radiotherapy

Their antiemetic effect results from blocking dopaminergic receptors (receptors for a chemical substance called dopamine) in the chemoreceptor trigger zone in the brain. This area of the brain stimulates the vomiting center in the medulla. Phenothiazines may also directly suppress the brain's vomiting center.

Phenothiazines may interact with several other medications.

- Similar to antihistamines, phenothiazines can also produce additive CNS depression and sedation when taken with barbiturates, tranquilizers, antidepressants, alcohol, or opioids.
- Droperidol used with phenothiazine antiemetics increases the risk of extrapyramidal effects (abnormal involuntary movements).
- Phenothiazine antiemetics taken with anticholinergic drugs increase the anticholinergic effect and decrease the antiemetic effects.

Chlorpromazine

Chlorpromazine is used to control nausea and vomiting. This drug is available by prescription only and may be administered by mouth in the form of tablets or by injection.

PROCEED WITH CAUTION

Adverse Reactions to Phenothiazines

Adverse effects of phenothiazines are usually dose related. They may include:

- hypotension
- orthostatic hypotension with an increased heart rate
- fainting
- dizziness
- drowsiness
- confusion
- anxiety
- euphoria
- agitation
- depression
- headache
- insomnia
- restlessness
- weakness

Patients taking phenothiazines over long periods of time are at increased risk for developing tardive dyskinesia, a syndrome characterized by involuntary movements.

In addition to the drug interactions typical of phenothiazines, the following drug interactions may occur:

- Chlorpromazine may reduce the effects of oral anticoagulants.
- Taking chlorpromazine with guanethidine may reduce the antihypertensive effects of guanethidine.
- Chlorpromazine increases the action of CNS depressants. Dosages of CNS depressants should be reduced when taken with chlorpromazine.
- Taking propranolol and chlorpromazine together may increase blood levels of both drugs.

Perphenazine

Perphenazine is a prescription-only medication used to control severe nausea and vomiting in adults. It's available as tablets.

Prochlorperazine

Prochlorperazine (Compro) is used to control severe nausea and vomiting. This drug is available by prescription only in various forms, including:

- tablets
- rectal suppositories
- vials for injection

Promethazine

Promethazine hydrochloride (Phenadoz, Phenergan) is used for:

- antiemetic therapy in patients after surgery
- prevention and control of nausea and vomiting associated with certain types of anesthesia
- treating symptoms of motion sickness

This drug is available by prescription only. Promethazine is manufactured as oral tablets, oral solution, rectal suppositories, and in vials for injection.

In addition to the adverse effects of other drugs in this class, promethazine may cause fatal respiratory depression.

TIP Promethazine shouldn't be given to children under two years old because of the risk of fatal respiratory depression.

Serotonin 5-HT₃ Receptor Antagonists

Serotonin 5-HT$_3$ receptor antagonists are used to prevent nausea and vomiting related to:

- cancer therapy
- surgery
- radiotherapy

These drugs work by blocking serotonin stimulation in the chemoreceptor trigger zone. They also block serotonin stimulation in certain nerve endings in the brain. Because both of these areas stimulate vomiting, blocking these receptors reduces the need to vomit.

PROCEED WITH CAUTION

Adverse Reactions to Serotonin 5-HT₃ Receptor Antagonists

There are several adverse reactions to serotonin 5-HT₃ receptor antagonists:

- confusion
- anxiety
- euphoria
- agitation
- depression
- headache
- insomnia
- restlessness
- weakness

Serotonin 5-HT₃ receptor antagonists may interact with other drugs. The specific drug interaction varies for different serotonin 5-HT₃ receptor antagonists.

Dolasetron

Dolasetron (Anzemet) is used in the following situations:

- to prevent nausea and vomiting associated with cancer chemotherapy
- to prevent nausea and vomiting after surgery

Dolasetron is available by prescription only as tablets or by injection.

Additional adverse reactions for patients taking dolasetron include bradycardia and tachycardia.

Granisetron

Granisetron (Kytril, Granisol) is a prescription drug used to prevent nausea and vomiting associated with cancer therapy and radiation. It's manufactured as tablets, oral solution, and single and multidose vials for injection.

In addition to the adverse reactions typical of other serotonin H₅ antagonists, granisetron may cause asthenia (weakness or loss of strength).

Ondansetron

Ondansetron (Zofran, Zofran ODT) is currently the antiemetic of choice in the United States. It's used to prevent nausea and vomiting in patients:

- undergoing cancer therapy
- undergoing radiotherapy
- after surgery

Ondansetron comes as tablets, orally disintegrating tablets, oral solution, and as vials or premixed containers for injection. It is available by prescription only.

Emetics

Emetics are used to induce vomiting in a person who has ingested a toxic substance. Ipecac syrup is used to induce vomiting in the early management of oral poisoning or drug overdose.

Ipecac syrup induces vomiting by stimulating the vomiting center located in the brain's medulla. However, little information exists concerning the absorption, distribution, and excretion of the drug. After administration of ipecac syrup, vomiting usually occurs within 30 minutes.

Ipecac syrup is manufactured in 30-mL bottles of oral syrup. It's available without a prescription; however, this drug is kept behind the counter in most pharmacies. It is no longer recommended to be kept at home. Pharmacies usually dispense ipecac syrup after a patient has called poison control and has been directed to use it.

TIP Ipecac syrup should be used only after a recommendation from the poison center. The national number is 1-800-222-1222. It will automatically direct you to your local poison control center. Every poison control center in the United States is staffed 24 hours a day.

Because ipecac syrup is used only in acute situations, drug interactions rarely occur.

- If poisoning is a result of ingesting a phenothiazine drug, the antiemetic effect of the phenothiazine may decrease the emetic effect of ipecac syrup.
- Ipecac syrup shouldn't be administered with activated charcoal. Activated charcoal will absorb the syrup and inactivate it.

Ipecac syrup shouldn't be used after the ingestion of the following substances:

- petroleum products
- volatile oils
- caustic substances, such as lye

These products increase the risk of additional esophageal injury or aspiration.

The use of ipecac syrup has become controversial. The American Academy of Pediatrics no longer recommends the routine use of ipecac syrup for several reasons.

- It delays the use of activated charcoal or antidotes to toxic substances.

PROCEED WITH CAUTION

Adverse Reactions to Ipecac Syrup

Ipecac syrup rarely produces adverse reactions when used in the recommended dosages. However, some people are very sensitive to the drug. Adverse reactions may include:

- prolonged vomiting (for longer than one hour)
- repeated vomiting (more than six episodes in one hour)
- lethargy (sluggishness, drowsiness)
- diarrhea

These reactions can occur even at regular dosages.

- There's a risk of potential abuse by individuals with eating disorders.

The first action parents or caregivers should take if a child has ingested a toxic substance is to call the National Capital Poison Center and emergency medical services.

QUICK QUIZ

Answer the following multiple-choice questions.

1. What is a common adverse reaction in patients receiving an antihistamine as an antiemetic?
   a. nausea
   b. hallucinations
   c. drowsiness
   d. tachycardia
2. Which of the following is a possible therapeutic use of bismuth subsalicylate?
   a. to prevent nausea from motion sickness
   b. as an adjunct to treatment for active duodenal ulcers
   c. to restore fluids and minerals lost in diarrhea and vomiting
   d. to treat constipation
3. Proton pump inhibitors are used:
   a. to treat erosive esophagitis
   b. to treat symptomatic GERD that doesn't respond to other therapies
   c. for long-term treatment of hypersecretory conditions
   d. all of the above
4. In what circumstances should activated charcoal be used?
   a. soon after ingestion of a toxic substance
   b. for acute poisoning with cyanide
   c. administered at the same time as ipecac syrup
   d. in a patient with a possible GI obstruction
5. Which of the following is a *not* a possible adverse effect for bulk-forming laxatives?
   a. indigestion
   b. esophageal obstruction
   c. gas
   d. severe diarrhea

Please answer each of the following questions in one to three sentences.

1. Describe a successful treatment plan for a patient with ulcers caused by *H. pylori*.

2. How does the action of proton pump inhibitors differ from the action of H_2 receptor antagonists?

3. Why do many antacid products contain both magnesium and aluminum?

4. Briefly explain the difference between hyperosmolar and stimulant laxatives.

5. Identify two situations in which phenothiazines are used as antiemetics.

Answer the following questions as either true or false.

1. ___ Tachycardia is an adverse reaction to opioid-related drugs.
2. ___ Ipecac syrup is a common antiemetic drug.
3. ___ Stool softeners are commonly prescribed after a Caesarean section, an episiotomy, or open heart surgery.
4. ___ Antacids should be taken at the same time as other oral drugs.
5. ___ Different digestive enzyme products shouldn't be substituted without the advice of a physician.

Match the generic name of each drug in the left column with the correct trade name from the right column.

1. lansoprazole   a. Antivert
2. meclizine   b. Gas-X
3. cimetidine   c. Axid
4. simethicone   d. Tagamet HB
5. nizatidine   e. Prevacid

DRUG CLASSIFICATION TABLE

Classification	Generic Name	Trade Name(s)
Antiulcer drugs	lansoprazole *(capsules)*, amoxicillin *(capsules)*, and clarithromycin *(tablets)* combination *lan-soe'-pra-zole a-mox'-i-sill'-in klar-ith-ro-my'-cin*	*tablets and capsules:* Prevpac Daily Administration Pack
	metronidazole *(tablets)*, tetracycline *(capsules)*, and bismuth subsalicylate *(tablets)* combination *meh-trow-nye'-dah-zoll tet-ra-sye'-kleen bis'-muth*	*tablets and capsules:* Helidac Therapy Kit
	bismuth subcitrate potassium, metronidazole, and tetracycline *bis'-muth meh-trow-nye'-dah-zoll tet-ra-sye'-kleen*	*capsules:* Pylera
	cimetidine *sye-met'-i-deen*	*tablets (Rx):* (no longer marketed under trade name) *tablets (OTC):* Tagamet HB *oral solution (Rx):* (no longer marketed under trade name) *oral solution (OTC):* Tagamet HB *injection (Rx):* (no longer marketed under trade name)
	famotidine *fa-moe'-ti-deen*	*powder for oral suspension (Rx):* Pepcid *injection (Rx):* Pepcid *tablets (Rx):* Pepcid *tablets (OTC):* Pepcid AC *chewable tablets (OTC):* Pepcid AC
	famotidine, calcium carbonate, and magnesium hydroxide *fa-moe'-ti-deen kal'-see-um mag-nee'-zee-um*	*chewable tablets:* Pepcid Complete
	nizatidine *ni-za'-ti-deen*	*capsules (Rx):* Axid *oral solution (Rx):* Axid *tablets (OTC):* Axid AR
	ranitidine *ra-nye'-te-deen*	*tablets (Rx):* Zantac *tablets (OTC):* Zantac *capsules (Rx):* (no longer marketed under trade name) *oral solution (Rx):* Zantac *effervescent tablets (Rx):* Zantac Efferdose *injection (Rx):* Zantac
	esomeprazole *ess-oh-me'-pra-zol*	*delayed-release capsules:* Nexium *powder for oral suspension:* Nexium *injection:* Nexium
	lansoprazole *lan-soe'-pra-zole*	*orally disintegrating delayed-release tablets:* Prevacid Solutab *delayed-release capsules:* Prevacid *granules for oral suspension:* Prevacid *injection:* Prevacid IV

continued

DRUG CLASSIFICATION TABLE (continued)

Classification	Generic Name	Trade Name(s)
Antiulcer drugs (continued)	lansoprazole (*capsules*) and naproxen (*tablets*) *lan-soe'-pra-zole na-prox'-en*	Prevacid NapraPAC
	omeprazole *oh-me'-pra-zol*	*delayed-release capsules (Rx):* Prilosec *delayed-release tablets (OTC):* Prilosec OTC
	omeprazole and sodium bicarbonate *oh-me'-pra-zol sow-dee'-um*	*capsules:* Zegerid *powder for oral suspension:* Zegerid
	pantoprazole *pan-toe'-pray-zol*	*delayed-release tablets:* Protonix *granules for oral suspension:* Protonix *injection:* Protonix
	rabeprazole *rah-beh'-pray-zol*	*delayed-release tablets:* Aciphex
	aluminum hydroxide *a-loo'-mi-num*	*oral suspension:* Alternagel
	aluminum hydroxide and magnesium carbonate *a-loo'-mi-num mag-nee'-zee-um*	*chewable tablets:* Gaviscon *oral solution:* Gaviscon *oral suspension:* (no longer marketed under trade name)
	aluminum hydroxide and magnesium hydroxide *a-loo'-mi-num mag-nee'-zee-um*	*oral suspension:* Mylanta Ultimate Strength
	aluminum hydroxide, magnesium hydroxide, and simethicone *a-loo'-mi-num mag-nee'-zee-um sigh-meth'-ih-kohn*	*chewable tablets:* Gelusil *oral suspension:* Maalox, Mylanta, Maalox Max, Mylanta Maximum Strength
	aluminum hydroxide and magnesium trisilicate *a-loo'-mi-num mag-nee'-zee-um*	*chewable tablets:* Gaviscon
	calcium carbonate *kal'-see-um*	*tablets:* Tums Ultra *chewable tablets:* Tums Ultra, Maalox Children's, Maalox Quick Dissolve, Mylanta Children's, Pepto-Bismol Children's, Titralac, Maalox Antacid Barrier Maximum Strength, Tums, Tums Lasting Effects, Tums Cool Relief, Tums E-X, Tums Smooth Dissolve, Tums Smoothies, Alka-Mints *soft chews:* Rolaids Extra Strength *oral suspension:* (no longer marketed under trade name)
	magnesium hydroxide *mag-nee'-zee-um*	*chewable tablets:* Phillips' Milk of Magnesia *soft chews:* Phillips' Laxative *oral suspension:* Ex-Lax Milk of Magnesia, Phillips' Milk of Magnesia
	calcium carbonate and magnesium hydroxide *kal'-see-um mag-nee'-zee-um*	*oral suspension:* Mylanta Supreme *oral tablets:* Mylanta *chewable tablets:* Rolaids, Rolaids Extra Strength, Mylanta Ultra
	calcium carbonate, magnesium hydroxide, simethicone *kal'-see-um mag-nee'-zee-um sigh-meth'-ih-kohn*	*chewable tablets:* Rolaids Multi-Symptom
	misoprostol *mye-soe-prost'-ol*	*tablets:* Cytotec
	sucralfate *soo-kral'-fate*	*tablets:* Carafate *oral suspension:* Carafate

continued

DRUG CLASSIFICATION TABLE (continued)

Classification	Generic Name	Trade Name(s)
Adsorbent drugs	activated charcoal *char'-kole*	*oral suspension:* Actidose-Aqua, EZ Char Pellets, Actidose with Sorbitol *enteric-coated tablets:* Charcoal Plus DS *capsules:* CharcoCaps
Antiflatulent drugs	simethicone *sigh-meth'-ih-kohn*	*chewable tablets:* Gas-X Extra Strength, Mylanta Gas, Phazyme *capsules:* Mylanta Gas, Phazyme *oral drops (solution):* Gas-X *oral drops (suspension):* Mylicon *orally disintegrating strips:* Gas-X
Digestive drugs	pancrelipase *pan-kre-li'-pase*	*delayed-release capsules:* Pancrease, Creon, Lipram, Ultrase, Dygase, Palcaps, Pangestyme, Panocaps, Pancrecarb, Dygase *tablets:* Panokase, Plaretase, Viokase *oral powder:* Viokase
Antidiarrheal drugs	diphenoxylate with atropine *di-fen-ox'-i-late a'-troe-peen*	*tablets:* Lomotil, Lonox *liquid:* Lomotil
	loperamide *loe-per'-a-mide*	*capsules (Rx):* (no longer marketed under trade name) *tablets (OTC):* Imodium A-D *oral suspension (OTC):* Imodium A-D *fast dissolving tablets (OTC):* Imodium A-D
	loperamide and simethicone *loe-per'-a-mide sigh-meth'-ih-kohn*	*caplets:* Imodium Advanced *chewable tablets:* Imodium Advanced
	alosetron *a-loe'-se-tron*	*tablets:* Lotronex
	bismuth subsalicylate *bis'-muth*	*tablets:* Kaopectate, Pepto-Bismol *chewable tablets:* Pepto-Bismol *oral suspension:* Kaopectate, Pepto-Bismol, Maalox Total Stomach Relief
Laxative drugs	glycerin *gli'-ser-in*	*rectal suppositories:* Colace *liquid suppositories:* Fleet Babylax *oral solution:* (no longer marketed under trade name)
	lactulose *lak'-tyoo-los*	*oral solution:* Acilac, Constulose, Cephulac, Enulose
	magnesium citrate *mag-nee'-zee-um*	*oral solution:* (no longer marketed under trade name)
	magnesium hydroxide *mag-nee'-zee-um*	*chewable tablets:* Phillips' Milk of Magnesia *soft chews:* Phillips' Laxative *oral suspension:* Ex-Lax Milk of Magnesia, Phillips' Milk of Magnesia
	sodium phosphate and sodium biphosphate *sow-dee'-um*	*oral tablets:* Osmo Prep, Visicol *oral solution:* no longer marketed under trade name *enema:* (no longer marketed under trade name)

continued

DRUG CLASSIFICATION TABLE *(continued)*

Classification	Generic Name	Trade Name(s)
Laxative drugs *(continued)*	polyethylene glycol *pol-e-eth'-i-leen*	*powder to be dissolved in water (Rx):* GlycoLax *powder to be dissolved in water (OTC):* MiraLax
	polyethylene glycol and electrolyte solution *pol-e-eth'-i-leen*	*powder for oral solution:* MoviPrep, GoLYTELY, NuLYTELY, TriLyte, Colyte
	polyethylene glycol with electrolytes *(powder for oral solution)* and bisacodyl *(tablets) pol-e-eth'-i-leen bis-a-koe'-dill*	*Delayed-Release Tablet Bowel Prep Kit:* HalfLytely and Bisacodyl
	methylcellulose *meth-ill-sell'-yoo-lose*	*tablets:* Citrucel *powder to be mixed with liquid:* Citrucel
	polycarbophil *pol-i-kar'-boe-fil*	*tablets:* Fibercon *chewable tablets:* Equalactin
	psyllium *sill'-i-um*	*powder for oral suspension:* Reguloid, GenFiber, Hydrocil, Metamucil *oral suspension:* Reguloid *chewable bar:* Metamucil *capsules:* Metamucil, GenFiber
	psyllium and calcium carbonate *sill'-i-um kal'-see-um*	*capsules:* Metamucil Plus Calcium
	docusate calcium *dok'-yoo-sate*	*capsules:* Sur-Q-Lax, Kaopectate
	docusate sodium *dok'-yoo-sate*	*capsules:* Colace, Correctol, Dulcolax, Phillips' Stool Softener, DocuLace, Doc-Q-Lace *oral solution:* Colace, Doc-Q-Lace, Diocto *oral suspension:* (no longer marketed under trade name) *syrup:* Silace, Colace, Diocto
	bisacodyl *bis-a-koe'-dill*	*tablets:* Dulcolax, Ex-Lax Ultra *capsules:* Doxidan *enteric-coated tablets:* Doxidan *rectal suppository:* Dulcolax
	cascara sagrada *kass-kar'-a sa-grad'-a*	*liquid:* (no longer marketed under trade name)
	castor oil *kas'-tor*	*liquid:* (no longer marketed under trade name)
	senna *sen'-a*	*tablets:* Black Draught, Ex-Lax, Perdiem, Senokot *chewable tablets:* Ex-Lax *syrup:* Black Draught *oral solution:* Fletcher's Laxative
	senna and docusate sodium *sen'-a dok'-yoo-sate*	*tablets:* Doc-Q-Lax, Peri-Colace, Senokot-S
	mineral oil *mihn'-er-uhl*	*oil to be administered orally or by enema:* (no longer marketed under trade name)

continued

DRUG CLASSIFICATION TABLE (continued)

Classification	Generic Name	Trade Name(s)
Antiemetic drugs	cyclizine hydrochloride *sye'-kli-zeen*	*tablets:* Marezine
	dimenhydrinate *dye-men-hye'-dri-nate*	*tablets (OTC):* Dramamine
		chewable tablets (OTC): Dramamine
		injection (Rx): (no longer marketed under trade name)
	diphenhydramine hydrochloride *dye-fen-hye'-dra-meen*	*tablets:* Simply Sleep, Sominex, Nytol
		chewable tablets: (no longer marketed under trade name)
		capsules: Nytol, Unisom Sleepgels
		orally disintegrating film: (no longer marketed under trade name)
		oral solution: Benadryl Allergy, PediaCare Night-time Cough
		oral suspension: (no longer marketed under trade name)
		syrup: (no longer marketed under trade name)
		orally dissolving tablets: (no longer marketed under trade name)
		elixir: (no longer marketed under trade name)
		injection (Rx): (no longer marketed under trade name)
	hydroxyzine *high-drox'-ih-zeen*	*tablets:* (no longer marketed under trade name)
		capsules: Vistaril
		oral solution: (no longer marketed under trade name)
		injection: (no longer marketed under trade name)
	meclizine *mek'-li-zeen*	*tablets (Rx):* Antivert
		tablets (OTC): Dramamine Less Drowsy Formula
		chewable tablets: (OTC): Bonine
	trimethobenzamide *trye-meth-oh-ben'-za-mide*	*capsules:* Tigan
		injection: Tigan
	chlorpromazine *klor-proe'-ma-zeen*	*tablets:* (no longer marketed under trade name)
		injection: (no longer marketed under trade name)
	perphenazine *per-fen'-a-zeen*	*tablets:* (no longer marketed under trade name)
	prochlorperazine *proe-klor-per'-a-zeen*	*tablets:* (no longer marketed under trade name)
		rectal suppositories: Compro
		injection: (no longer marketed under trade name)
	promethazine *proe-meth'-a-zeen*	*tablets:* (no longer marketed under trade name)
		oral solution: (no longer marketed under trade name)
		rectal suppositories: Phenadoz
		injection: Phenergan

continued

DRUG CLASSIFICATION TABLE (continued)

Classification	Generic Name	Trade Name(s)
Antiemetic drugs (continued)	dolasetron *doe-laz-e'-tron*	*tablets:* Anzemet *injection:* Anzemet
	granisetron *gran-iz'-e-tron*	*tablets:* Kytril *oral solution:* Granisol *injection:* Kytril
	ondansetron *on-dan'-sa-tron*	*tablets:* Zofran *orally disintegrating tablets:* Zofran ODT *oral solution:* Zofran *injection:* Zofran
Emetic drugs	ipecac syrup *ip'-e-kak*	*syrup:* (no longer marketed under trade name)

Anti-Infective Drugs

- Match brand and generic names of commonly used anti-infective drugs
- Identify the classification of commonly used anti-infective drugs
- Explain why resistance to antimicrobial drugs is increasing
- Explain the difference between bactericidal and bacteriostatic
- List serious adverse reactions to aminoglycosides
- Identify and justify anti-infective alternatives for patients who are allergic to penicillins, cephalosporins, or erythromycins
- List typical symptoms of a hypersensitivity reaction to commonly used anti-infectives
- List the general cautions and interactions that a patient should be aware of when taking a tetracycline, a fluoroquinolone, or a sulfonamide
- Compare the use of vancomycin with other anti-infectives
- Identify the uses of commonly used antivirals
- Explain the parameters for starting antiviral treatment for a patient with influenza
- Describe a typical treatment regimen for a patient being treated for HIV
- List the four-drug regimen recommended for initial treatment of tuberculosis
- Match the antifungal drugs with the conditions they are used to treat
- Identify the antifungal drugs that are available over the counter

KEY TERMS

aerobic bacteria—bacteria requiring oxygen to live

anaerobic bacteria—bacteria able to live without oxygen

antibacterial drugs—see *antibiotics*

antibiotics—natural or synthetic substances that kill or inhibit the growth of bacteria; also known as *antibacterial drugs*

antifungal drugs—drugs used to fight infections by various types of fungi; also known as *antimycotic drugs*

antimycotic drugs—see *antifungal drugs*

antiretroviral drugs—a group of antiviral drugs that are used to treat HIV infections

antitubercular drugs—drugs used to treat active cases of tuberculosis

bacteria—groups of round, spiral, or rod-shaped single-celled microorganisms that may live in soil, in water, and in dead or living organisms; usually live in colonies; can have beneficial or harmful (pathogenic) effects on humans

bactericidal—able to destroy bacteria

bacteriostatic—able to slow the multiplication of bacteria

bolus—the IV injection of a large amount of drug in a short amount of time, usually by syringe through a port in an existing IV line

diluent—fluid used to dilute a drug that is being reconstituted

fungicidal—able to destroy fungi

fungistatic—able to slow the multiplication of fungi

microbe—see *microorganism*

microorganism—a living thing, such as a virus or bacterium, that is too small to be seen with the naked eye

pathogen—a disease-causing microorganism

penicillinase—an enzyme that renders penicillin inactive

protozoa—any of a large group of moving, usually microscopic, single-celled organisms that are found throughout the environment that are pathogens in animals and humans

resistance—a microbe's ability to live and grow in the presence of an antimicrobial drug

virus—an infectious microorganism that is capable of growth and multiplication only in living cells and that causes various diseases in humans, animals, and plants

The human body is full of **bacteria**. Many of these bacteria are harmless or even beneficial. But other bacteria can cause disease. In this chapter, you'll learn about classes of drugs that are used to fight harmful bacteria that infect the body. You'll also learn about other drugs that combat **viruses**—infectious microorganisms capable of growth and multiplication—and fungi that also infect the body and cause harm.

SELECTING AN ANTIMICROBIAL DRUG

Antimicrobial drugs are used to kill pathogens. A **pathogen** is a disease-causing **microorganism**, an organism such as a bacterium or virus that is too small to be seen by the naked eye. Another term for microorganism is **microbe**.

In selecting the right drug to combat a microbial infection, several important factors must be considered, including:

- *The type of pathogen responsible for the infection.* The microbe is generally identified by growing a culture of it in a medical laboratory.
- *The pathogen's susceptibility to various drugs.* The culture is generally exposed to various drugs to see which ones kill the microorganism.
- *The location of the infection.* For therapy to be effective, an adequate concentration of the drug must reach the infection site.
- *The drug's cost, its potential adverse effects, and possible patient allergies.* Once the pathogen and location of the infection have been identified, these additional factors can help a physician choose the drug to best fit the patient's needs.

T I P Determining a microbe's drug sensitivity can take up to 48 hours, although some tests can be done in the physician's office with faster results. Treatment begins immediately and is adjusted, if necessary, when the sensitivity test results are in.

The usefulness of an antimicrobial drug is limited to the resistance that microorganisms may develop to the drug's action. **Resistance** is a microbe's ability to live and grow in the presence of an antimicrobial drug. It generally results from the genetic mutation of the microorganism.

ANTIBACTERIAL DRUGS

Antibacterial drugs are also called **antibiotics**, drugs that inhibit the growth of bacteria. An antibiotic drug may be **bacteriostatic** (slowing the growth or multiplication of a type of bacteria) or **bactericidal** (killing a type of bacteria).

The various classes of antibiotic drugs include:

- aminoglycosides
- penicillins
- cephalosporins
- tetracyclines
- lincomycin derivatives
- macrolides
- vancomycin
- carbapenems
- monobactams
- fluoroquinolones
- sulfonamides
- nitrofurantoin (nitrofuran)

Aminoglycosides

Aminoglycosides provide effective bactericidal activity against the following types of microbes:

- gram-negative bacilli bacteria
- some **aerobic** (oxygen-requiring) gram-positive bacteria
- mycobacteria
- some **protozoa** (any of a large group of moving, usually microscopic, single-celled organisms that are found throughout the environment that are pathogens in animals and humans)

Aminoglycosides do not work against **anaerobic bacteria**, however. Anaerobic bacteria do not need oxygen to survive.

T I P "Gram-positive" and "gram-negative" refer to the type of stain that highlights microbes on a slide when identifying them under a microscope.

However, because these drugs are absorbed poorly from the GI tract, they're usually given parenterally, by IV or IM injection. As with many IV drugs, IV injection can be either of two methods:

- *By infusion.* A bag of solution containing the drug is infused to a vein drop by drop over a long period of time.
- *By bolus.* The drug is injected from a syringe into a port in an existing IV line, either all at once or over a short period of time. A **bolus** is sometimes called an IV push.

Of course, IM injections place the drug directly into tissue rather than into the bloodstream.

Some gram-positive bacteria resist aminoglycosides' bactericidal effect. But when penicillin is used along with an aminoglycoside, it increases the aminoglycoside's effectiveness.

Each aminoglycoside is useful only against specific kinds of bacteria. But as a group, they are used in treating these conditions:

- infections caused by gram-negative bacilli
- urinary tract infections (UTIs) caused by bacteria that are resistant to less toxic antibiotics, such as penicillins and cephalosporins

- infections of the central nervous system (CNS) and eyes
- bacteremia (the abnormal presence of microbes in the bloodstream)
- peritonitis (inflammation of the peritoneum—the membrane that lines the abdominal cavity)
- pneumonia in critically ill patients

Aminoglycosides must always be administered with caution because a number of adverse reactions and drug interactions can occur. For example, these drugs may cause ototoxicity (damage to the organs or nerves affecting hearing and balance). Varying degrees of hearing loss may occur, which may be irreversible. This risk increases when loop diuretics are taken with aminoglycosides. In addition, taking antiemetic drugs with aminoglycosides may mask the symptoms of ototoxicity.

Aminoglycosides may also be toxic to the neurologic system, causing neurotoxicity (peripheral neuropathy with numbness and tingling of the extremities). Aminoglycosides may be toxic to the kidneys as well and may cause nephrotoxicity (renal failure). This risk increases when cyclosporine, amphotericin B, or acyclovir is taken with the following aminoglycosides:

- amikacin
- gentamicin
- kanamycin
- tobramycin

Here are some other drug interactions that apply to these four aminoglycosides, as well as to neomycin and streptomycin:

- The effects of these drugs are reduced if they are taken with the penicillins carbenicillin or ticarcillin. This is especially true if the aminoglycoside and the penicillin are mixed in the same container or IV line.
- Giving these drugs to patients taking neuromuscular blockers will increase neuromuscular blockade. Increased muscular relaxation and respiratory distress can result.

PROCEED WITH CAUTION

Adverse Reactions to Aminoglycosides

Serious adverse reactions limit the use of aminoglycosides. These reactions include:

- neurotoxicity
- ototoxicity
- nephrotoxicity

Additional adverse reactions to oral aminoglycosides include:

- nausea and vomiting
- diarrhea

Gentamicin

Gentamicin is available in several different forms, including:

- a solution for injection
- a topical ointment
- a topical cream
- an ophthalmic solution (Gentak)
- an ophthalmic ointment (Gentak)

Gentamicin is also available in combination with prednisolone as an ophthalmic ointment and suspension. This combination drug is sold under the brand name Pred-G.

The solution may be given via IV infusion or as a direct IM injection. The solution form is used to combat serious infections caused by certain bacteria. It is also given before certain procedures or surgeries to prevent endocarditis, an inflammation of the heart lining and valves.

Neomycin

Neomycin is available as tablets. Its major use is to combat infectious diarrhea caused by *Escherichia coli* bacteria and to suppress intestinal bacteria before surgery.

Neomycin is also available in combination with other drugs for topical, otic and ophthalmic use, as well as irrigation. These combination drugs are manufactured under various brand names, and include the following dosage forms:

- a topical ointment, lotion, and cream for local use (Cortisporin, Triple Antibiotic, Neosporin)
- an ophthalmic ointment, suspension, and solution (Maxitrol, AK-Trol, Neosporin, Poly-Pred)
- an otic solution and suspension (Cortisporin, Aural Otic, Oticin HC, Otimar, Otocidin, Cortomycin, Oticin HC, Otimar, Pediotic)
- an irrigation solution used to flush out the genitourinary (GU) tract (Neosporin GU)

Tobramycin

Tobramycin is available in several different forms, including:

- solution for injection
- ophthalmic ointment and solution (AK-Tob, Tobrex)
- nebulizer solution for inhalation (Tobi)

In combination with other drugs, it's manufactured in the form of an ophthalmic suspension and ointment (Tobradex, Zylet). Tobramycin is used against *Pseudomonas* species, *E. coli* infections, and serious infections caused by other bacteria.

T I P Be careful not to confuse tobramycin (Tobrex) with the combination drug tobramycin and dexamethason (Tobradex).

Other Aminoglycosides

Other aminoglycosides include:

- amikacin (Amikin)—injection used to treat serious infections and UTIs that don't respond to less toxic drugs; also used to treat tuberculosis
- kanamycin—injection
- paramomycin—oral capsule used to treat amoebic infections in the intestines
- streptomycin—injection used to treat various kinds of endocarditis; also used to treat tuberculosis

Penicillins

Although many other antibacterials are now available, penicillins remain one of the most important and useful classes of antibiotics. These drugs are usually bactericidal in action.

No other class of antibiotics provides as wide of a spectrum of antimicrobial activity as penicillins do. Specific penicillins are only effective against certain organisms. But as a class, they cover gram-positive, gram-negative, and anaerobic organisms.

Most penicillins can be given orally or by IM injection. Absorption of oral penicillin varies, depending on such factors as:

- the specific penicillin drug that is used
- the pH level of the patient's stomach and intestine (pH is a measure of acidity or alkalinity)
- the presence of food in the GI tract

Most penicillins should be taken on an empty stomach (one hour before or two hours after a meal) to increase absorption.

Penicillins are usually given by IM injection only when oral administration is inconvenient or when the patient cannot be counted on to take the drug properly by mouth. However, some long-acting penicillin must be administered via the IM route because they are very slowly absorbed.

Large doses of intravenous penicillins can increase the bleeding risk of anticoagulants by prolonging bleeding time. Here are some other important general drug interactions that involve penicillin:

- Probenecid increases the blood concentration of penicillins.
- Tetracyclines and chloramphenicol reduce the bactericidal action of penicillins.
- Penicillins reduce tubular secretion of methotrexate in the kidneys. This increases the risk of methotrexate toxicity.

Natural Penicillins

The molds that were originally identified and studied in the 1930s are known as natural penicillins. They have been used in treating infectious diseases for many years. As a

PROCEED WITH CAUTION

Adverse Reactions to Penicillins

Hypersensitivity reactions are the major adverse reactions to penicillins. These reactions may include:

- anaphylactic reactions such as itching, hives, and respiratory distress
- serum sickness
- drug fever
- various rashes

Adverse reactions associated with oral penicillins include:

- tongue inflammation
- nausea and vomiting
- diarrhea

Aminopenicillins and extended-spectrum penicillins can cause pseudomembranous colitis (diarrhea caused by a change in the flora of the colon or an overgrowth of a toxin-producing microbe).

result, over time, drug-resistant strains of some bacteria have developed. In addition, natural penicillins have a fairly narrow spectrum of activity. This means that they are effective against only a few strains of bacteria.

For these reasons, scientists have chemically altered some penicillin to produce new, more effective antibiotics. These other types of penicillins are discussed below.

Penicillin G

Penicillin G benzathine (Bicillin L-A) is administered in solution as an IM injection. Its main use is in treating syphilis and streptococcal upper respiratory tract infections and in preventing cholera and rheumatic fever.

Penicillin G potassium (Pfizerpen) is produced as a solution that is administered by IV or IM injection. It is used in treating moderate to severe systemic infections and to treat anthrax.

Penicillin G procaine is a solution that is administered by IM injection. It has the same uses as penicillin G potassium. Penicillin G benzathine and procaine are combined in an injection solution under the trade name of Bicillin C-R.

Penicillin G sodium is a solution that can be delivered by IM or IV injection. It is used to treat moderate to severe systemic infections and to treat neurologic syphilis, an advanced form of the disease.

Penicillin VK

Penicillin VK, often called pen VK, is available in tablet and oral solution form. It is used:

- to treat mild to moderate systemic infections
- to treat Lyme disease, an infection caused by ticks who carry the disease

- to prevent recurrent rheumatic fever
- to prevent inhalation of anthrax after possible exposure to anthrax spores

Female patients of childbearing age should be made aware that the effectiveness of hormonal contraceptives is reduced while they are taking penicillin VK. Also, neomycin increases the absorption of this antibiotic.

T I P Most penicillins end in the letters *-cillin*.

Penicillinase-Resistant Penicillins

As you learned earlier in this chapter, strains of bacteria have developed that are resistant to natural penicillins. One example of this resistance is some bacteria's ability to produce **penicillinase**, an enzyme that renders penicillins inactive. To overcome this problem, penicillinase-resistant penicillins have been developed. These include:

- dicloxacillin—capsule used to treat infections by penicillinase-producing staphylococcal bacteria
- nafcillin—injection used to treat staphylococcal infections, meningitis, certain types of osteomyelitis and heart-valve endocarditis
- oxacillin—injection

Dicloxacillin and nafcillin can cause resistance to warfarin. Oxacillin may cause liver toxicity.

T I P Reconstituted antibiotics have very specific reconstitution directions. It's your responsibility to make sure you are adding the correct amount of **diluent** (fluid used to dilute the drug) each time you reconstitute a medication.

Aminopenicillins

Like penicillinase-resistant penicillins, aminopenicillins have been chemically altered to prevent resistant bacteria from destroying the drug. But aminopenicillins are active against a wider range of bacteria than are penicillinase-resistant penicillins.

Amoxicillin

Amoxicillin is manufactured as oral capsules, conventional tablets, chewable tablets, and as a powder for oral suspension. It is mainly used in treating:

- ear, nose, throat, and sinus infections
- lower respiratory tract infections
- GU tract infections
- uncomplicated gonorrhea

Amoxicillin is also used to prevent endocarditis in patients having dental, oral, respiratory tract, GI, or GU procedures.

Amoxicillin and Clavulanate Potassium

Amoxicillin and clavulanate potassium (Augmentin, Augmentin XR) is amoxicillin mixed with clavulanic acid. It's available as tablets, chewable tablets, extended-release tablets, and a powder for oral suspension. This antibiotic is used to treat recurring ear infections as well as sinus, skin, and lower respiratory tract infections and UTIs. It's also used in treating pneumonia.

T I P When a physician prescribes amoxicillin and clavulanate potassium, the dosage form is especially important. Although one teaspoon of the oral suspension may contain the same amount of amoxicillin as one chewable tablet, the amount of clavulanic acid won't necessarily be the same.

Ampicillin

Ampicillin is administered by mouth in the form of capsules and oral suspension or by injection. It's used in treating:

- respiratory tract infections
- skin infections
- GI infections
- UTIs
- uncomplicated gonorrhea
- bacterial meningitis
- septicemia (a systemic infection of the blood, which is also called blood poisoning)

Like amoxicillin, this drug is also used to prevent endocarditis in patients having dental, GI, or GU procedures.

Advise female patients who are taking hormonal contraceptives that ampicillin reduces the effectiveness of these drugs.

Ampicillin and Sulbactam

The combination drug ampicillin and sulbactam (Unasyn) is administered by injection. It is used to treat skin infections, intra-abdominal infections, and gynecological infections.

Extended-Spectrum Penicillins

These drugs were developed to increase effectiveness against certain microbes. They are also effective against a wider range of bacteria than aminopenicillins. However, high doses of extended-spectrum penicillins inactivate aminoglycoside drugs.

Ticarcillin and Clavulanate Potassium

The combination product ticarcillin and clavulanate potassium (Timentin) is administered by injection. This drug is used to treat a number of infections, such as:

- septicemia
- lower respiratory tract infections
- bone and joint infections
- skin infections
- UTIs
- gynecologic infections
- intra-abdominal infections

Cephalosporins

Many of the antibacterial drugs introduced for clinical use in recent years have been cephalosporins. Like penicillins, cephalosporins are bactericidal.

Many cephalosporins aren't absorbed from the GI tract. These drugs are administered parenterally. Other cephalosporins can be administered orally; however, food usually decreases their absorption rate (although not the amount absorbed). Two cephalosporins (oral cefuroxime and cefpodoxime) actually have increased absorption when taken with food.

Patients who drink alcoholic beverages with cephalosporins or within 72 hours of taking a dose may experience acute alcohol intolerance. Symptoms may include:

- headache
- dizziness
- flushing
- nausea
- vomiting
- abdominal cramps

These symptoms may occur within 30 minutes of drinking alcohol. They also can occur up to three days after discontinuing the antibiotic.

Because penicillins and cephalosporins are chemically similar, cross-sensitivity occurs in 3 to 16 percent of patients.

! PROCEED WITH CAUTION

Adverse Reactions to Cephalosporins

Hypersensitivity reactions are the most common adverse reactions to cephalosporins. These reactions include:

- hives
- itching
- measles-like rash
- serum sickness
- anaphylaxis (in rare cases)

Other adverse reactions may include:

- confusion
- seizures
- bleeding
- nausea and vomiting
- diarrhea

The use of some cephalosporins can lead to an increased risk of bleeding. Patients with renal impairment, liver disease, or impaired vitamin K synthesis or storage are at greatest risk. This concern applies to the following cephalosporins:

- cefmetazole
- cefoperazone
- cefotetan
- ceftriaxone

This means that someone who has a reaction to penicillin is also at risk for a reaction to cephalosporins.

Cephalosporins are grouped into four "generations" according to their development, characteristics, and effectiveness against certain organisms.

First-Generation Cephalosporins

First-generation cephalosporins act mainly against gram-positive organisms. They may be used as alternative therapy in patients who are allergic to penicillin, depending on their level of sensitivity. They're also used to threat staphylococcal and streptococcal infections, including:

- pneumonia
- cellulitis (skin infection)
- osteomyelitis (bone infection)

Cefadroxil

Cefadroxil is available in capsules and tablets. It's also manufactured as a fruit-flavored powder for oral suspension. This drug is used to treat UTIs, skin infections, and tonsillitis or pharyngitis (commonly known as a sore throat).

Cefazolin

Cefazolin is a powder that is mixed with sterile water and then administered by IM injection or IV infusion. It's used to treat a wide variety of infections. Cefazolin is also given before and after some surgeries to help prevent infections that might result from the surgery.

Cephalexin

Cephalexin (Keflex, Panixine) is available as oral capsules and tablets and as a powder for oral suspension. This drug is mainly used to treat skin and bone infections, ear infections, GU tract infections, and respiratory tract infections.

Second-Generation Cephalosporins

Second-generation cephalosporins act against gram-negative bacteria. Only two of these cephalosporins, cefotetan and cefoxitin, are effective against anaerobic organisms.

Cefaclor

Cefaclor (Raniclor) is available as single-dose capsules, extended-release tablets, chewable tablets, and a fruit-flavored powder for oral suspension. The extended-release tablets provide a treatment for pharyngitis and tonsillitis, uncomplicated skin infections, and bacterial infections related to chronic bronchitis. The other dosage forms are used to treat ear infections, UTIs, lower respiratory tract infections, pharyngitis, and tonsillitis.

T I P Cephalosporins are easily recognizable. Most of these drug names begin with the letters *cef-* or *ceph-*.

Cefuroxime

Cefuroxime axetil (Ceftin) is supplied as tablets and as a powder for oral suspension, which is fruit flavored. This

HOW IT WORKS

How Cephalosporins Attack Bacteria

The antibacterial action of cephalosporins depends on their ability to penetrate the bacterial cell wall and bind with proteins on the cytoplasmic membrane. The process by which the drug kills the bacteria is illustrated in figure 9-1.

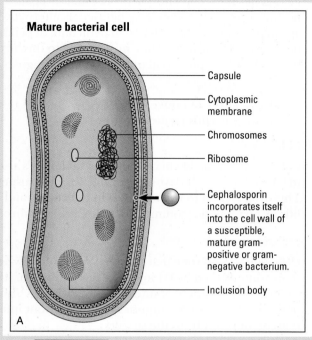

Mature bacterial cell

- Capsule
- Cytoplasmic membrane
- Chromosomes
- Ribosome
- Cephalosporin incorporates itself into the cell wall of a susceptible, mature gram-positive or gram-negative bacterium.
- Inclusion body

A

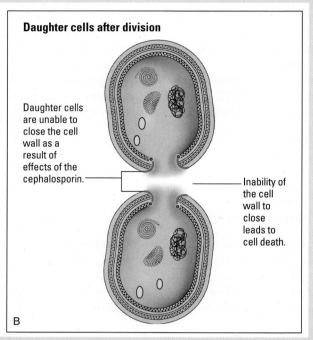

Daughter cells after division

Daughter cells are unable to close the cell wall as a result of effects of the cephalosporin.

Inability of the cell wall to close leads to cell death.

B

FIGURE 9-1 Mature bacterial cell (A) and daughter cells after division (B). (From *Clinical Pharmacology Made Incredibly Easy*. 2nd Ed. Philadelphia, PA: Lippincott Williams & Wilkins; 2005.)

drug is used mainly to treat ear and skin infections, pharyngitis, and tonsillitis. In addition, the tablets are prescribed for the treatment of sinus infections, UTIs, bronchitis, gonorrhea, and the early stages of Lyme disease.

Cefuroxime sodium (Zinacef) is available as a powder for solution or premixed solution that can be administered by IM injection, IV infusion, or injection into an existing IV line (IV push). This drug is used to treat UTIs, skin infections, bone and joint infections, gonorrhea, meningitis, and septicemia.

Other Second-Generation Cephalosporins

- cefotetan (Cefotan)—solution and injection used to treat bone and joint infections, pelvic inflammatory disease, and UTIs
- cefprozil (Cefzil)—tablets and powder for oral suspension used to treat ear, sinus, and skin infections; tonsilitis; and acute bronchitis
- ceftibuten (Cedax)—capsules and powder for oral suspension used to treat ear infections, bronchitis, tonsillitis, and pharyngitis
- cefoxitin—injection used to treat a wide variety of infections and to prevent infection in patients undergoing GI surgery, a hysterectomy, or a cesarean section

TIP A person with an allergy to penicillin may be allergic to cephalosporins, too. In cases like this, always make sure the pharmacist is aware of the patient's allergy.

Third-Generation Cephalosporins

Third-generation cephalosporins mainly act against gram-negative organisms. They are the drugs of choice for infections caused by:

- *Enterobacter* bacteria
- *Pseudomonas aeruginosa* bacteria
- anaerobic organisms

Cefdinir

Cefdinir (Omnicef) is supplied as capsules and as a powder for oral suspension. It's prescribed to treat pneumonia, bronchitis, sinus infections, skin infections, pharyngitis, and tonsillitis.

Cefotaxime

Cefotaxime (Claforan) is available as a premeasured powder that must be mixed in solution before being administered as an IM injection or by IV infusion. It's also offered as a premixed solution for IV administration. This drug is used to treat a wide variety of infections. In addition, cefotaxime is used to prevent infection during certain surgeries.

Cefpodoxime

Cefpodoxime (Vantin) is supplied as tablets and as granules that must be mixed with distilled water to create an oral suspension. It's used to treat skin infections, ear and sinus infections, pharyngitis and tonsillitis, pneumonia, bronchitis, UTIs, and gonorrhea.

Ceftazidime

Ceftazidime (Fortaz, Tazicef) is a powder for mixing to create a solution for IV or IM injection. A premixed solution is also available. This drug is used against a number of gynecological, abdominal, lower respiratory tract, skin, bone, joint, and CNS infections, as well as to treat UTIs.

Other Third-Generation Cephalosporins

Other third-generation cephalosporins with the same uses as ceftazidime include:

- ceftizoxime (Cefizox)—injection
- ceftriaxone (Rocephin)—injection

Fourth-Generation Cephalosporins

Fourth-generation cephalosporins are the most recently developed drugs in this class. They are active against many gram-positive and gram-negative bacteria.

Cefditoren

Cefditoren (Spectracef) is supplied as tablets. Like some other cephalosporins, this drug should be taken with meals. It's used in treating skin infections, chronic bronchitis, pneumonia, pharyngitis, and tonsillitis.

Cefepime

Cefepime (Maxipime) is supplied as a powder to be mixed with fluid to create a solution for IV administration. After being mixed with sterile water or some other appropriate fluid, the resulting solution can be injected intramuscularly or "piggybacked" on an existing IV line to be delivered along with another therapy. This drug is mainly used to treat complicated or moderate to severe UTIs, abdominal infections, and pneumonia.

Tetracyclines

Tetracyclines are primarily bacteriostatic, meaning they inhibit the growth or multiplication of bacteria. This class of drugs provides a broad spectrum of activity against the following types of microorganisms:

- gram-positive and gram-negative aerobic and anaerobic bacteria
- spirochetes
- mycoplasma
- rickettsiae
- chlamydiae
- some protozoa

Tetracyclines have a number of uses:

- They treat Rocky Mountain spotted fever, Q fever, and Lyme disease.
- They're the drugs of choice in treating GU infections caused by *Chlamydia* and *Ureaplasma* species.
- Taken in combination with streptomycin, they're the most effective treatment for brucellosis, a disease resulting from contact with infected animals or by consuming milk or meat from infected animals.
- Taken in low doses, they are an effective treatment for acne.

This class of drugs is organized into two groups:

- intermediate-acting compounds, such as demeclocycline hydrochloride
- long-acting compounds, such as doxycycline hyclate and minocycline hydrochloride

The long-acting compounds doxycycline and minocycline provide more action against various organisms than other tetracyclines.

Taking tetracyclines can reduce the effectiveness of hormonal contraceptives. Patients taking contraceptives should use another reliable method of contraception. Breakthrough bleeding may also occur. Other interactions commonly affect the ability of tetracycline to move through the body.

- Aluminum, calcium, and magnesium reduce the absorption of oral tetracyclines.
- Iron salts, bismuth subsalicylate, and zinc sulfate reduce the absorption of doxycycline, oxytetracycline, and tetracycline. This interaction can be prevented by separating doses of tetracyclines and these agents by two to three hours.
- Barbiturates, carbamazepine, and phenytoin increase the metabolism and reduce the effects of doxycycline.
- Except for doxycycline and minocycline, milk and milk products may bind to tetracyclines and prevent their absorption. This effect may be avoided if the drugs are administered one hour before or two hours after meals.

T I P Taking tetracyclines may decrease the bactericidal action of penicillin.

Doxycycline

Doxycycline is manufactured in a variety of dosage forms, which differ with each drug compound. Doxycycline hyclate is available in the following forms:

- injection
- powder for injection solution (Doxy)
- capsules and extended-release capsules (Vibramycin, Oraxyl)
- tablets and extended-release tablets (Vibra-Tabs, Alodox, Periostat, Doryx)

PROCEED WITH CAUTION

Adverse Reactions to Tetracyclines

Tetracyclines produce many of the same adverse reactions as other antibacterial drugs. These include:

- superinfection (the overgrowth of resistant organisms)
- nausea and vomiting
- abdominal distress and distention
- diarrhea

Other adverse reactions include:

- photosensitivity reactions (red rash on areas exposed to sunlight)
- liver toxicity
- renal toxicity

PROCEED WITH CAUTION

Adverse Reactions to Lincomycin Derivatives

Lincomycin derivatives may cause pseudomembranous colitis (a condition marked by severe diarrhea), which may lead to abdominal pain, fever, and mucus and blood in the stool. This syndrome can be fatal. If these symptoms occur, the drug should be discontinued immediately and followed with aggressive fluid and electrolyte management. Other less serious adverse reactions to lincomycin derivatives include:

- diarrhea
- stomatitis (inflammation of the mouth)
- nausea and vomiting
- hypersensitivity reactions

Doxycycline monohydrate is supplied as:

- capsules and biphasic capsules (Monodox, Adoxa, Oracea)
- tablets (Adoxa)
- oral suspension (Vibramycin)

Doxycycline calcium (Vibramycin) is available in the form of an oral suspension.

Minocycline

Minocycline is supplied as:

- single-dose capsules (Dynacin, Minocin)
- single-dose and extended-release tablets (Dynacin, Myrac, Solodyn)
- periodontal powder (for dental use) (Arestin)

Other Tetracyclines

The following tetracyclines should be taken with plenty of fluids:

- demeclocycline (Declomycin)—tablets
- tetracycline—capsules

In addition, food and some dairy products may interfere with the body's absorption of these drugs.

TIP Tetracyclines have many interactions with other drugs and food. Each bottle that is dispensed should have multiple auxiliary labels, including: take on an empty stomach; no iron or dairy products; no antacids.

Lincomycin Derivatives

Lincomycin derivatives are bacteriostatic. They're effective against many gram-positive and gram-negative organisms.

Lincomycin derivatives are sometimes used to treat staphylococcal infections in patients who are allergic to penicillin. But because they can cause serious toxicity and other serious adverse reactions, they generally aren't used unless there's no effective and safer antibiotic available.

Drugs in this class also have neuromuscular blocking properties. They may enhance the action of neuromuscular blockers, which can lead to profound respiratory depression.

Clindamycin

Clindamycin (Cleocin) is supplied as capsules, as granules for oral solution (for pediatric use), and as a solution for IM or IV administration. In addition, it's available in topical forms (Cleocin T, Clinda-Derm, Clindamax, Evoclin), such as pledgets (small pads or compresses that may be used to apply medication to the skin), solution, lotion, gel, and foam, which are used to treat acne. Clindamycin is also supplied as vaginal suppositories (Cleocin Ovules) and cream (Cleocin, Clindamax, Clindesse) to treat bacterial vaginosis (an infection caused by a disruption of the normal balance of bacteria in the vagina).

At therapeutic concentrations, clindamycin is bacteriostatic against most organisms. It is potent against most gram-positive organisms, including staphylococci, pneumococci, and most streptococci. This drug is also effective against many anaerobes and is used primarily to treat anaerobic intra-abdominal and lung infections.

Lincomycin

Lincomycin (Lincocin) is available as a solution for IM injection or IV infusion. This drug is less effective than clindamycin and is rarely used.

Lincomycin shouldn't be administered for minor infections. It is only indicated for serious respiratory or skin infections in patients who are allergic to other antibiotics that could be used.

Macrolides

Macrolides are used to treat a number of infections. These drugs are bacteriostatic and work in much the same manner as clindamycin.

PROCEED WITH CAUTION

Adverse Reactions to Macrolides

Erythromycin, a macrolide antibiotic, may produce adverse effects including:

- epigastric distress (reduced by taking the drug with food)
- nausea and vomiting
- diarrhea (especially with large doses)
- rash
- fever
- eosinophilia (an increase in the number of eosinophils, a type of white blood cell)
- anaphylaxis

Erythromycin and Its Derivatives

Erythromycin is one of the major macrolides. It's supplied in a number of dosage forms:

- tablets and extended-release tablets (Ery-Tab, PCE)
- capsules containing extended-release granules
- topical solution, ointment, gel, pads and pledgets (Eryderm, Akne-mycin, Emgel, Erygel, Emcin Clear, Ery Pad, T Stat). It is also available in combination with benzoyl peroxide in a powder and topical gel formulations (Benzamycin).
- ophthalmic ointment

Erythromycin and its derivatives are used to treat a variety of infections.

- It provides a broad spectrum of activity against gram-positive and gram-negative bacteria.
- For patients allergic to penicillin, it's effective against many infections generally treated by that class of antibiotic.
- It's used to treat gonorrhea and syphilis in patients who cannot tolerate tetracycline drugs or penicillin G.
- It's useful in treating minor staph infections of the skin.
- It's the drug of choice for treating certain types of pneumonia, including Legionnaires' disease.

Erythromycin is acid-sensitive. To prevent it from being destroyed by gastric acid in the stomach, tablets are buffered or coated. Erythromycin also may increase theophylline levels. Patients who are already receiving high doses of theophylline have an increased risk of developing theophylline toxicity.

TIP Allergies to antibiotics are always a concern, so you should understand the difference between an allergy and an adverse reaction. If a patient develops a rash or experiences difficulty breathing, then that is a true allergy. An upset stomach caused by erythromycin, however, is not a true allergy but rather an adverse reaction to the medication.

Other Erythromycins

Other erythromycins include:

- erythromycin ethylsuccinate (E.E.S., Eryped)—tablets, fruit-flavored liquid suspension, and granules for oral suspension
- erythromycin lactobionate (Erythrocin)—injection
- erythromycin stearate (My-E)—coated tablets

Other Macrolides

Some other macrolides also provide a broad spectrum of activity against various types of bacteria, such as microbes causing ear, respiratory, and skin infections.

Azithromycin

Azithromycin is supplied as:

- Tablets (Zithromax)
- a powder and extended-release powder that is mixed with water to create a suspension for oral administration (Zithromax, ZMax)
- a powder that is mixed for IV infusion (Zithromax)
- an ophthalmic solution (Azasite)

No other substances can be administered in the same IV bag or line with this drug. In addition, like erythromycin, it may increase theophylline to dangerous levels in patients taking theophylline. The tablets and the single-dose oral suspension can be taken with or without food. However, the extended-release suspension must be taken on an empty stomach.

Azithromycin is used to treat several different types of bacterial infections, including:

- ear infections
- conjunctivitis (pinkeye)
- respiratory tract infections (sinusitis, pneumonia)
- pharyngitis/tonsillitis
- skin infections
- other genital and urinary tract infections

Dosing varies depending on the brand prescribed. For example, Tri-Pak is usually dosed once daily for three days. With Z-Pak, however, two tablets are usually prescribed for the first day of treatment, followed by one tablet daily for the next four days. Zmax Oral Suspension is prescribed as a single dose.

Clarithromycin

Clarithromycin (Biaxin, Biaxin XL) is supplied in single-dose and extended-release tablets and as granules that are mixed in water to create a fruit-flavored oral suspension. It's used to treat:

- ear infections
- respiratory tract infections (pneumonia, sinusitis)
- tonsillitis
- skin infections
- bacteria-induced duodenal ulcers (in combination with antacids and other drugs)

AT THE COUNTER

Storing Suspensions and Solutions

A customer calls the pharmacy regarding the clarithromycin (Biaxin) oral suspension prescription that she had filled yesterday for her daughter. She didn't read the label or patient information yesterday and refrigerated the Biaxin overnight. Today, she tried to give her daughter the medication and she couldn't get it to come out of the bottle. Then she noticed the label that read, "Store at room temperature." What can she do?

Biaxin turns into a gelatin-like consistency when refrigerated, and there is nothing that can be done to reverse the effects. She will need to come in and get a new bottle.

When the patient comes in to get a new bottle, she is upset about the price and doesn't understand why it isn't covered by her insurance. What should you tell her?

Insurance companies usually will not pay for lost medication. The customer will need to pay full price for the prescription. *What can you do in the future to prevent such situations?*

Always be sure to point out storage directions for oral solutions or suspensions when you are giving the product to a customer.

Clarithromycin is also used to prevent mycobacterial disease in patients with advanced human immunodeficiency virus (HIV).

Clarithromycin may increase the concentration of carbamazepine when the two drugs are used together. It also can increase theophylline levels and should be used with the same precautions as erythromycin and azithromycin.

Vancomycin

Vancomycin (Vancocin) is supplied as capsules and as a powder that is mixed for IV solutions. It acts by damaging the bacteria's cell wall, which allows the body's natural defenses to attack the bacteria.

Because vancomycin is absorbed poorly from the GI tract, it must be given intravenously to treat systemic infections. Intravenous vancomycin is the drug of choice for patients with serious resistant infections who are hypersensitive to penicillins. When used with an aminoglycoside, intravenous vancomycin is also the treatment of choice for certain forms of endocarditis.

Oral vancomycin is generally used only to treat certain types of colitis. The oral forms are not effective for most other kinds of infections.

Vancomycin is used increasingly to treat methicillin-resistant bacteria. The development of such resistant strains has become a major concern in the United States and other countries. However, this drug must be used judiciously because vancomycin-resistant bacteria have also developed. As a rule of thumb, vancomycin should be

PROCEED WITH CAUTION

Adverse Reactions to Vancomycin

Although rare, adverse reactions to vancomycin include:

- hypersensitivity and anaphylactic reactions
- eosinophilia
- neutropenia (an increase in neutrophils, a type of white blood cell)
- hearing loss (temporary or permanent) especially with excessive doses (as when given with other ototoxic drugs)

Severe hypotension may occur with rapid IV administration of vancomycin and may be accompanied by a red rash on the face, neck, chest, and arms (also called *red man syndrome*). Dosages of one gram or less should be given over the course of one hour. Dosages of more than one gram should be given over one and a half to two hours.

used only when test results on bacteria confirm the need for this drug.

Vancomycin may increase the risk of toxicity when given with other drugs that are toxic to the kidneys and organs of hearing, such as:

- aminoglycosides
- amphotericin B
- bacitracin
- cisplatin
- colistin
- polymyxin B

Carbapenems

Carbapenems are a class of bactericidal antibiotics.

Imipenem-Cilastatin

The combination drug imipenem-cilastatin is available as a solution for IV infusion (Primaxin IV) and as a powder for suspension, which is administered by IM injection (Primaxin IM). This drug is one of the broadest-spectrum

PROCEED WITH CAUTION

Adverse Reactions to Carbapenems

Common adverse reactions to carbapenems include:

- nausea and vomiting
- diarrhea
- rashes and other hypersensitivity reactions (especially in patients sensitive to penicillin)

In patients with decreased or impaired kidney function, the dosage of these drugs may need to be adjusted.

antibiotics available. It's effective against bacteria that resist many other drugs. For this reason, it's used to treat serious or life-threatening infections.

Imipenem must be given with cilastatin because imipenem alone is metabolized rapidly in the kidneys, which renders the drug ineffective. Taking probenecid with imipenem-cilastatin increases blood levels of cilastatin although only slightly increasing imipenem levels in the blood.

Ertapenem

Ertapenem (Invanz) is supplied as a powder that is mixed with water for IV infusion or with lidocaine for IM injection. Its spectrum of activity includes skin, intra-abdominal, urinary tract, and gynecological infections, and several types of pneumonia. Taking probenecid with this drug may cause ertapenem to accumulate to toxic levels.

T I P Carbapenems all end in the letters *-penem*.

Meropenem

Meropenem (Merrem) is a powder that is mixed with sterile water for IV bolus or infusion. It is not indicated for IM or SubQ injection. In addition, no other drugs may be mixed into a solution that contains meropenem. This drug is used to treat intra-abdominal infections and to manage bacterial meningitis.

Monobactams

Aztreonam (Azactam) is the first member of a class of antibiotic drugs called monobactams, and it is the only monobactam currently available. It's a synthetic monobactam with a narrow spectrum of activity that's effective against many gram-negative bacteria. Aztreonam is a bactericidal drug that is used to treat:

- UTIs
- septicemia
- lower respiratory tract infections
- skin infections
- intra-abdominal infections
- gynecological infections

Aztreonam is supplied in vials of powder to which sterile water or another diluent is added and the contents are shaken to create a solution. The solution is then administered by IM injection or by IV bolus injection or infusion. Intravenous administration is the preferred method if the infection is severe or systemic. Aztreonam shouldn't be used alone if a patient may have a gram-positive bacterial infection or a mixed aerobic-anaerobic bacterial infection.

This drug may interact with several other drugs.

- Probenecid increases the level of aztreonam in the blood by slowing the rate at which it is excreted by the kidneys.

PROCEED WITH CAUTION

Adverse Reactions to Aztreonam

Aztreonam can cause the following adverse reactions:

- diarrhea
- hypersensitivity and skin reactions
- hypotension
- nausea and vomiting
- temporary electrocardiogram changes (including ventricular arrhythmias)
- temporary increases in liver enzyme levels in the blood

- Additive effects occur when aztreonam is used with aminoglycosides or other antibiotics such as cefoperazone, cefotaxime, clindamycin, and piperacillin.
- Cefoxitin and imipenem may inactivate aztreonam and shouldn't be used by patients taking this drug.
- Taking aztreonam with clavulanic acid-containing antibiotics may produce additive or antagonistic effects, depending on the microorganism involved.

Fluoroquinolones

Fluoroquinolones are synthetic antibiotics. They are all structurally similar. These drugs are bacteriostatic.

Fluoroquinolones are primarily used to treat UTIs, upper respiratory tract infections, pneumonia, and gonorrhea. Each drug in this class also has other specific uses.

Taking antacids that contain magnesium or aluminum hydroxide with a fluoroquinolone will decrease the antibiotic's absorption.

T I P Caution patients to avoid mixing their fluoroquinolone with antacids, which may decrease the effectiveness of their antibiotic.

PROCEED WITH CAUTION

Adverse Reactions to Fluoroquinolones

Fluoroquinolones are well tolerated in most patients. But some adverse reactions may occur. These include:

- dizziness
- nausea and vomiting
- diarrhea
- abdominal pain

Moderate to severe phototoxic reactions have occurred with exposure to direct and indirect sunlight and artificial ultraviolet light. These reactions have occurred with and without the use of sunscreen. Unecessary exposure to light should be avoided for several days after stopping fluoroquinolone therapy.

Ciprofloxacin

Ciprofloxacin (Cipro) is available as tablets, extended-release tablets, oral liquid suspension, and as a solution for IV infusion. This drug is used to treat lower respiratory tract infections, infectious diarrhea, and skin, bone, and joint infections. An ophthalmic solution and an ophthalmic ointment (Ciloxan) provide treatment for certain eye infections.

Be aware of these interactions when dispensing this drug:

- Ciprofloxacin interacts with xanthine derivatives, such as aminophylline and theophylline. This interaction can result in increased theophylline levels in the blood and can increase the risk of theophylline toxicity.
- Taking probenecid with ciprofloxacin reduces this antibiotic's elimination through the kidneys. This interaction increases the serum level and half-life of the antibiotic.

Levofloxacin

Levofloxacin (Levaquin) is supplied as tablets, oral solution, and solution for IV infusion. This drug is indicated for lower respiratory tract infections, skin infections, and UTIs. Levofloxacin ophthalmic solution (Quixin, Iquix) is prescribed for the treatment of bacterial conjunctivitis (pinkeye) and other eye infections.

T I P You can recognize fluoroquinolones by looking at their generic names. Each of these drugs ends in the letters -*floxacin*.

Moxifloxacin

Moxifloxacin is available in tablets (Avelox), in bags of premixed solution for IV infusion (Avelox I.V.), and as an ophthalmic solution (Vigamox) with a dropper for use in treating several types of bacterial eye infections. The oral and IV forms are used in treating acute sinus infections and mild to moderate cases of pneumonia. Similar to other fluoroquinolones, parenteral administration of this drug should be by IV infusion only.

Ofloxacin

Ofloxacin is supplied as tablets and coated tablets, as an ophthalmic solution (eye drops) for treating eye infections (Ocuflox), and as an otic solution (ear drops) for treating ear infections (Floxin). The tablets are used to treat some sexually transmitted diseases, lower respiratory tract infections, skin infections, and prostatitis.

Other Fluoroquinolones

Other fluoroquinolones include:

- gatifloxacin (Zymar)—ophthalmic solution
- norfloxacin (Noroxin)—coated tablets for treating prostatitis (inflammation of the prostate gland) and UTIs

Sulfonamides

Sulfonamides were the first systemic antibacterial drugs. They are bacteriostatic. Sulfonamides are active against a wide range of gram-positive and gram-negative bacteria. They're commonly used to treat acute UTIs.

As a class, sulfonamides have few significant interactions. However, crystals and stones may form in the kidneys as some of these drugs are excreted. Therefore, it's important for patients to have adequate fluid intake while taking sulfonamides. Oral doses should be taken with eight ounces of water, and patients should drink two to three liters of fluids per day during therapy.

- When taken with methenamine, sulfonamides may lead to the development of crystals in urine.
- Sulfonamides increase the hypoglycemic effects of diabetes medications, which may lower blood sugar levels.

Sulfamethoxazole and Trimethoprim

Sulfamethoxazole and trimethoprim (Bactrim, Septra, Sulfatrim, Sultrex), commonly abbreviated SMX-TMP, is supplied for oral administration as tablets and as a fruit-flavored oral suspension. An IV solution is also available for treating acute infections or when oral therapy is not possible. This solution must be infused and not injected intramuscularly or as an IV bolus.

This drug is a combination of a sulfa drug and a folate antagonist. In addition to treating UTIs, it's used for a variety of other infections, including pneumonia, acute ear infections, and acute chronic bronchitis.

SMX-TMP may increase the anticoagulant effect of coumarin anticoagulants. When taken with cyclosporine, SMX-TMP increases the risk of kidney toxicity.

T I P Sulfonamides become easier to spot once you know that these drug names all begin with the letters *sulfa*-.

 PROCEED WITH CAUTION

Adverse Reactions to Sulfonamides

Adverse reactions to sulfonamides include:

- hypersensitivity reactions, which appear to increase as dosage increases
- photosensitivity reactions
- a reaction resembling serum sickness, producing fever, joint pain, hives, bronchospasm, and leukopenia (reduced white blood cell count)
- crystals in urine and crystal deposits in the renal tubes (with high doses of older, non—water-soluble sulfonamides)

Sulfadiazine

Sulfadiazine is prescribed as tablets. A topical cream known as silver sulfadiazine (Silvadene, SSD, Thermazene) is also available for use in preventing infection in patients with second- and third-degree burns.

Erythromycin Ethylsuccinate and Sulfisoxazole

This combination drug (Pediazole, E.S.P.) is available as a fruit-flavored oral suspension. It's used to treat acute ear infections in children.

Nitrofurantoin

Because it concentrates in urine, nitrofurantoin (Macrobid, Macrodantin, Furadantin, Urotoin) is used to treat severe and chronic UTIs. This drug is usually bacteriostatic; however, depending on its concentration level and the infecting organism's susceptibility, it may be bactericidal. Nitrofurantoin also has higher antibacterial activity in acid urine. Exactly how this drug works is unknown.

Nitrofurantoin is available as capsules, tablets, and as an oral suspension. All forms are more effective when taken with food.

This drug has only a few significant interactions:

■ Probenecid and sulfinpyrazone inhibit nitrofurantoin's excretion by the kidneys. This reduces its effectiveness and increases the risk for toxicity.
■ Magnesium salts and magnesium-containing antacids can decrease the rate and extent of nitrofurantoin absorption.
■ Nitrofurantoin may decrease the antibacterial activity of norfloxacin and nalidixic acid.

Adverse reactions to nitrofurantoin include:

■ GI irritation
■ anorexia
■ nausea and vomiting
■ diarrhea
■ dark yellow or brown urine
■ abdominal pain
■ joint pain
■ chills
■ fever
■ anaphylaxis
■ hypersensitivity reactions involving the skin, lungs, blood, and liver

T I P It's important for patients to complete an antibiotic regimen. Always make sure that the directions and quantities match so that the patient has enough medication for the entire regimen. Often, the physician leaves it up to the pharmacy to determine the quantity based on her directions. For example, the physician may write "1 po tid × 10 days" and expect you to be able to calculate the correct number of tablets or capsules to be dispensed.

ANTIVIRAL DRUGS

Antiviral drugs are used to prevent or treat viral infections ranging from influenza to HIV. The major classes of antiviral drugs include:

■ synthetic nucleosides
■ pyrophosphate analogs
■ influenza A and syncytial virus drugs
■ nucleoside analog reverse transcriptase inhibitors
■ non-nucleoside reverse transcriptase inhibitors
■ nucleotide analog reverse transcriptase inhibitors
■ protease inhibitors

T I P Antiviral drugs often end in the letters -vir.

Synthetic Nucleosides

Synthetic nucleosides are used to treat many of the viral syndromes that can occur in patients with compromised immune systems. These viruses include herpes simplex virus (HSV) and cytomegalovirus (CMV), another type of herpes virus.

There are several interactions associated with the drugs in this class.

■ Probenecid reduces kidney excretion of all synthetic nucleosides. This interaction increases drug levels in the blood, resulting in greater risk for drug toxicity.
■ Taking ganciclovir with drugs that are damaging to tissue cells (such as dapsone, pentamidine isethionate, flucytosine, vincristine, vinblastine, doxorubicin, amphotericin B, and SMX-TMP) inhibits the replication of rapidly dividing cells in the bone marrow, GI tract, skin, and sperm-producing cells.
■ Imipenem-cilastatin increases the risk of seizures when taken with ganciclovir or valganciclovir.
■ Zidovudine increases the risk of granulocytopenia (a reduced number of granulocytes, or a type of white blood cell filled with microscopic granules containing enzymes digest microorganisms) when taken with ganciclovir.

Acyclovir

Acyclovir (Zovirax) is available as tablets, capsules, oral suspension, and an injection solution and injection powder that are diluted for IV infusion. The drug works by entering virus-infected cells, where it inhibits an enzyme that the virus needs for growth and replication.

Intravenous acyclovir is used to treat severe HSV type 2 infections in patients with normal immune systems. It's also used to treat certain herpes-related infections in patients with compromised immune systems. These infections include:

■ initial and recurring skin and mucous membrane HSV type 1 and 2 infections, such as genital herpes
■ severe cases of genital herpes

- varicella-zoster infections, such as shingles and chickenpox

Oral acyclovir is used to treat these same conditions in patients with normal immune systems. A topical ointment is also used in managing genital herpes, and a topical cream is available for the treatment of recurring herpes labialis (cold sores).

Common adverse reactions to acyclovir include:

- hypersensitivity reactions
- headache, nausea, vomiting, and diarrhea (with oral administration)
- reversible kidney impairment (with rapid infusion or IV injection)

Famciclovir

Famciclovir (Famvir) is available in tablet form only. This drug is used to treat acute herpes zoster (shingles), genital herpes, and recurrent HSV infections in patients with HIV. It works by entering viral cells (herpes simplex 1 and 2 and varicella zoster), where it inhibits their DNA synthesis and replication. Common adverse reactions to famciclovir include headache and nausea.

Ganciclovir

Ganciclovir is supplied as oral capsules, as a reconstittutable powder for IV infusion (Cytovene), and as a pellet (Vitasert) that is surgically implanted in the eye and releases the drug over a six- to eight-month period of time.

This drug is used to treat CMV retinitis (a herpes infection of the eye) in immunocompromised patients with AIDS or other CMV infections such as encephalitis. Ganciclovir enters CMV-infected cells and is believed to inhibit the virus' DNA synthesis.

Common adverse reactions to ganciclovir include granulocytopenia and thrombocytopenia (low blood platelet count).

Valacyclovir

Valacyclovir (Valtrex) is available as tablets. Once in the body, it rapidly converts to acyclovir, inserts itself into viral DNA, and inhibits the multiplication of the virus. It is used to treat shingles, genital herpes, and cold sores. Like famciclovir, common adverse reactions to this drug include headache and nausea.

Valganciclovir

Valganciclovir (Valcyte) is also supplied as tablets. It is used to treat CMV retinitis. When taken, it converts to ganciclovir and has the same mechanism of action as that drug.

Common adverse reactions to valganciclovir include:

- hypersensitivity reactions
- headache, nausea, vomiting, and diarrhea
- abdominal pain
- insomnia
- seizures
- retinal detachment

- neutropenia, pancytopenia, and thrombocytopenia
- anemia and aplastic anemia
- bone marrow depression
- sepsis

Pyrophosphate Analogs

The antiviral drug foscarnet (Foscavir) is mainly used to treat CMV retinitis in AIDS patients. It is also used:

- in combination therapy with ganciclovir for patients who have relapsed while taking either drug
- to treat acyclovir-resistant HSV infections in patients with compromised immune systems

Foscarnet is available only as an injection solution for IV infusion. It has few interactions with other drugs.

- When administered with pentamidine, the risk of hypocalcemia (low blood calcium levels) and toxicity to the kidneys is increased.
- Its use with other drugs that alter serum calcium levels may result in hypocalcemia.
- The risk of kidney impairment increases when drugs toxic to the kidneys (such as aminoglycosides and amphotericin B) are taken with foscarnet. Because of this risk, the patient must be well hydrated during treatment.

Influenza A and Syncytial Virus Drugs

This group of antiviral drugs is used to prevent or treat influenza A infections. These drugs can reduce the severity and duration of fever and other symptoms in patients infected with influenza A.

These drugs also can protect patients who have received the flu vaccine during the two weeks it takes for immunity to develop and those who can't receive the flu vaccine for some medical reason.

T I P If you have flu symptoms, such as fever, headache, and achiness, you have 12 to 48 hours to begin taking a flu drug to combat the effects of the flu. It works by helping to stop the spread of the virus within the body.

! **PROCEED WITH CAUTION**

Adverse Reactions to Foscarnet

Adverse reactions to foscarnet may include:

- fatigue, depression, and confusion
- dizziness, headache, fever, numbness, and tingling
- nausea and vomiting, diarrhea, and abdominal pain
- granulocytopenia and leukopenia
- seizures, involuntary muscle contractions, and neuropathy
- rash and difficulty breathing
- altered kidney function

CHAPTER 9 ■ Anti-Infective Drugs   187

Oseltamivir

Oseltamivir (Tamiflu) is supplied as capsules for oral administration and as a fruit-flavored powder that is mixed with water to create an oral suspension. Taking this drug with probenecid slows its excretion through the kidneys. The result is increased levels of oseltamivir in the body.

Adverse reactions to oseltamivir include:

- headaches and dizziness
- fatigue and insomnia
- diarrhea, nausea, vomiting, and abdominal pain
- coughing and bronchitis
- vertigo

Ribavirin

Ribavirin is available as tablets (Copegus, RibaTab) and capsules (Rebetol), as an oral solution (Rebetol), and as a powder from which an inhalation solution is mixed (Virazole). The drug is administered by aerosol inhalation to treat respiratory syncytial virus infections in children. The oral dosage forms are used in combination with other drugs to treat hepatitis C virus infections. Its mechanism of action is not completely known.

Like amantadine, ribavirin has interactions with other drugs:

- It reduces the antiviral activity of zidovudine. In addition, the use of these drugs together may cause blood toxicity.
- Taking ribavirin and digoxin can cause digoxin toxicity, which can produce effects such as GI distress, CNS abnormalities, and cardiac arrhythmias.

Adverse reactions to ribivarin include:

- apnea (lack of breathing)
- cardiac arrest
- hypotension
- pneumothorax (air in the pleural space, causing the lung to collapse)
- worsening of respiratory function

Zanamivir

Zanamivir (Relenza) is produced as a powder that is inhaled through the mouth using an inhaler supplied with the drug. There are no known drug interactions associated with zanamivir.

Adverse reactions to this drug include:

- headaches and dizziness
- nausea, vomiting, and diarrhea
- cough, bronchitis, and sinusitis
- ear, nose, and throat infections

Other Influenza A and Syncytial Virus Drugs

Amantadine (Symmetrel) is administered orally as tablets, capsules, and oral solution. It seems to inhibit an early stage of viral replication. In addition to its antiviral uses, amantadine is used to treat parkinsonism and drug-induced involuntary movements. Amantadine interacts with several other drugs:

- anticholinergics
- hydrochlorothiazide/triamterene
- SMX-TMP

Adverse reactions to amantadine include:

- anorexia
- anxiety and nervousness
- confusion, forgetfulness, hallucinations, and psychosis
- depression and irritability
- insomnia and fatigue
- nausea
- hypersensitivity reactions

Rimantadine (Flumadine) is taken orally in tablet form. It's a derivative of amantadine and inhibits viral RNA and protein synthesis. No clinically significant drug interactions have been documented with rimantadine. Adverse reactions to rimantadine are similar to those for amantadine; however, they tend to be less severe.

Nucleoside Analog Reverse Transcriptase Inhibitors

Nucleoside analog reverse transcriptase inhibitors (NRTIs) are used to treat patients with advanced HIV infection and AIDS. Each of these drugs has its own pharmacokinetic

AT THE COUNTER

Aiding in the War on AIDS

When a patient is diagnosed as HIV-positive, he is placed on a regimen that contains several different drugs. If a patient is not compliant and stops taking his medication, the entire regimen may need to be changed when he starts taking medication again. As a pharmacy technician, what can you do to help these patients?

First, the antivirals often have several different names: a generic name, a brand name, and an abbreviated name. For example, lamivudine is also known as Epivir and 3TC. It is critical that you become familiar with all the names for each medication.

Second, you can help the pharmacist monitor patients for compliance. As a technician, you are often the person taking refill requests from patients and calling physicians for refill authorizations. As a result, you are on the frontline for monitoring patients' compliance with any medication.

Third, you can remind each patient how many refills he has left when he picks up the medication. You can also stress to patients the importance of taking the medication exactly as prescribed.

properties, but they all must undergo a conversion to produce their action. Most act on the HIV virus in some way to inhibit its replication.

NRTIs may be responsible for a variety of drug interactions. Specific interactions are discussed below. But when patients take NRTIs alone or with other **antiretroviral drugs** (antivirals used to treat HIV infection), potentially fatal lactic acidosis (increased lactic acid production in the blood)

and severe hepatomegaly (liver enlargement) with steatosis can occur. Most of these reactions have occurred in women. Obesity and prolonged NRTI exposure may also be risk factors.

TIP Although privacy is an issue with all patients, make sure to interact *very* discreetly with patients who are receiving antiretrovirals.

HOW IT WORKS

How Zidovudine Works

Zidovudine inhibits replication of HIV in the body. See figure 9-2. The top two panels depict how HIV invades human cells and then replicates itself. The bottom panel shows how zidovudine blocks viral transformation.

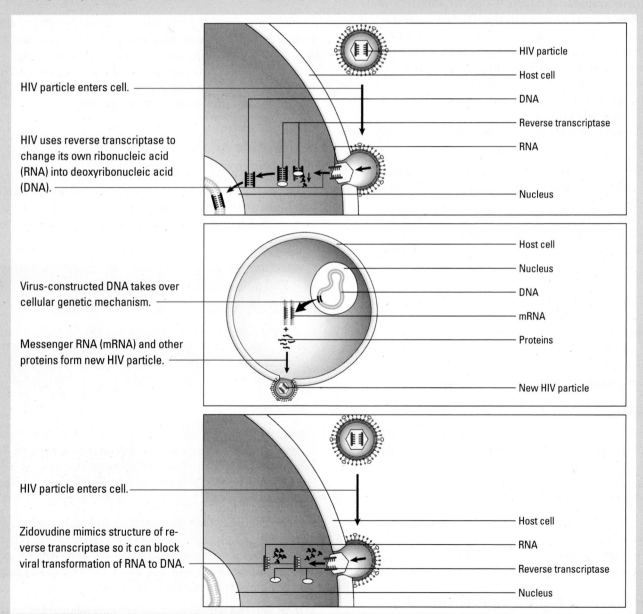

FIGURE 9-2 How zidovudine works. (From *Clinical Pharmacology Made Incredibly Easy.* 2nd Ed. Philadelphia, PA: Lippincott Williams & Wilkins; 2005.)

Zidovudine

Zidovudine (Retrovir), abbreviated ZDV, was the first drug to receive approval by the Food and Drug Administration for treating AIDS and AIDS-related complex. It can be prescribed as tablets, capsules, or fruit-flavored syrup for oral administration. An injection solution is also available for IV infusion.

Intravenous zidovudine is used to prevent transmission of HIV from an infected mother to her fetus and to treat AIDS-related dementia. It's also used to treat hospitalized patients who can't take oral medication. Oral zidovudine, like all drugs for HIV infection, is used as part of a multidrug regimen.

- Combivir is a combination therapy that includes zidovudine and lamivudine.
- Trizivir is a combination therapy that includes zidovudine, lamivudine, and abacavir.

Giving zidovudine in combination with stavudine, however, will inhibit the metabolite-forming process that both drugs use to act on the HIV virus. Here are some other drug interactions of which you should be aware:

- There's an increased risk of cellular and kidney toxicity when zidovudine is taken with such drugs as dapsone, pentamidine, isethionate, flucytosine, vincristine, vinblastine, doxorubicin, interferon, and ganciclovir.
- Taking zidovudine with probenecid, aspirin, acetaminophen, indomethacin, cimetidine, or lorazepam increases both drugs' risk of toxicity.
- Zidovudine taken with acyclovir may produce profound lethargy and drowsiness.

Adverse reactions to zidovudine may include:

- headache and dizziness
- muscle pain, fever, and rash
- nausea, vomiting, abdominal pain, and diarrhea
- bone marrow toxicity and other blood-related disorders

Other Nuceloside Analog Reverse Transcriptase Inhibitors

Abacavir (Ziagen) is produced as tablets and as a solution for oral administration. This drug is part of the Trizir combination therapy you read about earlier in this section. Abacavir is also taken in combination with lamivudine. The combination product is an oral tablet called Epzicom. Abacavir should not be combined with alcohol. In addition, it can cause potentially fatal hypersensitivity reactions.

Didanosine, abbreviated ddI, is supplied as extended-release capsules (Videx EC) and as a powder to be mixed as an oral solution (Videx). Used in combination with other antiretrovirals, it is an alternative initial treatment for HIV. However, didanosine may reduce the absorption of tetracyclines, fluoroquinolones, and delavirdine. Adverse reactions to didanosine may include:

- headache, dizziness, and peripheral neuropathy
- muscle pain and muscle weakness
- rash and itching
- nausea, vomiting, abdominal pain, diarrhea, and constipation
- dry mouth, unusual taste or loss of taste, and stomatitis
- pancreatitis
- hair loss

Emtricitabine (Emtriva) is available as capsules and as an oral solution. It is used with efavirenz and tenofovir in treating HIV infections. These combination products are sold under the trade names Atripla and Truvada. There are no significant drug interactions associated with emtricitabine.

Lamivudine (Epivir, EPivir HBV), abbreviated 3TC, is produced as tablets and as an oral solution. This drug is part of the Combivir, Trizivir, and Epzicom combination therapies. However, lamivudine shouldn't be used in combination with stavudine because doing so will inhibit the antiviral action of both drugs.

Stavudine (Zerit), abbreviated d4T, is supplied as capsules and as a powder that is mixed with purified water to create an oral solution. It is used in combination with other antiretrovirals. However, it should not be used with lamivudine or didanosine.

Non-Nucleoside Reverse Transcriptase Inhibitors

Non-nucleoside reverse transcriptase inhibitors (NNRTIs) are another class of antiviral drugs that are used to treat HIV infection. NNRTIs are used in combination with other antiretrovirals.

Delavirdine

Delavirdine (Rescriptor) is prescribed as tablets. It binds to the virus's reverse transcriptase enzyme, which prevents the virus from gaining control of the invaded cell and using it to replicate.

PROCEED WITH CAUTION

Adverse Reactions to Non-nucleoside Reverse Transcriptase Inhibitors

Adverse reactions to NNRTIs include:

- headache
- dizziness
- muscle weakness
- nausea and vomiting
- diarrhea
- rash

In administering delavirdine, it's important to know that this drug may increase levels of the following drugs:

- benzodiazepines
- the antibiotic clarithromycin
- rifabutin
- warfarin
- two other antiretroviral drugs, saquinavir and indinavir

Increases in indinavir concentrations may be so great that the dosage of indinavir may need to be decreased.

Other Non-Nucleoside Reverse Transcriptase Inhibitors

Nevirapine (Viramune) is marketed as tablets and as an oral suspension. Its action is similar to that of delavirdine. This drug may decrease the effectiveness of hormonal contraceptives. It also may decrease the activity of another class of antiretrovirals called protease inhibitors and should never be used in combination with them. The use of nevirapine has been associated with a severe rash that may be life threatening. If a rash develops, the drug should be discontinued.

A final NNRTI, efavirenz (Sustiva) is supplied in both capsule and tablet form.

Nucleotide Analog Reverse Transcriptase Inhibitors

Like other classes of HIV drugs, nucleotide analog reverse transcriptase inhibitors are used in combination with other antiretrovirals in treating HIV. To date, the only drug in this class is tenofovir (Viread), abbreviated PMPA. It works much like the NRTIs. Tenofovir is used in combination with the NNRTI drug efavirenz and the NRTI drug emtricitabine.

Tenofovir is prescribed as tablets. It is absorbed best when taken after a high-fat meal. It also may interact with certain other drugs.

- Didanosine levels increase when this NRTI drug is given with tenofovir. Patients should be alerted to watch even more carefully for didanosine-based adverse effects.
- Drugs that are eliminated through the kidneys or that decrease kidney function may increase tenofovir levels when they are taken together.
- Potentially fatal lactic acidosis and severe liver enlargement have occurred in patients taking tenofovir, either in combination with other antiretrovirals or alone. Most of these cases occurred in women, and obesity and previous NRTI exposure may be risk factors. Patients with existing liver disease should take this drug with caution. Treatment should be suspended if liver toxicity is suspected.

PROCEED WITH CAUTION

Adverse Reactions to Tenofovir

Adverse reactions to tenofovir include:

- nausea and vomiting
- diarrhea
- abdominal pain
- anorexia
- severe hepatomegaly
- lactic acidosis

Protease Inhibitors

Protease inhibitors are drugs that inhibit the activity of HIV protease, an enzyme the virus needs in order to develop. When the enzyme is blocked by the drug, the result is an immature, noninfectious virus.

The drugs in this class have different pharmacokinetic properties and are absorbed, metabolized, and eliminated from the body in different ways. However, they are all used in combination with other antiretroviral drugs in treating HIV infections.

Each of the drugs in this class has its own interactions with other drugs. These are noted in the discussion of the individual drugs that follow. However, rifampin markedly reduces the blood level of most protease inhibitors. In addition, each of the protease inhibitors may increase levels of sildenafil, a drug used to treat male sexual dysfunction. This may cause adverse reactions associated with sildenafil, including hypotension, vision changes, and priapism (an abnormally prolonged erection).

Fosamprenavir

Fosamprenavir (Lexiva) comes in the form of tablets and oral suspension. The following drugs may interact with this drug:

- When taken with fosamprenavir, cisapride, ergotamine, erythromycin, H1 antagonists, and pimozide may cause seizures, blood vessel problems, or heart problems.
- Fosamprenavir may cause increased or prolonged sedation and breathing problems when taken with benzodiazepines.
- Amprenavir may increase the risk of adverse reactions associated with fosamprenavir.

The effectiveness of fosamprenavir may be decreased if it is taken with rifampin or St. John's wort.

The most common adverse reactions to fosamprenavir include:

- diarrhea
- headache
- nausea

- rash
- vomiting

Atazanavir

Atazanavir (Reyataz) is available as oral capsules. It is often used in combination with indinavir sulfate, another protease inhibitor.

Atazanavir is associated with a number of drug interactions:

- Atazanavir shouldn't be given with benzodiazepines, such as midazolam and triazolam, because of the risk of increased sedation or respiratory depression.
- Drugs that prolong the heart's PR interval, such as calcium-channel blockers and beta-adrenergic blockers, should be used cautiously with atazanavir, because this drug may prolong the PR interval.
- Atazanavir shouldn't be given with other drugs that are metabolized by the same pathway in the liver (the CYPA3A pathway), such as HMG-CoA reductase inhibitors (including lovastatin, simvastatin, and atorvastatin). Using atazanavir with such drugs may increase the risk of myopathy (muscle weakness) and rhabdomyolysis (a degenerative muscle disease).
- Atazanavir shouldn't be given to patients taking ergot derivatives. Administering atazanavir to such patients creates the potential for life-threatening ergot toxicity.
- Taking St. John's wort may reduce a patient's blood levels of atazanavir.

Indinavir

Indinavir (Crixivan) is another drug that's available only in capsule form. For maximum absorption, it should be taken without food but with plenty of water or other liquids.

Important interactions that involve this drug include the following:

- It inhibits the metabolism of midazolam and triazolam, which increases the risk of potentially fatal events such as cardiac arrhythmias.
- Taking it in combination with didanosine, another antiretroviral, decreases its gastric absorption. The two drugs should be administered at least one hour apart.
- Taking it with nelfinavir, another protease inhibitor, may increase levels of nelfinavir in the blood.

Common adverse reactions include the following:

- nausea and vomiting
- diarrhea
- abdominal pain
- back pain
- flank pain
- muscle weakness
- fatigue
- insomnia
- headache
- dizziness
- anorexia
- dry mouth and taste perversion
- acid regurgitation

Other Protease Inhibitors

Nelfinavir (Viracept) is supplied as tablets and a powder for oral suspension. This drug should be taken with food. Its presence in the body may greatly increase blood levels of amiodarone, ergot derivatives, midazolam, rifabutin, quinidine, and triazolam. At the same time, nelfinavir's effectiveness may be reduced by the presence of carbamazepine, phenobarbital, and phenytoin.

Ritonavir (Norvir) is available in a gel cap or as an oral solution for use in combination therapy with other antiretrovirals. Ritonavir increases blood levels of lopinavir and nelfinavir when either one is used in combination with ritonavir. In addition, ritonavir may increase the effects of the following drugs and types of drugs, including:

- alpha-blockers
- antiarrhythmics
- antidepressants
- antiemetics
- antifungals
- antilipemics
- antimalarials
- beta-blockers
- calcium-channel blockers
- cimetidine
- corticosteroids
- erythromycin
- immunosuppressants
- methylphenidate
- pentoxifylline
- phenothiazines
- warfarin

Saquinavir (Invirase) is available in both tablet and capsule form. This drug is used only in combination with ritonavir. The action of saquinavir may be reduced by phenobarbital, phenytoin, dexamethasone, and carbamazepine.

Lopinavir and ritonavir (Kaletra) are given as a combination tablet or oral solution that contains both drugs. They are used in combination because of their positive effects on HIV RNA levels and CD4 counts.

ANTITUBERCULAR DRUGS

Antitubercular drugs are used to treat tuberculosis (TB), which is caused by a bacterium called *Mycobacterium tuberculosis*. Although these drugs can't always cure TB, they can halt the progression of the infection. They are also effective against other less common mycobacterial infections.

Unlike most other antibiotics, antitubercular drugs may need to be administered over a period of many months. This creates a special set of problems that can include:

- patient noncompliance
- development of bacterial resistance
- drug toxicity

First-Line Therapy

Because of the current incidence of drug-resistant TB strains, a four-drug regimen is now recommended for initial treatment of TB:

- isoniazid
- rifampin
- pyrazinamide
- ethambutol or streptomycin

This regimen should be modified if testing shows resistance to one or more of these drugs. For example, if local outbreaks of TB resistant to isoniazid and rifampin occur, such as in health care or correctional facilities, then five- or six-drug regimens are recommended as initial therapy.

Antitubercular drugs may interact with many other drugs. Individual interactions are discussed with each specific drug that follows. However, when they are given together, isoniazid, rifampin, pyrazinamide, and ethambutol increase the risk of damage to the liver.

Isoniazid

Isoniazid (Nydrazid), abbreviated INH, is taken orally as tablets or solution. Oral administration is the typical route, but an injection solution is also available for IV administration, if necessary. This drug is tuberculostatic, meaning that it inhibits the growth of TB bacteria rather then killing them.

Although isoniazid is the most important drug for treating patients with TB, bacterial resistance develops quickly if it's used alone. For this reason, it's often administered with rifampin, ethambutol, or streptomycin. A combination capsule with rifampin is available, as is a combination tablet with rifampin and pyrazinamide. However, isoniazid can be used alone to prevent TB from developing in someone who's been exposed to the disease.

Drug interactions with isoniazid include:

- increased levels of phenytoin, carbamazepine, diazepam, ethosuximide, primidone, theophylline, and warfarin in patients who are taking any of these drugs
- reduced blood levels of ketoconazole, itraconazole, and oral antidiabetic agents
- reduced effectiveness of isoniazid and increased effectiveness of corticosteroids when these drugs are taken together
- additive CNS effects (such as drowsiness, dizziness, headache, lethargy, depression, tremor, anxiety, confusion, and ringing in the ears) when isoniazid is administered with cycloserine and ethionamide

Peripheral neuropathy is the most common adverse reactions associated with isoniazid. Severe and occasionally fatal hepatitis can occur even months after treatment has stopped. For this reason, patients must be monitored carefully.

Rifampin

Rifampin (Rifadin) is supplied in capsules for oral administration and as a powder that must be diluted and infused intravenously. This drug is tuberculocidal. But as with isoniazid, bacterial resistance to rifampin can develop rapidly. For this reason, it is seldom used in treating nonmycobacterial infections and should always be used with other antitubercular drugs in treating TB. A combination capsule with isoniazid (IsonaRif, Rifamate) and a combination tablet with isoniazid and pyrazinamide (Rifater) are available.

The following adverse reactions may occur with rifampin use:

- anorexia
- nausea and vomiting
- abdominal cramps and epigastric pain
- flatulence and diarrhea
- reddish-orange or reddish-brown discoloration of urine, stool, saliva, perspiration, and tears

TIP Rifampin can change urine, stool, saliva, sweat, and tears to a reddish-orange or reddish-brown color. Be sure to tell patients that these discolored substances can stain clothing.

Pyrazinamide

Pyrazinamide, abbreviated PZA, is supplied as tablets for oral administration. It's a highly specific drug that's active only against *M. tuberculosis*. Pyrazinamide is recommended as a frontline TB drug in combination with ethambutol, isoniazid, and rifampin. As you read earlier in this chapter, a combination tablet containing this drug with isoniazid and rifampin is available. Resistance to pyrazinamide may develop rapidly when it's used alone. When combined with phenytoin, pyrazinamide may increase phenytoin levels.

Pyrazinamide may cause the following adverse reactions:

- serious liver toxicity
- nausea and vomiting
- anorexia

Ethambutol

Ethambutol (Myambutol) is prescribed as tablets. Like isoniazid, it is tuberculostatic. This drug is used with isoniazid and rifampin to treat patients with uncomplicated pulmonary TB. It's also used to treat other mycobacterial infections.

Although they are rare, hypersensitivity reactions such as rash, fever, and anaphylaxis may occur with ethambutol use. Other adverse reactions include:

■ GI distress
■ itching
■ numbness and tingling of the extremities
■ joint pain
■ headache, dizziness, and confusion
■ leukopenia
■ malaise

Other Antitubercular Drugs

Other antitubercular drugs include:

■ *Streptomycin.* As you learned earlier in this chapter, streptomycin is administered by injection. It was the first drug recognized as effective in treating TB. However, its route of administration limits its usefulness in long-term therapy. Most patients tolerate it well, but persons receiving large doses may exhibit ototoxicity.
■ *Fluoroquinolones.* Some fluoroquinolones are also effective against TB. They're often used in combination with first-line drugs. But because they have a greater incidence of toxicity, they're mainly used for patients who are resistant or allergic to less toxic antitubercular drugs.
■ *Ofloxacin.* This drug is administered orally as tablets when used in treating TB. It is more potent than ciprofloxacin and may be the first choice in retreatment.
■ *Ciprofloxacin.* Ciprofloxacin is supplied as tablets, extended-release tablets, and as a powder for mixing an oral suspension.

ANTIFUNGAL DRUGS

Antifungal, or **antimycotic**, **drugs** are used to fight infections by various types of fungi. The major antifungal drugs and drug groups include:

■ polyenes
■ imidazole
■ synthetic triazoles
■ glucan synthesis inhibitors
■ synthetic allylamine derivatives

T I P Many antifungal drug names end in the letters *-azole.*

Polyenes

The polyenes include:

■ amphotericin B
■ nystatin

Amphotericin B

Amphotericin B is supplied as a premixed liquid suspension for administration by slow IV infusion. This powerful drug is the most widely used antifungal for severe systemic and potentially life-threatening fungal infections. It works by altering the cell membrane of fungal cells, which causes the cells' internal parts to leak out.

Amphotericin B is usually **fungistatic**, inhibiting the growth of a fungus. But in high doses it can be **fungicidal** and destroy the fungus. It's only used under close medical supervision and is almost never used for noninvasive forms of fungal disease because it's highly toxic. However, it is sometimes used in combination with flucytosine to treat candidal or cryptococcal infections, especially cryptococcal meningitis.

Magnesium levels, potassium levels, and kidney function must be frequently monitored in patients who receive amphotericin B. The risk of kidney toxicity increases when the drug is taken with aminoglycosides, cyclosporine, or acyclovir. Other important drug interactions also exist.

■ Corticosteroids, extended-spectrum penicillins, and digoxin may worsen the hypokalemia (low potassium levels) produced by amphotericin B, leading to possible heart problems. The risk of digoxin toxicity is also increased.
■ Amphotericin B will increase muscle relaxation in patients who are taking nondepolarizing muscle relaxers
■ Electrolyte solutions may inactivate amphotericin B when diluted in the same solution. Therefore, amphotericin B can't be mixed with saline solution. Amphotericin B must be mixed with dextrose 5% in water.

Almost all patients receiving intravenous amphotericin B, particularly at the beginning of low-dose therapy, experience:

■ fever and chills
■ indigestion, nausea, and vomiting
■ anorexia
■ muscle and joint pain

In addition, more serious adverse reactions occur in most patients:

■ normochromic anemia (inadequate hemoglobin in each red blood cell) or normocytic anemia (too few red blood cells)
■ dangerously low magnesium and potassium levels, causing ECG changes and requiring electrolyte replacement therapy
■ some degree of kidney toxicity (in up to 80 percent of patients), causing the kidneys to lose their ability to concentrate urine

T I P Amphotericin B is a potent weapon against fungi, but it's highly toxic and must be used carefully.

Nystatin

Nystatin is mainly used to treat fungal skin infections. But different forms are available for treating other kinds of infections, including:

- oral capsules (Bio-Statin) and tablets that are swallowed to treat GI infections
- a liquid suspension and a powder that is dissolved in water for treating fungal infections of the mouth or intestines
- a topical powder (Mycostatin, Nyamyc, Pedi-Dri) that can be sprinkled on an affected area of the skin or into clothing that is covering the area
- a cream and an ointment for topical use in treating mucous membrane infections, skin infections, or fungus between skin folds
- tablets that are inserted in the vagina to treat yeast infections

Nystatin works in much the same way as amphotericin B and can be fungistatic or fungicidal, depending on the organism that is present. But unlike amphotericin B, nystatin has no significant interactions with other drugs.

Adverse reactions to nystatin are rare, but high doses may produce:

- nausea and vomiting
- abdominal pain and diarrhea
- a bitter taste in the mouth
- skin irritation (with topical nystatin)
- hypersensitivity reaction (with oral or topical nystatin)

Flucytosine

Flucytosine (Ancobon) is prescribed as capsules for oral administration. It works by penetrating fungal cells and altering their protein synthesis, which causes them to die.

Flucytosine is used primarily with other antifungal drugs, such as amphotericin B, to treat systemic fungal infections. This allows the dose of amphotericin B to be reduced, which reduces the risk of toxicity. Flucytosine can be used alone to treat candidal infections of the lower urinary tract because it reaches a high urinary concentration. It's also effective in treating some other types of fungal infections.

Cytarabine may antagonize the antifungal activity of flucytosine, possibly by competing with flucytosine. Blood, liver, and kidney function must be closely monitored while patients are taking flucytosine because of the drug's serious risk of toxicity.

Imidazoles

Ketoconazole is the most commonly used imidazole. It may be prescribed as tablets for oral administration or as a cream (Kuric), foam (Extina), gel (Xolegel), or shampoo (Nizoral) for topical use. This drug has a broad spectrum of

 PROCEED WITH CAUTION

Adverse Reactions to Flucytosine

Flucytosine may produce unpredictable adverse reactions, including:

- nausea, vomiting, and diarrhea
- anorexia
- abdominal distention
- rash
- headache, drowsiness, and vertigo
- confusion and hallucinations
- difficulty breathing and respiratory arrest

activity and is used against topical and systemic infections caused by a large number of fungi. It works by damaging the membrane of the fungal cell, which leads to the cell's loss of essential internal elements. Ketoconazole is usually fungistatic, but it can be fungicidal under certain conditions.

Ketoconazole can have some significant interactions with other drugs:

- Drugs that decrease gastric activity (such as cimetidine, ranitidine, famotidine, nizatidine, antacids, and anticholinergic drugs) may decrease the absorption of ketoconazole. After taking any of these drugs, patients should wait two hours before taking ketoconazole.
- Taking ketoconazole with phenytoin may alter metabolism and increase blood levels of both drugs.
- Using ketoconazole with other drugs that are toxic to the liver may increase the risk of liver disease.
- When combined with cyclosporine, ketoconazole may increase cyclosporine and serum creatinine levels.
- Ketoconazole increases the effects of oral anticoagulants and can cause hemorrhage.

 PROCEED WITH CAUTION

Adverse Reactions to Ketoconazole

The most common adverse reactions to ketoconazole are nausea and vomiting. Less common reactions include:

- anaphylaxis
- joint pain
- chills
- fever
- ringing in the ears
- photophobia (light sensitivity)
- liver toxicity (which is rare and reversible when the drug is stopped)

■ Ketoconazole can inhibit the metabolism of quinidine, sulfonylureas, carbamazepine, and protease inhibitors. This interaction can increase the levels of these drugs in the body.

■ Ketoconazole should not be given with rifampin because blood levels of ketoconazole may decrease.

Synthetic Triazoles

Synthetic triazoles are a class of broad-spectrum antifungal drugs that are used to treat a number of serious or systemic fungal infections. They work by weakening the fungal cell wall, which makes the cell unstable.

Fluconazole

Fluconazole (Diflucan) is supplied as tablets, as a powder for mixing an oral suspension, and as an injection solution for IV infusion. It is used to treat:

■ fungal infections of the mouth, throat, and esophagus
■ UTIs, peritonitis, and vaginal yeast infections
■ serious systemic infections
■ pneumonia
■ cryptococcal meningitis

Fluconazole can interact with several other drugs.

■ Using fluconazole with warfarin may increase the risk of bleeding.
■ Fluconazole may increase levels of phenytoin and cyclosporine in persons taking those drugs.
■ Fluconazole may increase blood levels of oral antidiabetic drugs (such as glyburide, tolbutamide, and glipizide), increasing the risk of hypoglycemia.
■ Fluconazole may increase the activity of zidovudine.
■ Rifampin and cimetidine may enhance the metabolism of fluconazole, reducing its levels in the bloodstream.

Adverse reactions to fluconazole include:

■ nausea and vomiting
■ abdominal pain
■ diarrhea
■ headache
■ dizziness
■ elevated liver enzymes
■ rash

Other Synthetic Triazoles

Itraconazole (Sporanox) is supplied as capsules, an oral solution, and an injection solution for IV infusion. It's used to treat blastomycosis, nonmeningeal histoplasmosis, candidiasis, aspergillosis, and fungal nail disease. Itraconazole may interact with oral anticoagulants, antacids, H_2-receptor antagonists, phenytoin, and rifampin. Adverse reactions include nausea, headache, dizziness, impaired liver function, and hypertension.

Voriconazole (Vfend) is available as tablets and as a powder for oral suspension. An injection powder is also available and is mixed to create a solution for IV infusion. Voriconazole is used to treat invasive aspergillosis and serious infections caused by certain other types of fungi. This drug may interact with oral anticoagulants, phenytoin, benzodiazepines, calcium-channel blockers, sulfonylureas, tacrolimus, sirolimus, ergot alkaloids, quinidine, and pimozide. Advesrse reations include nausea and vomiting, headache, chills, fever, vision disturbances, elevated liver enzymes, rash, and tachycardia.

Glucan Synthesis Inhibitors

Caspofungin (Cancidas) is a drug in a new class of antifungal agents called glucan synthesis inhibitors. It works against fungi by inhibiting the synthesis of (1,3)-beta-D-glucan, which is an important component of the fungal cell wall.

Caspofungin is supplied as a powder that is mixed to create a solution for IV infusion. It is mainly used to treat invasive aspergillosis in patients who haven't responded to or can't tolerate other antifungal drugs.

Some important drug interactions occur with this drug:

■ Patients taking tacrolimus with caspofungin may need higher doses of tacrolimus because caspofungin decreases the blood level of tacrolimus.
■ Inducers of drug clearance (such as phenytoin, carbamazepine, efavirenz, nevirapine, and nelfinavir) may lower caspofungin clearance.
■ The use of caspofungin with cyclosporine may result in elevated liver enzyme levels and decreased caspofungin clearance. The use of these two drugs together is not recommended.

Synthetic Allylamine Derivatives

Terbinafine (Lamisil) is the most commonly used synthetic allylamine derivative. This drug inhibits fungal cell growth by inhibiting an enzyme responsible for the manufacture of ergosterol. As you read earlier, ergosterol is an important component of the fungal cell membrane.

 PROCEED WITH CAUTION

Adverse Reactions to Caspofungin

Adverse reactions to caspofungin may include:

■ nausea and vomiting
■ diarrhea
■ rash
■ facial swelling
■ tachycardia
■ tachypnea (rapid breathing)
■ paresthesia (burning or prickling sensation)

Terbinafine's main use is in treating fungal infections of fingernails or toenails. For oral administration, it is available as tablets or as granules that are sprinkled on food. The granules should not be sprinkled on applesauce or any fruit-based food and should be swallowed whole. Taking the tablet with food also increases the drug's absorption. It is available OTC (Lamisil AT) as a cream, gel, or spray for topical use.

Rare cases of liver failure have occurred with terbinafine use, even in patients with no known history of liver disease. Baseline liver enzyme test results should be obtained before terbinafine is used, and use should be avoided altogether if liver disease is suspected. There are also a few drug interactions to watch out for:

- Terbinafine clearance is decreased when it's taken with cimetidine and is increased when it's taken with rifampin.
- Terbinafine use increases plasma levels of caffeine and dextromethorphan and decreases levels of cyclosporine.

Other Antifungal Drugs

Several other drugs offer alternative forms of treatment for topical fungal infections.

Clotrimazole

Clotrimazole (Gyne-Lotrimin, Cruex, Lotrimin AF) is available OTC as a vaginal cream for internal and external treatment of candidiasis (yeast) infections. Prescription and OTC topical creams and solutions are also available to relieve external itching. These creams are also used to treat tinea cruris (jock itch), tinea pedis (athlete's foot), and ringworm. Prescription clotrimazole (Mycelex) troches (small lozenges) are used for treating candidiasis of the mouth and throat.

Clotrimazole is also available by prescription only in combination with betamethasone (topical corticosteroid) in a topical lotion and a topical cream (Lotrisone).

Griseofulvin

Griseofulvin (Grifulvin V, Gris-PEG) is supplied by prescription only as tablets and as an oral suspension. It is best

PROCEED WITH CAUTION

Adverse Reactions to Terbinafine

Adverse reactions to terbinafine include:

- headache
- visual disturbances
- nausea
- abdominal pain
- neutropenia
- Stevens-Johnson syndrome

taken with a fatty meal. It is used to treat severe fungal infections of the:

- skin (tinea corporis)
- feet (tinea pedis)
- groin (tinea cruris)
- beard area of the face and neck (tinea barbae)
- nails (tinea unguium)
- scalp (tinea capitis)

The use of griseofulvin is not indicated when the infection can be successfully treated by topical drugs. To prevent a relapse, griseofulvin therapy must continue until the fungus is eradicated and the infected skin or nails are replaced.

Miconazole

Miconazole is used to treat local fungal infections, such as vaginal and vulvar candidiasis, and topical fungal infections, such as chronic candidiasis of the skin and mucous membranes. It is supplied OTC as:

- vaginal suppositories and a vaginal cream, and combination packages that contain both dosage forms (Vagistat-3)
- a topical cream (Neosporin AF, Baza)
- a topical powder and spray powder (Desenex, Lotrimin AF, Zeasorb-AF, Cruex, Micatin, Neosporin AF)
- a topical spray solution and topical solution (Desenex, Lotrimin AF, Micatin, Neosporin AF, Fungoid)
- a topical gel (Zeasorb-AF), lotion (Zeasorb-AF), and ointment

Miconazole may be administered:

- locally to treat vaginal infections
- topically to treat topical infections

Other Topical Antifungal Drugs

The following antifungals are available only as topical drugs:

- ciclopirox (Loprox, Loprox TS, Penlac Nail Lacquer), supplied as a prescription cream, gel, shampoo, topical suspension, and topical solution
- econazole nitrate, available by prescription as a topical cream
- butoconazole nitrate (Gynazole-1) is available by prescription in the form of a vaginal cream
- naftifine (Naftin, Naftin-MP), manufactured as a prescription cream and gel
- tioconazole (Vagistat-1), supplied as an OTC vaginal ointment
- terconazole (Terazol-3, Terazol-7, Zazole), available by prescription in the form of vaginal cream and suppositories
- tolnaftate (Absorbine Athlete's Foot, Absorbine Jr., Fungi-Guard, Tinactin, Lamisil AF, Termin8, Tinaderm), manufactured as an OTC cream, solution, gel, powder, spray powder, and spray solution

- butenafine (Mentax, Lotrimin Ultra), supplied as an OTC topical cream
- sulconazole (Exelderm), available as a prescription cream and solution
- oxiconazole (Oxistat), manufactured as a prescription cream and lotion
- clioquinol with hydrocortisone (Ala-Quin, Dofscort), supplied as a prescription cream
- undecylenic acid with zinc undecylenate, supplied as an OTC ointment, and undecylenic acid with chloroxylenol (Gordochom), which is available as a prescription topical solution

QUICK QUIZ

Answer the following multiple-choice questions.

1. Which of the following conditions would typically *not* be treated with an antiviral drug?
   a. HIV/AIDS
   b. UTIs
   c. herpes infections
   d. chickenpox
2. Which of the following serious adverse reactions is *not* a danger when taking aminoglycosides?
   a. liver failure
   b. neuromuscular blockade
   c. ototoxicity
   d. renal toxicity
3. Common hypersensitivity reactions to anti-infective drugs include:
   a. anorexia, nausea, vomiting, and diarrhea.
   b. headache, dizziness, and vision disturbances.
   c. itching, rashes, hives, and respiratory distress.
   d. chills, fever, and muscle weakness.
4. Which person would be the *least* likely candidate for treatment with an influenza A antiviral drug?
   a. a person infected with influenza A
   b. a person who cannot take the flu vaccine
   c. a person who had a flu shot last week
   d. a person who had a flu shot a month ago
5. What rationale justifies using some antitubercular drugs together when treating TB?
   a. They're second-line drugs and are effective only when used together.
   b. The risk of drug toxicity is reduced.
   c. Combination therapy can prevent or delay bacterial resistance.
   d. Single-drug therapy is never effective.

Please answer each of the following questions in one to three sentences.

1. Why is resistance to antimicrobial drugs increasing?

   _____

   _____

2. What is the recommended four-drug regimen for initial treatment of tuberculosis? When and how should it be modified?

   _____

   _____

3. Describe a typical treatment regimen for a patient being treated for HIV.

   _____

   _____

4. What general precautions should a patient be aware of when taking a tetracycline?

   _____

   _____

5. What general instruction should be given to a patient who's about to start taking an oral sulfonamide?

   _____

   _____

Answer the following questions as either true or false.

1. ____ A bacteriostatic drug is more effective against bacterial pathogens than a bactericidal drug is.
2. ____ Vancomycin is the IV drug of choice for patients with serious resistant bacterial infections who are allergic to penicillin.
3. ____ A broad-spectrum antibiotic is effective against several kinds of bacteria.
4. ____ Persons who are allergic to penicillins are more likely to be allergic to cephalosporins than to other classes of antibiotics.
5. ____ Fewer antifungal drugs are available over the counter than any other type of anti-infective drug.

Match each antifungal drug in the left column with the fungal infection it treats in the right column.

1. amphotericin B   a. athlete's foot
2. clotrimazole   b. bladder infections
3. miconazole   c. fingernail and toenail infections
4. nystatin   d. skin infections
5. terbinafine   e. systemic infections

DRUG CLASSIFICATION TABLE

Classification	Generic Name	Trade Name(s)
Antibacterial drugs (aminoglycosides)	gentamicin *jen-ta-mye'-sin*	*injection:* (no longer marketed under trade name) *ointment:* (no longer marketed under trade name) *cream:* (no longer marketed under trade name) *ophthalmic ointment:* Gentak *ophthalmic solution:* Gentak
	gentamicin and prednisolone *jen-ta-mye'-sin pred-niss'-oh-lone*	*ophthalmic ointment:* Pred-G *ophthalmic suspension:* Pred-G
	neomycin *nee-o-mye'-sin*	*tablets:* (no longer marketed under trade name)
	neomycin, bacitracin, hydrocortisone, and polymyxin B *knee-oh-my'-sin ba-ci-tra'-sin hye-droe-kor'-ti-zone pol-ee-mix'-in*	*ophthalmic ointment:* (no longer marketed under trade name) *topical ointment:* Cortisporin
	neomycin, bacitracin, and polymyxin B *knee-oh-my'-sin ba-ci-tra'-sin pol-ee-mix'-in*	*topical ointment:* Triple Antibiotic, Neosporin *topical lotion:* Neosporin To Go *ophthalmic ointment:* (no longer marketed under trade name)
	neomycin, dexamethasone, and polymyxin B *knee-oh-my'-sin dex-a-meth'-a-sone pol-ee-mix'-in*	*ophthalmic suspension:* Maxitrol *ophthalmic ointment:* AK-Trol, Maxitrol
	neomycin, gramicidin, and polymyxin B *knee-oh-my'-sin gram-i-sye'-din pol-ee-mix'-in*	*ophthalmic solution:* Neosporin
	neomycin, hydrocortisone, and polymyxin B *knee-oh-my'-sin hye-droe-kor'-ti-zone pol-ee-mix'-in*	*ophthalmic suspension:* Cortisporin *otic solution:* Cortisporin, Aural Otic, Oticin HC, Otimar, Otocidin, Cortomycin *otic suspension:* Cortisporin, Cortomycin, Oticin HC, Otimar, Padiotic *topical cream:* Cortisporin
	neomycin and polymyxin B *knee-oh-my'-sin pol-ee-mix'-in*	*bladder irrigation:* Neosporin GU
	neomycin, polymyxin B, and prednisolone *knee-oh-my'-sin pol-ee-mix'-in pred-niss'-oh-lone*	*ophthalmic suspension:* Poly-Pred
	tobramycin *toe-bra-mye'-sin*	*injection:* (no longer marketed under trade name) *ophthalmic solution:* AK-Tob, Tobrex *ophthalmic ointment:* Tobrex *nebulizer solution:* Tobi
	dexamethasone and tobramycin *dex-a-meth'-a-sone toe-bra-mye'-sin*	*ophthalmic suspension:* Tobradex *ophthalmic ointment:* Tobradex
	loteprednol and tobramycin *loe-te-pred'-nol toe-bra-mye'-sin*	*ophthalmic suspension:* Zylet
	amikacin *am-i-kay'-sin*	*injection:* Amikin
	kanamycin *kan-a-mye'-sin*	*injection:* (no longer marketed under trade name)
	paromomycin *par-oh-moe-mye'-sin*	*capsules:* (no longer marketed under trade name)
	streptomycin *strep-toe-mye'-sin*	*injection:* (no longer marketed under trade name)

continued

DRUG CLASSIFICATION TABLE (continued)

Classification	Generic Name	Trade Name(s)
Antibacterial drugs (penicillins)	penicillin G benzathine *pen-i-sill'-in*	*injection:* Bicillin L-A
	penicillin G benzathine and procaine *pen-i-sill'-in pro'-cane*	*injection:* Bicillin C-R
	penicillin G potassium *pen-i-sill'-in*	*injection:* Pfizerpen
	penicillin G procaine *pen-i-sill'-in*	*injection:* (no longer marketed under trade name)
	penicillin G sodium *pen-i-sill'-in*	*injection:* (no longer marketed under trade name)
	penicillin V potassium *pen-i-sill'-in*	*tablets:* (no longer marketed under trade name) *oral solution:* (no longer marketed under trade name)
	dicloxacillin *dye-klox-a-sill'-in*	*capsules:* (no longer marketed under trade name)
	nafcillin *naf-sill'-in*	*injection:* (no longer marketed under trade name)
	oxacillin *ox-a-sill'-in*	*injection:* (no longer marketed under trade name)
	amoxicillin *a-mox-i-sill'-in*	*capsules:* (no longer marketed under trade name) *tablets:* (no longer marketed under trade name) *chewable tablets:* (no longer marketed under trade name) *oral suspension:* Amoxil
	amoxicillin and clavulanate potassium *a-mox-i-sill'-in klah-view-lan'-ate*	*tablets:* Augmentin *extended-release tablets:* Augmentin XR *chewable tablets:* Augmentin *oral suspension:* Augmentin
	ampicillin *am-pi-sill'-in*	*capsules:* (no longer marketed under trade name) *injection:* (no longer marketed under trade name) *oral suspension:* (no longer marketed under trade name)
	ampicillin and sulbactam *am-pi-sill'-in sull-back'-tam*	*injection:* Unasyn
	ticarcillin and clavulanate potassium *ty-kar-sill'-in klav'-ue-la-nate*	*injection:* Timentin
Antibacterial drugs (cephalosporins)	cefadroxil *saf-a-drox'-ill*	*capsules:* (no longer marketed under trade name) *tablets:* (no longer marketed under trade name) *oral suspension:* (no longer marketed under trade name)
	cefazolin *sef-a'-zoe-lin*	*injection:* (no longer marketed under trade name)
	cephalexin *sef'-a-lex-in*	*capsules:* Keflex *tablets:* (no longer marketed under trade name) *oral suspension:* Panixine
	cefaclor *sef'-a-klor*	*capsules:* (no longer marketed under trade name) *extended-release tablets:* (no longer marketed under trade name) *chewable tablets:* Raniclor *oral suspension:* (no longer marketed under trade name)

continued

DRUG CLASSIFICATION TABLE (continued)

Classification	Generic Name	Trade Name(s)
Antibacterial drugs (cephalosporins) (continued)	cefuroxime axetil *sef-yoor-ox'-eem*	*tablets:* Ceftin *oral suspension:* Ceftin
	cefuroxime sodium *sef-yoor-ox'-eem*	*injection:* Zinacef
	cefotetan *sef-oh-tee'-tan*	*injection:* Cefotan
	cefprozil *sef-proe'-zil*	*tablets:* Cefzil *oral suspension:* Cefzil
	ceftibuten *sef-ta-byoo'-ten*	*capsules:* Cedax *oral suspension:* Cedax
	cefoxitin *sef-ox'-i-tin*	*injection:* (no longer marketed under trade name)
	cefdinir *sef'-din-er*	*capsules:* Omnicef *oral suspension:* Omnicef
	cefotaxime *sef-oh-taks'-eem*	*injection:* Claforan
	cefpodoxime *sef-poed-ox'-eem*	*tablets:* Vantin *oral suspension:* (no longer marketed under trade name)
	ceftazidime *sef-taz'-i-deem*	*injection:* Fortaz, Tazicef
	ceftizoxime *sef-ti-zox'-eem*	*injection:* Cefizox
	ceftriaxone *sef-try-ax'-on*	*injection:* Rocephin
	cefditoren *sef-di-tor'-en*	*tablets:* Spectracef
	cefepime *sef'-ah-pime*	*injection:* Maxipime
Antibacterial drugs (tetracyclines)	doxycycline hyclate *dox-i-sye'-kleen*	*injection:* Doxy *capsules:* Vibramycin, Oraxyl *tablets:* Vibra-Tabs, Alodox, Periostat *extended-release tablets:* Doryx *extended-release capsules:* (no longer marketed under trade name)
	doxycycline monohydrate *dox-i-sye'-kleen*	*capsules:* Monodox, Adoxa *tablets:* Adoxa *oral suspension:* Vibramycin *biphasic capsules:* Oracea
	doxycycline calcium *dox-i-sye'-kleen*	*oral suspension:* Vibramycin
	minocycline *min-oh-sye'-kleen*	*capsules:* Dynacin, Minocin *tablets:* Dynacin, Myrac *extended-release tablets:* Solodyn *periodontal powder:* Arestin
	demeclocycline *deh-meh-kloe-sye'-kleen*	*tablets:* Declomycin
	tetracycline *tet-ra-sye'-kleen*	*capsules:* (no longer marketed under trade name)

continued

DRUG CLASSIFICATION TABLE (continued)

Classification	Generic Name	Trade Name(s)
Antibacterial drugs (lincomycin derivatives)	clindamycin *klin-da-my'-sin*	*capsules:* Cleocin *oral solution:* Cleocin *injection:* Cleocin *topical solution:* Cleocin T, Clinda-Derm *topical pledget:* Cleocin T *topical gel:* Cleocin T, Clindagel, Clindamax *topical foam:* Evoclin *topical lotion:* Cleocin T, Clindamax *vaginal suppository:* Cleocin Ovules *vaginal cream:* Cleocin, Clindamax, Clindesse
	lincomycin *lin-koe-my'-sin*	*injection:* Lincocin
Antibacterial drugs (macrolides)	erythromycin *er-ith-roe-my'-sin*	*tablets:* (no longer marketed under trade name) *extended-release capsules:* (no longer marketed under trade name) *extended-release tablets:* Ery-Tab, PCE *topical solution:* Eryderm *topical ointment:* Akne-mycin *topical gel:* Emgel, Erygel *topical pledget:* Emcin Clear, Ery Pad *topical pad:* T Stat *ophthalmic ointment:* (no longer marketed under trade name)
	erythromycin ethylsuccinate *er-ith-roe-my'-sin*	*tablets:* E.E.S. *oral suspension:* E.E.S., Eryped
	erythromycin lactobionate *er-ith-roe-my'-sin*	*injection:* Erythrocin
	erythromycin stearate *er-ith-roe-my'-sin*	*tablets:* My-E
	erythromycin and benzoyl peroxide *er-ith-roe-my'-sin been'-zoyl per-ox'-ide*	*powder:* Benzamycin *topical gel:* Benzamycin
	azithromycin *ay-zi-thro-my'-sin*	*tablets:* Zithromax *oral suspension:* Zithromax *injection:* Zithromax *ophthalmic solution:* Azasite *extended-release oral suspension:* ZMax
	clarithromycin *klar-ith-ro-my'-sin*	*tablets:* Biaxin *extended-release tablets:* Biaxin XL *oral suspension:* Biaxin
Antibacterial drugs (vancomycin)	vancomycin *van-koe-mye'-cin*	*injection:* Vancocin *capsules:* Vancocin
Antibacterial drugs (carbapenems)	imipenem-cilastatin *ih-mih-pen'-em sigh-lah-stat'-in*	*injection solution:* Primaxin IV *injection suspension:* Primaxin IM
	ertapenem *er-ta-pen'-em*	*injection:* Invanz
	meropenem *meh-row-pen'-em*	*injection:* Merrem

continued

DRUG CLASSIFICATION TABLE *(continued)*

Classification	Generic Name	Trade Name(s)
Antibacterial drugs (monobactams)	aztreonam *azz-tree'-oh-nam*	*injection:* Azactam
Antibacterial drugs (fluoroquinolones)	ciprofloxacin *si-proe-flox'-a-sin*	*tablets:* Cipro *extended-release tablets:* Cipro XR *oral suspension:* Cipro *injection:* Cipro *ophthalmic solution:* Ciloxan *ophthalmic ointment:* Ciloxan
	ciprofloxacin and dexamethasone *si-proe-flox'-a-sin dex-a-meth'-a-sone*	*otic suspension:* Ciprodex
	ciprofloxacin and hydrocortisone *si-proe-flox'-a-sin hye-droe-kor'-ti-zone*	*otic suspension:* Cipro HC
	levofloxacin *lee-voe-flox'-a-sin*	*tablets:* Levaquin *oral solution:* Levaquin *injection:* Levaquin *ophthalmic solution:* Quixin, Iquix
	moxifloxacin *mocks-ah-flox'-a-sin*	*tablets:* Avelox *injection:* Avelox I.V. *ophthalmic solution:* Vigamox
	ofloxacin *oe-flox'-a-sin*	*tablets:* (no longer marketed under trade name) *ophthalmic solution:* Ocuflox *otic solution:* Floxin
	gatifloxacin *ga-tah-flox'-a-sin*	*ophthalmic solution:* Zymar
	norfloxacin *nor-flox'-a-sin*	*tablets:* Noroxin
Antibacterial drugs (sulfonamides)	sulfamethoxazole and trimetho-prim (SMX-TMP) *sul-fa-meth-ox'-a-zole trye-meth'-oh-prim*	*tablets:* Bactrim, Septra *oral suspension:* Sulfatrim, Sultrex *injection:* (no longer marketed under trade name)
	sulfadiazine *sul-fa-dye'-a-zeen*	*tablets:* (no longer marketed under trade name)
	silver sulfadiazine *sil'-ver sul-fa-dye'-a-zeen*	*topical cream:* Silvadene, SSD, Thermazene
	erythromycin ethylsuccinate and sulfisoxazole *er-ith-roe-my'-sin sul-fi-sox'-a-zole*	*oral suspension:* Pediazole, E.S.P.
Antibacterial drugs (nitrofurantoin)	nitrofurantoin *nye-troe-fyoor-an'-toyn*	*capsules:* Macrobid, Macrodantin *oral suspension:* Furadantin
Antiviral drugs	acyclovir *ay-sye'-kloe-ver*	*tablets:* Urotoin *tablets:* Zovirax *capsules:* Zovirax *oral suspension:* Zovirax *injection:* (no longer marketed under trade name) *topical ointment:* Zovirax *topical cream:* Zovirax

continued

DRUG CLASSIFICATION TABLE (continued)

Classification	Generic Name	Trade Name(s)
Antiviral drugs (continued)	famciclovir *fam-sye'-kloe-vir*	*tablets:* Famvir
	ganciclovir *gan-sye-kloe-vir*	*capsules:* (no longer marketed under trade name) *injection:* Cytovene *ophthalmic insert:* Vitasert
	valacyclovir *val-ah-sye'-kloe-ver*	*tablets:* Valtrex
	valganciclovir *val-gan-si'-klo-veer*	*tablets:* Valcyte
	foscarnet *foss-car'-net*	*injection:* Foscavir
	oseltamivir *oh-sell-tam'-ih-veer*	*capsules:* Tamiflu *oral suspension:* Tamiflu
	ribavirin *rye-ba-vye'-rin*	*tablets:* Copegus, RibaTab *capsules:* Rebetol *oral solution:* Rebetol *powder for nebulizer solution:* Virazole
	zanamivir *zan-am'-ah-ver*	*inhalation powder:* Relenza
	amantadine *a-man'-ta-deen*	*tablets:* Symmetrel *capsules:* (no longer marketed under trade name) *oral solution:* (no longer marketed under trade name)
	rimantadine *ri-man'-ta-deen*	*tablets:* Flumadine
	zidovudine (ZDV) *zid-o-vew'-den*	*tablets:* Retrovir *capsules:* Retrovir *syrup:* Retrovir *injection:* Retrovir
	lamivudine and zidovudine *la-mi'-vyoo-deen zid-o-vew'-den*	*tablets:* Combivir
	abacavir, lamivudine, and zidovudine *ab-ah-kav'-ear la-mi'-vyoo-deen zid-o-vew'-den*	*tablets:* Trizivir
	abacavir *ab-ah-kav'-ear*	*tablets:* Ziagen *oral solution:* Ziagen
	abacavir and lamivudine *ab-ah-kav'-ear la-mi'-vyoo-deen*	*tablets:* Epzicom
	didanosine (ddI) *dye-dan'-oh-sin*	*extended-release capsules:* Videx EC *oral solution:* Videx
	emtricitabine *em-trye-sye'-ta-been*	*capsules:* Emtriva *oral solution:* Emtriva
	efavirenz, emtricitabine, and tenofovir *ef-ah-vi'-renz em-trye-sye'-ta-been te-noe'-fo-veer*	*tablets:* Atripla

continued

DRUG CLASSIFICATION TABLE *(continued)*

Classification	Generic Name	Trade Name(s)
Antiviral drugs *(continued)*	emtriciabine and tenofovir *em-trye-sye'-ta-been te-noe'-fo-veer*	*tablets*: Truvada
	lamivudine (3TC) *la-mi'-vyoo-deen*	*tablets:* Epivir, Epivir HBV *oral solution:* Epivir, Epivir HBV
	stavudine (d4T) *stay-vew'-den*	*capsules:* Zerit *oral solution:* Zerit
	delavirdine *dell-ah-vur'-den*	*tablets:* Rescriptor
	efavirenz *ef-ah-vi'-renz*	*tablets:* Sustiva *capsules:* Sustiva
	nevirapine *neh-vear'-ah-peen*	*tablets:* Viramune *oral suspension:* Viramune
	tenofovir (PMPA) *te-noe'-fo-veer*	*tablets:* Viread
	fosamprenavir *fos-am-pren'-a-veer*	*tablets:* Lexiva *oral suspension:* Lexiva
	atazanavir *a-ta-zan'-a-vir*	*capsules:* Reyataz
	indinavir *in-din'-ah-ver*	*capsules:* Crixivan
	nelfinavir *nell-fin'-a-veer*	*tablets:* Viracept *oral suspension:* Viracept
	ritonavir *rih-ton'-ah-veer*	*capsules:* Norvir *oral solution:* Norvir
	saquinavir *sa-kwen'-a-veer*	*tablets:* Invirase *capsules:* Invirase
	lopinavir and ritonavir *low-pin'-ah-veer rih-ton'-ah-veer*	*tablets:* Kaletra *oral solution:* Kaletra
Antitubercular drugs	isoniazid (INH) *eye-soe-nye'-a-zid*	*tablets:* (no longer marketed under trade name) *oral solution:* (no longer marketed under trade name) *injection:* Nydrazid
	rifampin *rif-am'-pin*	*capsules:* Rifadin *injection:* Rifadin
	isoniazid and rifampin *eye-soe-nye'-a-zid rif-am'-pin*	*capsules:* IsonaRif, Rifamate
	pyrazinamide (PZA) *peer-a-zin'-a-mide*	*tablets:* (no longer marketed under trade name)
	isoniazid, rifampin, and pyrazinamide *eye-soe-nye'-a-zid rif-am'-pin peer-a-zin'-a-mide*	*tablets:* Rifater
	ethambutol *eth-am'-byoo-tole*	*tablets:* Myambutol

continued

DRUG CLASSIFICATION TABLE (continued)

Classification	Generic Name	Trade Name(s)
Antifungal drugs	amphotericin B *am-fo-ter'-eye-sin*	*injection:* (no longer marketed under trade name)
	nystatin *nye-stat'-in*	*capsules:* Bio-Statin *tablets:* (no longer marketed under trade name) *oral suspension:* (no longer marketed under trade name) *topical powder:* Mycostatin, Nyamyc, Pedi-Dri *topical ointment:* (no longer marketed under trade name) *topical cream:* (no longer marketed under trade name) *vaginal tablets:* (no longer marketed under trade name)
	flucytosine *floo-sye'-toe-seen*	*capsules:* Ancobon
	ketoconazole *kee-toe-koe'-na-zole*	*tablets:* (no longer marketed under trade name) *cream:* Kuric *foam:* Extina *gel:* Xolegel *shampoo:* Nizoral
	fluconazole *floo-kon'-a-zole*	*tablets:* Diflucan *oral suspension:* Diflucan *injection:* Diflucan
	itraconazole *eye-tra-kon'-a-zole*	*capsules:* Sporanox *oral solution:* Sporanox *injection:* Sporanox
	voriconazole *vor-i-kon'-a-zole*	*tablets:* Vfend *oral suspension:* Vfend *injection:* Vfend
	caspofungin *kass-poe-fun'-jin*	*injection:* Cancidas
	terbinafine *ter-ben'-a-feen*	*tablets (Rx):* Lamisil oral granules (Rx): Lamisil *topical cream (OTC):* Lamisil AT *topical gel (OTC):* Lamisil AT *topical spray (OTC):* Lamisil AT
	clotrimazole *kloe-trye'-ma-zole*	*troche (Rx):* Mycelex *vaginal cream (OTC):* Gyne-Lotrimin *topical cream (OTC):* Anti-Fungal, Cruex, Lotrimin AF *topical solution (OTC):* Lotrimin AF *topical solution (Rx):* (no longer marketed under trade name)

continued

DRUG CLASSIFICATION TABLE *(continued)*

Classification	Generic Name	Trade Name(s)
Antifungal drugs *(continued)*	betamethasone and clotrimazole *bay-ta-meth'-a-zone kloe-trye'-ma-zole*	*topical lotion:* (no longer marketed under trade name) *topical cream:* Lotrisone
	griseofulvin *griz-ee-oh-full'-vin*	*tablets:* Grifulvin V, Gris-PEG *oral suspension:* Grifulvin V
	miconazole *mi-kon'-a-zole*	*vaginal suppositories:* (no longer marketed under trade name) *vaginal cream:* (no longer marketed under trade name) *vaginal cream and suppository combination pack:* Vagistat-3 *topical cream:* Micatin, Neosporin AF, Baza *topical powder:* Desenex, Lotrimin AF, Zeasorb-AF *spray powder:* Cruex, Desenex, Lotrimin AF, Micatin, Neosporin AF
	ciclopirox *sic-lo-peer'-ox*	*topical cream:* Loprox *gel:* Loprox *shampoo:* Loprox *topical solution:* Penlac Nail Lacquer *topical suspension:* Loprox TS
	econazole nitrate *ee-con'-uh-zole nye'-trate*	*topical cream:* (no longer marketed under trade name)
	butoconazole nitrate *byoo-toe-koe'-nuh-zole*	*vaginal cream (Rx):* Gynazole-1
	naftifine *naf'ti-feen*	*topical cream:* Naftin, Naftin-MP *gel:* Naftin
	tioconazole *tee-o-kon'-a-zole*	*vaginal ointment:* Vagistat-1
	terconazole *ter-kon'-a-zole*	*vaginal suppositories:* Terazol-3, Zazole *vaginal cream:* Terazol-3, Terazol-7, Zazole
	tolnaftate *tole-naf'-tate*	*topical cream:* Absorbine Athlete's Foot, Fungi-Guard, Tinactin *topical powder:* Lamisil AF, Tinactin *spray powder:* Lamisil AF, Tinactin, Aftate *spray solution:* Tinactin *topical solution:* Fungi-Guard, Termin8, Tinaderm *topical gel:* Absorbine Jr.
	butenafine *beu-ten'-ah-feen*	*topical cream:* Mentax, Lotrimin Ultra
	sulconazole *sul-kon'-a-zole*	*topical cream:* Exelderm *topical solution:* Exelderm
	oxiconazole *ox-ee-kon'-ah-zole*	*topical cream:* Oxistat *lotion:* Oxistat

continued

DRUG CLASSIFICATION TABLE *(continued)*

Classification	Generic Name	Trade Name(s)
Antifungal drugs *(continued)*	clioquinol and hydrocortisone *kli-oh-qwe'-knol hye-droe-kor'-ti-zone*	*topical cream:* Ala-Quin, Dofscort
	undecylenic acid and zinc undecylenate *un-deh-sil-en'-ik zink un-deh-sil-en'-ate*	*topical ointment:* (no longer marketed under trade name)
	undecylenic acid and chloroxylenol *un-deh-sil-en'-ik klor-oh-zye'-le-nole*	*topical solution:* Gordochom

CHAPTER 10

Anti-Inflammatory, Anti-Allergy, and Immunosuppressant Drugs

CHAPTER OBJECTIVES

- Match brand and generic names of commonly used anti-inflammatory, anti-allergy, and immunosuppressant drugs
- Identify the classification of commonly used anti-inflammatory, anti-allergy, and immunosuppressant drugs
- Identify the uses of commonly used respiratory drugs
- Explain the mechanism of action and effects of sedating and nonsedating antihistamines
- Describe the differences in how antihistamines, mast cell stabilizers, and leukotriene receptor antagonists work to treat allergies
- Explain the mechanism of action and effects of glucocorticoids
- Identify common adverse reactions to noncorticosteroid immunosuppressants
- Explain how immunosuppressants work in transplant patients
- Compare and contrast the use of uricosurics and other antigout drugs in treating gout

KEY TERMS

allergic reaction—an immune system response to a substance the body doesn't normally attack

antibodies—proteins that are specialized to fight specific invading organisms

antihistamines—drugs that block the effects of histamine on body organs and structures

conjunctivitis—inflammation of the mucous membrane lining the inner surfaces of the eye

corticosteroids—hormones secreted from the adrenal cortex that suppress immune responses and reduce inflammation; the collective name for *glucocorticoids* and *mineralocorticoids*

glucocorticoids—natural or synthetic hormones with anti-inflammatory, metabolic, and immunosuppressant effects

gout—a type of arthritis (gouty arthritis) in which uric acid accumulates in increased amounts in the blood and is often deposited in the joints

histamine—a substance in various body tissues, such as the heart, lungs, gastric mucosa, and skin, that is produced in response to injury

mineralocorticoids—hormones that regulate the balance of potassium, sodium, and water in the body

osteoarthritis—a noninflammatory joint disease resulting in degeneration of the articular cartilage and changes in the synovial membrane

phagocytosis—the process of destroying foreign cells and bacteria by digestion

rheumatoid arthritis—a chronic disease characterized by inflammatory changes within the body's connective tissue

rhinitis—inflammation of the nasal passages resulting in increased nasal secretions

uricosurics—drugs that act to increase the excretion of uric acid from the body

Immune and inflammatory responses protect the body from invading foreign substances. When the body encounters a virus or injury, the immune system acts immediately by producing a generalized inflammatory response. This response is like an artillery attack. Fighters go after any viruses, bacteria, or other microorganisms in range. The immune response gradually becomes more specific as it continues. White blood cells called lymphocytes produce **antibodies**, special fighter proteins that search for and destroy specific invading organisms.

There are several key fighters in the immune system defense.

- **Histamine** is a substance released in the body when tissues are injured. It causes blood (including white blood cells) and fluids to enter the tissues, resulting in swelling and inflammation.
- B cells produce antibodies, which are proteins that are specialized to fight specific invading organisms.
- Phagocytes are a type of white blood cell (leukocyte) that surrounds invading organisms and antigens. They break into and digest foreign cells, destroying the invader.
- T cells are a type of lymphocyte that recruits fighter cells, such as macrophages, to destroy invading organisms.

In this chapter, you'll learn about drugs that modify immune or inflammatory system responses. These drugs are used in the following ways:

- to block the effects of histamine on target tissues
- to suppress immune responses and reduce inflammation
- to prevent the rejection of transplanted organs
- to treat autoimmune disease
- to prevent or control the frequency of gouty arthritis attacks

ANTIHISTAMINES

Antihistamines are used to block the effects of histamine that occur during what is commonly known as an **allergic reaction** (an immediate hypersensitivity reaction). An allergic reaction occurs when the immune system responds to a normally harmless substance such as pollen or dust. Histamine is a chemical released by the body during allergic reactions that increases swelling, inflammation, itching, and other body responses to allergy. Antihistamines are typically used to treat the symptoms of the following reactions:

- allergic **rhinitis** (runny nose and itchy eyes caused by local sensitivity reaction)
- vasomotor rhinitis (rhinitis not caused by allergy or infection)
- allergic **conjunctivitis** (inflammation of the membranes of the eye)

- urticaria (hives)
- angioedema (submucosal swelling in the hands, face, and feet)

Antihistamines are histamine-1 (H_1) receptor antagonists. They work by competing with histamine for binding to H_1-receptor sites throughout the body. H_1-receptor sites are found on effector cells, the cells that cause allergic symptoms. When antihistamines bind with the H_1-receptor sites, they stop histamine from producing its effects. However, these drugs can't displace histamine that is already bound to the receptor.

TIP The prefix *anti-* means "opposing." That's exactly what antihistamines are—opposing forces against allergic reactions.

In general, H_1-receptor antagonists produce their effects by:

- blocking the action of histamine on the small blood vessels
- decreasing dilation of arterioles (small branches of arteries) and engorgement of tissues
- reducing the leakage of plasma proteins and fluids from capillaries, which lessens edema
- stopping smooth muscle responses to histamine (especially blocking the constriction of bronchial, GI, and vascular smooth muscle)
- relieving symptoms by acting on terminal nerve endings in the skin that flare and itch when stimulated by histamine
- suppressing adrenal medulla stimulation (part of the adrenal gland that releases epinephrine)
- suppressing autonomic ganglia stimulation (nerve cells that stimulate the organs and muscles in the autonomic nervous system response)
- suppressing exocrine gland secretion, such as the glands that produce tears and saliva

Antihistamines may interact with many drugs, sometimes with life-threatening consequences.

- They may block or reverse the vasopressor effects of epinephrine, producing vasodilation, increased heart rate, and very low blood pressure.
- They may mask the toxic signs and symptoms of ototoxicity (a damaging effect on hearing) related to aminoglycosides or large dosages of salicylates.

When filling a prescription for a H_1-receptor antagonists, it's important to know whether the drug is sedating or nonsedating.

Antihistamines can have other therapeutic uses.

- As you learned in Chapter 3, the antihistamine diphenhydramine can help treat the symptoms of Parkinson disease.
- As you learned in Chapter 8, some antihistamines are used primarily to control nausea and vomiting. Examples include dimenhydrinate and meclizine.

- Antihistamines may also be used as adjunctive therapy to treat an anaphylactic reaction after life-threatening symptoms are controlled.
- Because of its antiserotonin qualities, the antihistamine cyproheptadine may be used to treat Cushing disease, serotonin-associated diarrhea, vascular cluster headaches, and anorexia nervosa.
- Antihistamines may be used as a sleep aid for patients with insomnia.

Sedating H₁-Receptor Antagonists

Sedating H₁-receptor antagonists affect the CNS and other areas of the body. They cross the blood-brain barrier and act on H₁-receptor sites in the brain. As a result, they often produce drowsiness and other CNS-depressing symptoms.

Sedating H₁-receptor antagonists may cause the following drug interactions:

- Sedating H₁-receptor antagonists may have additive effects with other CNS depressants, such as hypnotics, sedatives, tranquilizers, and alcohol.
- MAO inhibitors may lengthen and intensify the effects of sedating H₁-receptor antagonists.

Brompheniramine

Brompheniramine is a prescription medication used to relieve symptoms of hay fever or other respiratory allergies, including:

- sneezing
- itchy nose or throat

! PROCEED WITH CAUTION

Adverse Reactions to Sedating H₁-Receptor Antagonists

The most common adverse reaction to sedating H₁-receptor antagonists is drowsiness. Other CNS reactions may include:

- disturbed coordination
- dizziness
- sleepiness and fatigue
- muscle weakness

GI reactions may include:

- dryness of the mouth, nose, and throat
- constipation
- epigastric distress
- loss of appetite
- nausea and/or vomiting

Antihistamines may also affect the heart. Cardiovascular reactions may include:

- hypotension
- hypertension
- rapid heart rate
- arrhythmias

- watery eyes
- runny nose

Some formulations may also be used to relieve sneezing and runny nose related to the common cold and to relieve simple cases of urticaria and angioedema.

Brompheniramine is available as chewable tablets (Brovex CT), extended-release tablets (Bidhist, BPM, Lo-Hist 12), extended-release capsules (Lodrane 12), oral solution (J-Tan PD, Vazol) and oral suspension (J-Tan, B-Vex, Brovex, TanaCof-XR). Brompheniramin and A similar compound, dexbrompheniramine, are found in combination with decongestants, acetaminophen, and/or cough suppressants. Some common trade names for these combination products include Drixoral and Comtrex. These combination products are available both OTC and by prescription. Brompheniramine is normally taken with food, water, or milk to reduce gastric irritation.

TIP Because many OTC products contain multiple ingredients, it's your responsibility as a technician to know all the generic names of the active ingredients. This way, you can help a patient determine whether she is buying products that contain a duplication in therapy.

Chlorpheniramine

Chlorpheniramine is used to treat symptoms of hay fever and other respiratory allergies, as well as the common cold. These symptoms include:

- sneezing
- itching, watery eyes
- scratchy throat
- runny nose

In OTC formulations, chlorpheniramine is manufactured as tablets (Aller-Chlor, Chlor-Trimeton Allergy), extended-release tablets (Chlor-Trimeton Allergy), and oral solution (Aller-Chlor, Diabetic Tussin Allergy Relief). By prescription, it's available as extended-release capsules (CPM 12 mg), extended-release tablets (ED-Chlor-Tan) and oral suspension (ED-Chlor Ped, TanaHist-PD, Chlor-Tan, P-Tann, PediaTan). Chlorpheniramine is also found in many combination products.

TIP Of the sedating antihistamines, brompheniramine, dexbrompheniramine, and chlorpheniramine are the *least* sedating.

Cetirizine

Cetirizine is used to treat chronic urticaria and perennial and seasonal allergic rhinitis. It is available OTC in the form of tablets (Zyrtec Allergy, Zyrtec Hives Relief), chewable tablets (Children's Zyrtec Allergy), and syrup (Zyrtec Children's Alelrgy, Zyrtec Children's Hives Relief). It is also available in a combination product with pseudoephedrine (Zyrtec-D).

A similar compound, levocetirizine, is available to treat the same conditions. Levocetirizine (Xyzal) is a prescription drug that is manufactured in the form of tablets.

Cyproheptadine

Cyproheptadine is used to treat the following hypersensitivity reactions:

- perennial and seasonal allergic rhinitis
- vasomotor rhinitis
- allergic conjunctivitis caused by inhalant allergens and foods
- mild urticaria and angioedema

- allergic reactions to blood or plasma
- cold urticaria
- dermatographism (chronic hives that result from touch and pressure on the skin)
- anaphylactic therapy (as an adjunct to standard therapy)

Cyproheptadine is available by prescription only. It's manufactured as tablets or oral solution.

Clemastine

Clemastine is used to treat allergic rhinitis, urticaria, and angioedema in adults and children aged 6 to 12 years old.

HOW IT WORKS

How Diphenhydramine Stops an Allergic Response

Although diphenhydramine can't reverse symptoms of an allergic response, it can stop the response from progressing. Here's what happens (see figure 10-1).

1. Mast cells play an important role in the allergic response. They are found in most body tissues. Mast cells become sensitized to specific antigens (foreign substances that cause the immune system to act). When they are exposed to the antigen many times, mast cells release chemical mediators. One of

these mediators, histamine, binds to H_1 receptors on the effector cells (the cells that are responsible for allergic symptoms). This starts an allergic response that affects the respiratory, cardiovascular, GI, endocrine, and integumentary (skin) systems.

2. Diphenhydramine competes with histamine for H_1-receptor sites on the effector cells. By attaching to these sites first, the drug prevents more histamine from binding to the effector cells.

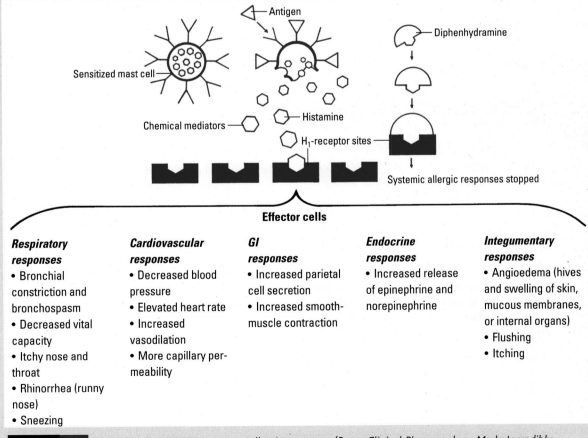

Respiratory responses
- Bronchial constriction and bronchospasm
- Decreased vital capacity
- Itchy nose and throat
- Rhinorrhea (runny nose)
- Sneezing

Cardiovascular responses
- Decreased blood pressure
- Elevated heart rate
- Increased vasodilation
- More capillary permeability

GI responses
- Increased parietal cell secretion
- Increased smooth-muscle contraction

Endocrine responses
- Increased release of epinephrine and norepinephrine

Integumentary responses
- Angioedema (hives and swelling of skin, mucous membranes, or internal organs)
- Flushing
- Itching

FIGURE 10-1 How chlorpheniramine stops an allergic response. (From *Clinical Pharmacology Made Incredibly Easy.* 2nd Ed. Philadelphia, PA: Lippincott Williams & Wilkins; 2005.)

Clemastine is sold over the counter as tablets (Tavist Allergy). It is also sold by prescription as tablets and syrup.

Dimenhydrinate

Dimenhydrinate is used to treat nausea. It's manufactured as tablets, and chewable tablets, OTC sale as Dramamine. It's also available by prescription as vials for injection. Dimenhydrinate is highly attracted to H_1 receptors in the brain and may have strong CNS effects.

Diphenhydramine

Diphenhydramine is used to treat the following reactions:

- perennial and seasonal allergic rhinitis
- vasomotor rhinitis
- allergic conjunctivitis caused by inhalant allergens and food
- mild, uncomplicated cases of urticaria and angioedema
- allergic reactions to blood or plasma in patients with a history of these reactions

It's also used as an adjunct to anaphylactic therapy, a cough suppressant for patients with colds or allergies, and a sleep aid for patients with insomnia.

Diphenhydramine is available OTC and by prescription. It's also found in many combination products. For OTC use, diphenhydramine is manufactured in many different forms, including:

- tablets, chewable tablets, and orally disintegrating tablets (Bendaryl Allergy)
- capsules (Benadryl Allergy)
- orally disintegrating strips (Benadryl Allergy, Benadryl Children's Allergy)

AT THE COUNTER

Double Duty for Diphenhydramine

A patient comes to the register with the store brand of a popular sleep aid medication and the store version of Benadryl, which she knows is for allergies. The patient seems somewhat puzzled because the two products appear to have the same active ingredient, diphenhydramine. What should you tell the patient when she asks what the difference is between them, other than price?

Diphenhydramine is an antihistamine for allergies; however, one of the most common adverse reactions to diphenhydramine is drowsiness. Therefore, diphenhydramine and other sedating antihistamines are often used in OTC sleep aids.

What would you tell the patient never to combine with diphenhydramine?

Alcohol and diphenhydramine should never be consumed together. The combination of the two increases the sedative and respiratory depressant effects of the central nervous system.

- oral solution, elixir, suspension, and syrup (Benadryl Allergy, PediaCare Nighttime Cough)
- topical cream, gel, solution, and spray (Benadryl)

By prescription, diphenhydramine comes in the form of cartridges and vials for parenteral injection.

Meclizine

Meclizine is an antihistamine that is sold OTC and by prescription. It's mainly used to treat nausea and vertigo. For OTC sales, it's manufactured as tablets (Dramamine Less Drowsy) and chewable tablets (Bonine). By prescription, meclizine is available in the form of tablets (Antivert). Children under 12 years of age shouldn't be given this medication without consultation with a physician.

TIP You learned about dimenhydrinate and meclizine in Chapter 8. These drugs are useful for treating nausea and vomiting.

Promethazine

A common drug for treating nausea, vomiting, and motion sickness is promethazine. It's also used to treat:

- perennial or seasonal allergic rhinitis
- vasomotor rhinitis
- allergic conjunctivitis due to allergens or food
- mild cases of urticaria and angioedema
- allergic reactions to blood or plasma
- anaphylactic reactions (used as an adjunct therapy)

Promethazine is available by prescription only. It's given as tablets, oral solution, suppositories (Phenadoz, Promethegan), and by injection (Phenergan). This drug is also found in combination with meperidine, dextromethorphan, phenylephrine, or codeine. These combination products are available by prescription only.

Injectable forms of promethazine are given by deep IM injection. This medication is associated with increased hazards when used for IV injections. Oral therapy should be resumed as soon as possible.

Promethazine may interact with other medications:

- Taking promethazine with anticholinergic drugs may increase the effects of the anticholinergics.
- Promethazine may increase or lengthen the sedative action of CNS depressants, including general anesthetics, narcotic analgesics, sedatives or hypnotics (such as barbiturates), tranquilizers, and tricyclic antidepressants.
- When taken with epinephrine, promethazine may reverse the vasopressor effect.
- Taking this drug with MAO inhibitors may increase extrapyramidal effects (involuntary movements).

In addition to the adverse reactions common to other sedating H_1-receptor antagonists, taking promethazine may also result in stimulation. (Hyperexcitability has been reported in children.) This medication shouldn't be used in children under two years of age because of the risk of fatal respiratory depression. Patients with compromised respiratory function (for example, sleep apnea, chronic obstructive pulmonary disease) should avoid using promethazine. Promethazine is highly attracted to H_1 receptors in the brain and may have strong CNS effects.

Nonsedating H_1-Receptor Antagonists

Nonsedating H_1-receptor antagonists have fewer effects on the CNS than other antihistamines. That's because they act a bit differently. They compete for H_1-receptor sites in peripheral areas of the body, but they don't cross the blood-brain barrier easily. As a result, these drugs have little action on H_1 receptors in the brain. They don't commonly produce drowsiness or other CNS symptoms.

Many nonsedating H_1-receptor antagonists also come in combination products with a decongestant, such as pseudoephedrine. These combination products are easy to identify because the letter D usually follows the trade name.

The most common adverse reaction to these drugs is headache.

T I P It's easy to recognize nonsedating H_1-receptor antagonists by their generic names: they all end in the letters *-adine*.

Desloratadine

Desloratadine (Clarinex, Clarinex RediTabs) is used to treat:

- chronic idiopathic urticaria
- perennial allergic rhinitis
- seasonal allergic rhinitis

Desloratadine is available by prescription only. It's manufactured as tablets, orally disintegrating tablets, and syrup. It's typically taken once a day. In addition to the adverse reactions common to other nonsedating antihistamines, desloratadine may cause:

- drowsiness
- dry mouth, nose, and throat
- fatigue

T I P Allegra comes in three strengths: 30-, 60-, and 180-mg tablets. Allegra 30 mg is for children who are 6 to 11 years old; Allegra 60 mg is dosed twice a day; Allegra 180 mg is a sustained-release tablet that is dosed once daily. Be careful to select the right product when preparing a prescription.

Fexofenadine

Fexofenadine (Allegra) is sold by prescription only. It's used for uncomplicated cases of chronic urticaria and for seasonal allergic rhinitis. It may be prescribed for adults and children older than two years of age.

This drug is manufactured as tablets, orally disintegrating tablets and oral suspension. Tablets should be taken with water. Fexofenadine may interact with other drugs.

- The effectiveness of fexofenadine is reduced if taken within 15 minutes of aluminum or magnesium antacids.
- Taking fexofenadine with azole antifungals or erythromycin may increase blood concentrations of fexofenadine.
- Administering fexofenadine with rifampin may reduce the effectiveness of fexofenadine.

Fruit juices such as apple juice, grapefruit juice, or orange juice may reduce the effect of fexofenadine.

In addition to headache, adverse reactions to this drug may include:

- drowsiness
- nausea
- back pain
- upper respiratory tract infection

T I P Forms of Allegra-D can result in excretion of something that looks very similar to the original tablet in the feces. This makes it look as if the tablet went all the way through the GI tract without being absorbed. You can inform patients that they may occasionally notice the tablet shell in their stool. Reassure them that this is normal and not a cause for concern.

Loratadine

Loratadine is mainly used to relieve symptoms of seasonal allergic rhinitis in children and adults. It may also be used to relieve chronic idiopathic urticaria. Loratadine is an OTC medication. It's manufactured as tablets (Claritin, Tavist ND), extended-release tablets (Alavert, Claritin Hives Relief), orally disintegrating tablets (Alavert, Claritin RediTab, Dimetapp Children's Non-Drowsy Allergy), oral solution (Claritin), and syrup (Claritin Children's, Dimetapp Children's Non-Drowsy Allergy).

Loratadine may cause serious cardiac effects when taken with macrolide antibiotics (such as erythromycin), fluconazole, ketoconazole, itraconazole, miconazole, cimetidine, ciprofloxacin, and clarithromycin.

In addition to the adverse reactions for nonsedating antihistamines, adverse reactions specific to loratadine include:

- blurred vision
- changes in salivation
- conjunctivitis
- dizziness
- migraine headache
- tremors

LEUKOTRIENE RECEPTOR ANTAGONISTS

Leukotriene is a substance released during the inflammation response by the immune system. It causes smooth muscle contractions in the airways, increased secretions, and other inflammatory responses. Leukotriene receptor antagonists block the action of leukotrienes, relieving airway inflammation.

As you learned in Chapter 7, leukotriene receptor antagonists are often used to treat asthma. However, because these drugs act to reduce inflammation in the airways, they may also be prescribed to treat allergic rhinitis.

Adverse reactions to these drugs include headache and nausea.

Montelukast

Montelukast (Singulair) is used to relieve the symptoms of allergic rhinitis. It's typically taken once a day. Forms of this drug include tablets, chewable tablets, and oral granules (for young children).

Montelukast may interact with other drugs.

- CYP450 inducers such as phenobarbital and rifampin may reduce blood concentrations of montelukast.
- Montelukast may increase the adverse effects of prednisone.

TIP Montelukast granules may be dissolved in a teaspoon of baby formula, breast milk, or soft food such as applesauce, carrots, rice, or ice cream. Once mixed, however, the granules can't be stored for future use.

Zafirlukast

Zafirlukast (Accolate) is an anti-inflammatory drug that's used to prevent and treat asthma. It's available by prescription in the form of oral tablets. It should be taken one hour before or two hours after meals. Zafirlukast may interact with other drugs.

- Taking zafirlukast with aspirin increases the effects of zafirlukast.
- Zafirlukast taken with erythromycin or theophylline decreases the effects.
- Taking zafirlukast with warfarin increases blood clotting time.

MAST CELL STABILIZERS

Like leukotriene receptor antagonists, mast cell stabilizers are often used to prevent and treat asthma. However,

PROCEED WITH CAUTION

Adverse Reactions to Cromolyn Sodium

The most common adverse reactions to cromolyn sodium include:

- sneezing
- nasal stinging
- nasal irritation

because of their anti-inflammatory action, they may also be used to treat allergic rhinitis. The main mast cell stabilizer used in this way is cromolyn sodium. It works by inhibiting the release of histamine and other chemical mediators from mast cells.

To treat allergic rhinitis, cromolyn sodium is sold over the counter as a nasal solution (Nasalcrom). Using the nasal spray at regular intervals is necessary for effective therapy. By prescription, cromolyn sodium is available in the form of an oral solution (Gastrocrom), an oral inhalation (Intal), a nebulizer solution (Intal), and an ophthalmic solution (Crolom). This drug is also used in treating symptoms of mastocytosis (a group of rare conditions involving excessive mast cells in the body).

MISCELLANEOUS ANTI-ALLERGY AGENTS

Some medications are not chemically related to antihistamines, but are effective for relieving symptoms of allergic reactions. They work by blocking inflammatory responses or by blocking the effects of histamine. These medications may interact with other drugs, but their effects vary depending on the specific medication.

Adverse reactions to other anti-allergy agents vary depending on the specific medication and method of administration. Inhaled anti-allergy agents may cause nasal burning and irritation.

Epinephrine

Epinephrine is used:

- to provide fast relief of hypersensitivity reactions due to drugs and other allergens
- to treat mucosal congestion of hay fever, rhinitis, and acute sinusitis
- to provide emergency treatment of allergic reactions (anaphylaxis) to foods, drugs, insect bites or stings, or other allergens

Epinephrine is manufactured in several different forms. It's sold over the counter as a solution for inhalation (Primatene Mist) to treat asthma symptoms. It's also available by prescription as a nasal spray (Adrenalin) and as a solution for SubQ or IM injection (Twinject, EpiPen, EpiPen Jr., Adrenalin).

Epinephrine works by relaxing smooth muscles of the bronchi and acting as an antagonist to histamine.

Hydroxyzine

Hydroxyzine hydrochloride and hydroxyzine pamoate (Vistaril) are not chemically related to antihistamines, but act as antihistamines do on the body. These drugs are used to relieve itching caused by chronic urticaria or other skin defects or lesions. These drugs are available by prescription only. Hydroxyzine is manufactured as tablets, capsules, oral suspension, oral solution, and vials for injection. Effects are usually observed within 30 minutes of administration. The injectable form of the drug is given by deep IM injection only.

Hydroxyzine may interact with other medications.

- Taking hydroxyzine with anticholinergics may result in additive anticholinergic effects.
- Hydroxyzine may increase CNS depression.
- Hydroxyzine shouldn't be taken with epinephrine, because it may reverse the vasopressor effects of epinephrine.

Adverse reactions to hydroxyzine may include drowsiness and dry mouth.

CORTICOSTEROIDS

Corticosteroids suppress immune responses and reduce inflammation. They are available as natural or synthetic steroids. Natural corticosteroids are hormones produced by the adrenal cortex, a part of a small gland located above the kidney. Synthetic corticosteroids, however, are man-made forms of natural hormones. Both natural and synthetic corticosteroids are classified according to the way they act on the body. There are two main types of corticosteroids.

- **Glucocorticoids** affect carbohydrate and protein metabolism.
- **Mineralocorticoids** regulate electrolyte and water balance.

 PROCEED WITH CAUTION

Adverse Reactions to Corticosteroids

Corticosteroids affect almost all body systems. Their widespread adverse effects include:

- insomnia
- increased sodium and water retention
- increased potassium excretion
- suppressed immune and inflammatory responses
- osteoporosis
- intestinal perforation
- peptic ulcers
- impaired wound healing

Endocrine system reactions may include:

- diabetes mellitus
- hyperlipidemia
- adrenal atrophy
- hypothalamic-pituitary axis suppression
- cushingoid signs and symptoms (such as buffalo hump, moon face, and elevated blood glucose levels)

Glucocorticoids

Most glucocorticoids are synthetic copies of hormones naturally secreted by the adrenal cortex. These drugs have anti-inflammatory, metabolic, and immunosuppressant effects. Glucocorticoids are used to treat:

- inflammation associated with asthma, **osteoarthritis** (a form of arthritis resulting in the degeneration of cartilage in the joints), and inflammatory bowel disease
- adrenocortical insufficiency conditions, such as Addison disease
- rheumatic disorders such as osteoarthritis, acute gouty arthritis, or ankylosing spondylitis
- collagen diseases such as systemic lupus erythematosus (a disease that affects the immune system)
- dermatologic diseases such as Stevens-Johnson syndrome and severe psoriasis
- allergic states, including contact dermatitis
- GI diseases, including ulcerative colitis and regional enteritis
- respiratory diseases
- hematologic disorders, such as acquired hemolytic anemia
- neoplastic diseases, such as lymphomas and leukemias
- transplant patients (by providing immunosuppressive effects)

These drugs are sometimes used in high doses to treat shock.

Glucocorticoids suppress hypersensitivity and immune responses through a process that isn't well understood. Glucocorticoids block the redness, edema, heat, and tenderness related to the inflammatory response. Glucocorticoids also:

- prevent plasma from leaking out of capillaries
- block the migration of polymorphonuclear leukocytes (cells that kill and digest microorganisms)
- stop **phagocytosis** (the process of destroying foreign cells and bacteria by digestion)

To ensure a job well done, glucocorticoids reduce the formation of antibodies in injured or injected tissues. They also disrupt several key processes:

- histamine synthesis
- fibroblast development
- depositing of collagen
- dilation of capillaries
- capillary permeability (the ability of capillary membranes to allow fluid in and out)

Many drugs interact with glucocorticoids.

- Aminoglutethimide, barbiturates, phenytoin, and rifampin may reduce the effects of glucocorticoids.
- The potassium-wasting effects of glucocorticoids may be enhanced by amphotericin B, chlorthalidone, ethacrynic acid, furosemide, and thiazide diuretics.

- Erythromycin and troleandomycin may increase the effects of glucocorticoids by reducing their metabolism.
- Glucocorticoids may reduce the serum concentration and effects of salicylates.
- The risk of peptic ulcers associated with NSAIDs and salicylates increases when these drugs are taken with glucocorticoids.
- The response to vaccines and toxoids may be reduced when patients are taking glucocorticoids.
- Estrogen and hormonal contraceptives that contain estrogen increase the effects of glucocorticoids.
- Taking glucocorticoids with antidiabetic drugs may reduce the effects of antidiabetic drugs, resulting in increased blood glucose levels.

Prolonged use of glucocorticoids can cause "moon face" or Cushing disease.

Taking glucocorticoids (steroids), administered either orally or intravenously, can affect the natural production of hormones in the body. The adrenal glands lose their ability to make natural glucocorticoids such as cortisol. The chance of suppressing the adrenal gland grows when glucocorticoids are used for long periods of time.

Doses of glucocorticoids should be tapered or gradually reduced to the smallest dose that provides results for the patient. Abruptly stopping the use of glucocorticoids can lead to flare-ups of the disease. Patients who have been taking glucocorticoids for long periods of time, such as a year, may need several months of tapering before they can stop taking the medication. This gives the body time to start producing glucocorticoids on its own again.

Beclomethasone

Beclomethasone (QVAR, Beconase AQ) is available by prescription only. It comes in an aerosol form, which is used to treat chronic asthma. It's also available as a nasal spray for relieving symptoms of seasonal or perennial allergic and vasomotor rhinitis. Additionally, the spray may be used to prevent the recurrence of nasal polyps after surgery.

T I P Glucocorticoids don't act instantly. It may take several days to see their effects.

Betamethasone

Betamethasone (Celestone) is available by prescription only. For systemic immunosuppressant effects, it's manufactured as a syrup or in vials for injection. The injectable forms are betamethasone sodium phosphate and betamethasone acetate injection. These forms should be administered by IM injection.

After the patient begins to respond to treatment, a maintenance dose may be determined by gradually decreasing the initial dosage. The patient should be given the lowest dosage that provides an effective response.

Other betamethasone compounds are available in topical forms. These forms are used to treat dermatologic conditions such as contact dermatitis, eczema, and psoriasis.

Cortisone

Cortisone is a prescription drug manufactured in the form of tablets.

Dexamethasone

Dexamethasone is sold by prescription only. It's manufactured in several different forms. For oral administration, dexamethasone is sold as tablets (Decadron, DexPak) and oral solution. When oral therapy isn't possible, dexamethasone sodium phosphate can be given by IV or IM injection. Infusions for IV administration should be used within 24 hours. Dexamethasone is also available in the form of an ophthalmic solution and suspension (Maxidex).

The injectable forms of the drug may contain sodium bisulfite, a sulfite that can cause allergic-type reactions in susceptible people.

In addition to the adverse reactions related to all glucocorticoids, dexamethasone may cause euphoria.

T I P Glucocorticoids may be administered by mouth or by injection. Be sure to check the correct administration route when filling a prescription or medication order.

Hydrocortisone

Hydrocortisone is a naturally occurring glucocorticoid. It can cause elevated blood pressure, salt and water retention, and increased excretion of potassium.

This drug is available in several different forms. For oral administration, hydrocortisone is sold by prescription as tablets (Cortef). A prescription-strength rectal enema

AT THE COUNTER

A Rash Decision

A patient comes to the pharmacy counter looking for an OTC drug to treat a rash on his arm. The pharmacist asks you to help the patient find Cortizone. Where is this product likely to be found in your store?

Cortizone is a topical steroid that contains hydrocortisone. Most pharmacies will stock it with other topical drugs or in the first aid section of the store.

What are the available strengths of Cortizone?

There are two available strengths. Hydrocortisone 0.5% is Cortizone-5. Hydrocortisone 1% is Cortizone-10.

The patient asks you if there is a stronger steroid available over the counter. What should you tell him?

Hydrocortisone 1% is the strongest topical steroid available without a prescription.

(Anusol HC, Proctocream HC, Proctosol-HC, Proctozone-HC, Procto-Kit, Proctocort) is available for rectal administration. Topical forms of hydrocortisone are sold over the counter in 0.5% and 1% strengths (Cortaid, Cortizone). Higher strengths are available by prescription only (Hytone). Forms of hydrocortisone for topical use include cream, ointment, lotion, spray, solution, and rectal cream under a variety of trade names. These topical forms are used in treating itching and rashes related to allergies or dermatologic conditions.

Adverse reactions to topical forms of the drug are usually local, rather than systemic. They include:

- burning
- itching
- irritation
- dryness

However, large quantities of topically applied corticosteroids over large body surface areas can lead to systemic effects. Children may absorb larger amounts of topical corticosteroids and are more susceptible to systemic toxicity.

Methylprednisolone

Methylprednisolone is a prescription medication used for severe inflammation or immunosuppression. For oral administration, this drug is sold in tablet form (Medrol).

Methylprednisolone tablets also come in packages of 21 tablets with specific dosing instructions. These "dose paks" are used to help patients taper their dosage of the drug over a period of six days.

In addition, methylprednisolone is manufactured in injectable forms. Methylprednisolone acetate, an injection suspension (Depo-Medrol), is used as a temporary substitute for oral therapy. The daily dose is given as a single IM injection.

Methylprednisolone sodium succinate is manufactured as an injection solution (A-Methapred, Solu-Medrol) for IV or IM administration when oral therapy can't be used. This form of the drug may also be used to treat shock.

Prednisolone

Prednisolone is available by prescription as tablets (Prednoral), orally disintegrating tablets (Orapred ODT), oral solution (Orapred, Pediapred, Prelone, Millipred), ophthalmic suspension (Pred Mild, Econopred, Econopred Plus, Omnipred, Pred-Forte), and ophthalmic solution. Dosage is individualized depending on the severity of the condition and the patient's response. Constant monitoring is needed to ensure that the patient is taking the lowest dosage that will produce the desired effect. When the drug has been administered for more than a few days, the dosage should be gradually decreased. Similarly, after long-term

HOW IT WORKS

How Methylprednisolone Works

Tissue trauma normally leads to tissue irritation, inflammation, and production of scar tissue. Methylprednisolone counteracts the effects of tissue trauma and promotes healing (figure 10-2).

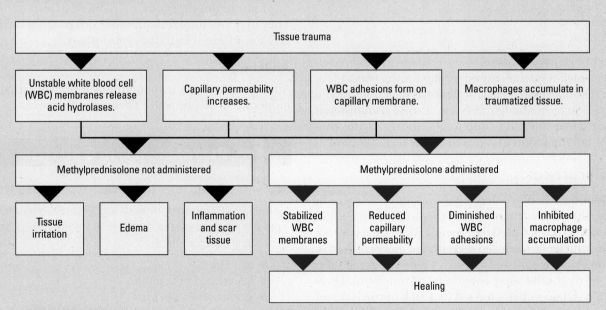

FIGURE 10-2 How methylprednisolone works. (From *Clinical Pharmacology Made Incredibly Easy.* 2nd Ed. Philadelphia, PA: Lippincott Williams & Wilkins; 2005.)

therapy, the drug should be withdrawn gradually rather than stopped abruptly.

Prednisone

Prednisone (Sterapred) is used to treat severe inflammation and for immunosuppression. It's also used for acute episodes of multiple sclerosis. It's sold as tablets of varying strengths and oral solution.

Triamcinolone

Triamcinolone is available by prescription only. It's manufactured in several different forms. Triamcinolone acetonide comes as a nasal spray (Nasacort AQ) and an aerosol (Azmacort) to relieve symptoms of perennial and seasonal rhinitis. It may be used for children older than six years of age. The aerosol form of this drug is also used in treating asthma.

In addition, triamcinolone acetonide is manufactured as vials for injection (Kenalog, Tac-3). It may be used locally to treat lesions or joints. For systemic therapy, IM injection should be used. This form of the drug contains benzyl alcohol, which can cause CNS depression, especially in children.

Topical forms of triamcinolone are prescribed for treating local inflammation and itching associated with dermatologic conditions. Available forms are topical spray (Kenalog), cream (Cinalog, SP Rx, Triderm), lotion, and ointment (Triderm). Triamcinolone is also available in the form of a dental paste (Kenalog in Orabase, Oralone) for relieving inflammation, ulcers, and lesions in the mouth caused by injury to the skin. Topically applied triamcinolone may cause local adverse effects, such as:

- burning
- itching
- irritation
- dryness

Another form of triamcinolone is triamcinolone hexacetonide, which is manufactured in vials for injection (Aristospan). It's administered by intralesional injection (near a lesion) to treat dermatologic diseases. It's also administered by intra-articular injection (into joints) to treat acute conditions of inflammation in joints for short-term therapy.

Mineralocorticoids

Mineralocorticoids affect electrolyte and water balance. In the body, the primary mineralocorticoid is aldosterone. Mineralocorticoids are used therapeutically to treat adrenocortical insufficiency (reduced secretion of glucocorticoids, mineralocorticoids, and androgens). These drugs may also be used to treat salt-losing congenital adrenogenital syndrome (a condition characterized by a lack of cortisol and deficient aldosterone production) after the patient's electrolyte balance has been restored.

The most commonly used mineralocorticoid drug is fludrocortisone acetate. This drug is manufactured in tablet form. Fludrocortisone affects fluid and electrolyte

PROCEED WITH CAUTION

Adverse Reactions to Fludrocortisone

Most adverse reactions to fludrocortisone are related to the body's retention of sodium and water. These effects are not usually a problem unless fludrocortisone is used over long periods of time or in conjunction with another glucocorticoid, such as cortisone. Less common adverse reactions may include:

- hypertension
- edema
- hypokalemia
- sweating
- urticaria
- allergic rash

balance by acting on the distal renal tubule. It increases sodium reabsorption and the secretion of potassium and hydrogen.

The drug interactions associated with mineralocorticoids are similar to those associated with glucocorticoids.

OTHER IMMUNOSUPPRESSANTS

Several drugs are used for their immunosuppressant effects in patients undergoing allograft transplantation (transplantation between people who are not identical twins). These drugs are also used experimentally to treat autoimmune diseases (diseases resulting from an inappropriate immune response directed toward the self).

Immunosuppressants act in different ways on the body. They may also interact with other drugs. Drug interactions vary for different immunosuppressants.

Anakinra

Anakinra (Kineret) is an immunosuppressant used to treat moderate to severe active **rheumatoid arthritis** (a chronic

PROCEED WITH CAUTION

Adverse Reactions to Immunosuppressants

All noncorticosteroid immunosuppressants may cause hypersensitivity reactions. Many of these drugs also have the following adverse effects:

- diarrhea
- nausea and/or vomiting
- stomach pain or upset

Because of the potential for adverse reactions, immunosuppressant drugs for organ transplants should only be prescribed by physicians who are experienced in immunosuppression therapy and the management of transplant patients.

disease characterized by inflammatory changes within the body's connective tissue) in adults who have not responded to at least one disease-modifying antirheumatic drug. It's administered by SubQ injection only. Anakinra works by blocking the action of interleukin. It binds to the interleukin-1 receptors, stopping the interleukin from binding. This reduces inflammation.

Anakinra shouldn't be given to patients with active infections or neutropenia. However, it causes fewer adverse reactions than most other drugs in this group. The most common adverse reaction to anakinra is pain or swelling at the injection site. Other adverse reactions include:

- upper respiratory tract infection
- stomach pain
- sinus inflammation

Azathioprine

Azathioprine (Azasan, Imuran) is a prescription medication manufactured as tablets and as vials for injection. It's used to treat severe rheumatoid arthritis and to prevent allograft rejection in kidney transplants. The exact mechanism of action for azathioprine is unknown. In patients receiving kidney allografts, azathioprine suppresses cell-mediated hypersensitivity reactions. It produces a variety of changes in antibody production.

This drug may interact with other medications.

- Allopurinol increases blood levels of azathioprine.
- Drugs that affect leukocyte production, such as cotrimoxazole, may lead to leukopenia when taken with azathioprine.
- Taking angiotensin-converting enzyme inhibitors with azathioprine may lead to anemia and severe leukopenia.
- Azathioprine may decrease the effects of anticoagulants.
- Azathioprine may decrease blood levels of cyclosporine.

The frequency and severity of adverse reactions to azathioprine depend on the dosage and length of treatment. In addition to the adverse effects common to all immunosuppressants, taking azathioprine may cause:

- bone marrow suppression
- liver toxicity
- leukopenia (reduced number of white blood cells)
- thrombocytopenia (reduced number of blood platelets)

Basiliximab

Basiliximab (Simulect) is used to suppress the immune system and prevent allograft rejection in patients receiving kidney transplants. It's typically used as part of a treatment regimen that includes cyclosporine and corticosteroids.

Basiliximab is administered by IV injection only. It's manufactured as a powder, which is gently mixed with sterile water for injection. The mixed solution can be stored for up to 24 hours if refrigerated.

Basiliximab works by blocking the activity of interleukin. This blocking reduces the immune system response and stops white blood cells from attacking the transplanted organ.

This drug has no known interactions with other medications. However, it does have many possible adverse reactions in addition to those already mentioned for immunosuppressants. These adverse reactions include:

- anemia
- constipation
- headache
- tremor
- fever
- hypertension
- leg or peripheral edema
- rhinitis
- pharyngitis
- dyspnea
- upper respiratory tract infection
- acne
- viral infection
- surgical wound complications

Potential adverse metabolic effects include:

- hypercholesterolemia
- hyperglycemia
- hyperkalemia
- hyperuricemia
- hypokalemia
- hypophosphatemia

Cyclosporine

Cyclosporine (Sandimmune, Gengraf, Neoral, Restasis) is used in several different situations:

- to prevent allograft rejection in kidney, liver, and heart transplants
- to treat severe, active rheumatoid arthritis that hasn't responded to treatment
- to treat severe cases of psoriasis that haven't responded to at least one other systemic therapy

This prescription medication is manufactured as capsules, oral solution, and vials for injection. The injectable form is usually given to patients only if they're unable to take oral medication. The oral solution should be stored at room temperature and used within the time allotted by the pharmacist. It is also manufactured as an ophthalmic suspension (Restasis) to increase tear production.

TIP Different brands and forms of cyclosporine are not interchangeable and may have different effects. It's important to read prescribing information carefully.

It's not known exactly how cyclosporine works to suppress the immune system. It's believed to inhibit helper T cells (white blood cells that activate other immune cells) and suppressor T cells (white blood cells that work to suppress the immune system response).

Cyclosporine may interact with other drugs and substances.

- Cyclosporine levels may increase if cyclosporine is taken with ketoconazole, calcium-channel blockers, cimetidine, anabolic steroids, hormonal contraceptives, erythromycin, or metoclopramide.
- The risk of toxicity to the kidneys increases when cyclosporine is taken with acyclovir, aminoglycosides, or amphotericin B.
- Barbiturates, rifampin, phenytoin, sulfonamides, and trimethoprim decrease blood levels of cyclosporine.
- Serum digoxin levels may increase when cyclosporine is taken with digoxin.
- Grapefruit and grapefruit juices may increase drug level and cause toxicity.

Patients who have psoriasis shouldn't take this medication if they are undergoing ultraviolet therapy or radiation or are taking other immunosuppressants.

Adverse reactions to cyclosporine include:

- kidney toxicity
- hyperkalemia
- infection
- liver toxicity

These are in addition to the adverse reactions common to other immunosuppressants.

Cyclophosphamide

Cyclophosphamide (Cytoxan), classified as an alkylating drug, is also used as an immunosuppressant. It's primarily used to treat cancer, often with antineoplastic drugs (drugs that block the growth of tumor cells). It may also be used to treat severe rheumatologic conditions or multiple sclerosis. This prescription drug is manufactured as tablets and as powder for injection.

Cyclophosphamide may interact with other drugs.

- The effects of cyclophosphamide may be increased if taken with allopurinol or phenobarbital.
- Cyclophosphamide increases the effects of succinylcholine, thiazide diuretics, and anticoagulants.
- Cyclophosphamide may decrease serum levels of digoxin.

Cyclophosphamide can cause potentially serious adverse reactions, including:

- hemorrhagic cystitis
- cardiac toxicity
- difficulties with wounds healing
- sterility
- secondary malignancies

Other adverse effects include:

- alopecia
- skin rash
- changes in skin pigmentation

- nausea and/or vomiting
- leukopenia
- interstitial pneumonitis

Daclizumab

Daclizumab (Zenapax) is administered by IV injection only. This drug is given to prevent allograft rejection in patients receiving kidney transplants. It's used as part of a regimen with cyclosporine and corticosteroids. Daclizumab must be diluted in sterile sodium chloride solution before IV administration. The IV bag should be mixed gently to avoid foaming. If the prepared solution is not administered within four hours, it can be refrigerated for up to 24 hours.

This drug works by blocking the action of interleukin. It competes for receptor sites with interleukin and keeps interleukin from binding. This suppresses the immune system response. There are no known drug interactions for daclizumab.

There is an increased mortality for patients taking this drug as part of treatment involving cyclosporine, mycophenolate mofetil, and corticosteroids. Other adverse reactions may include:

- hypertension
- hypotension
- chest pain
- tachycardia
- edema
- dyspnea
- pulmonary edema
- thrombosis
- bleeding
- renal tubular necrosis

Antithymocyte Globulin

Antithymocyte globulin, or ATG, is used to treat organ rejection in kidney transplant patients. It's administered by IV infusion only. In addition to the adverse reactions common to all immunosuppressants, ATG may cause:

- fever and chills
- reduced white blood cell (leukopenia) or platelet (thrombocytopenia) count
- chest pain
- infection
- dyspnea
- headache
- dizziness

ATG is made from one of two different animal sources: equine (horse) or rabbit. It's unclear exactly how ATG works to suppress the immune system.

In addition to its use for kidney transplant patients, ATG [equine] (ATGAM) is used:

- to treat moderate to severe aplastic anemia in patients who can't have bone marrow transplants
- to suppress the immune system in liver, bone marrow, heart, and other organ transplants

ATG [equine] must be diluted with sterile solution for IV infusion. Dextrose or solutions with low salt concentrations are not recommended. If necessary, the diluted mixture may be stored in the refrigerator, but the total time that the drug is diluted shouldn't be longer than 24 hours. It's recommended that patients be given a skin test before this drug is first administered to check for allergic reactions.

ATG [rabbit] (Thymoglobulin) comes in two vials, one containing the drug and a second vial containing sterile water for dilution. The vials should be mixed immediately before use.

Muromonab-CD3

Muromonab-CD3 (Orthoclone OKT) is administered by IV bolus injection only. It's used to treat:

- acute allograft rejection in kidney transplant patients
- steroid-resistant allograft rejection in cardiac and liver transplant patients
- acute graft-versus-host disease in bone marrow transplantation

Muromonab-CD3 works by blocking the action of T cells. It may interact with other drugs.

- This drug may increase the risk of infection when used with other immunosuppressant drugs.
- Indomethacin may increase levels of muromonab-CD3, increasing the risk of CNS effects such as encephalopathy.

In addition to the adverse reactions noted for other immunosuppressants, muromonab-CD3 may result in the following:

- fever and chills
- tremor
- pulmonary edema
- infection

Patients may be pretreated with an antipyretic to reduce fever and chills.

Mycophenolate

Mycophenolate (CellCept, Myfortic) is given to prevent allograft rejection in kidney, heart, or liver transplants, along with cyclosporine and corticosteroids. It's manufactured as capsules, tablets, gastro-resistant tablets, and oral suspension. It's also available as a powder for injection solution. The powder must be mixed with dextrose 5% solution.

T I P Protect your skin and mucous membranes from mycophenolate mofetil.

Mycophenolate works by inhibiting responses of T and B lymphocytes. It stops B lymphocytes from producing antibodies. It may also reduce inflammatory responses and graft rejection by stopping the site from recruiting leukocytes. This drug may interact with other medications.

- When mycophenolate is taken with antacids or cholestyramine, mycophenolate levels decrease.
- Taking mycophenolate with acyclovir may increase concentrations of both drugs, especially in patients with impaired kidney function.
- Mycophenolate may increase levels of phenytoin or theophylline.
- Probenecid and salicylates may increase levels of mycophenolate.
- Mycophenolate shouldn't be taken with azathioprine, cholestyramine, or live vaccines.

Mycophenolate can cause many adverse reactions in addition to those common to all immunosuppressants. Adverse reactions may include:

- leukopenia
- headache
- weakness
- urinary frequency
- leg cramps or pain
- liver function test abnormalities
- rash

Using this drug increases the patient's susceptibility to infection as well as the risk of developing lymphoma. It's also associated with increased risk of miscarriage and birth defects.

Sirolimus

Sirolimus (Rapamune) is an immunosuppressant that stops T lymphocytes from being activated and multiplying. This drug also stops the formation of antibodies. It's used to prevent and treat allograft rejection in patients receiving kidney transplants. This drug should be used initially in a regimen with cyclosporine and corticosteroids.

Sirolimus is manufactured as tablets and oral solution. It's typically given once a day. It may interact with medications and other substances.

- The risk of toxicity to the kidneys increases when sirolimus is taken with acyclovir, aminoglycosides, or amphotericin B.
- Barbiturates, rifampin, phenytoin, sulfonamides, and trimethoprim decrease blood plasma levels of sirolimus.
- Verapamil increases blood levels of sirolimus.
- Voriconazole shouldn't be given with sirolimus because the combination blocks CYP3A4 enzymes, leading to increased sirolimus levels.
- Grapefruit juice may decrease metabolism of sirolimus.

In addition to the adverse reactions for all immunosuppressants, taking sirolimus may result in the following:

- anemia
- thrombocytopenia
- hyperlipidemia
- hypertension

T I P Transplant recipients should take immunosuppressants regularly. As a technician, your job is to help the pharmacist monitor compliance for immunosuppressant therapy.

Temsirolimus

Temsirolimus (Torisel) is used to treat advanced renal cell carcinoma. It's administered once a week by IV infusion. The most common adverse reactions to temsirolimus include:

- anorexia
- asthenia (weakness or loss of strength)
- edema (accumulation of excess water in the body)
- mucositis (mucous membrane inflammation)
- nausea
- skin rash

Tacrolimus

Tacrolimus (Prograf) is used to prevent allograft rejection in patients receiving liver, kidney, or heart transplants. It's administered orally in capsule form, or by IV infusion. Diluted infusion may be stored up to 24 hours in glass or polyethylene containers. However, the solution isn't stable in a PVC container.

T I P Because of the risk of anaphylaxis, the injection form of tacrolimus is used only for patients who can't take the oral capsules.

Tacrolimus is also manufactured as a topical ointment (Protopic) for treating moderate to severe atopic dermatitis. The ointment may cause local adverse reactions such as burning or itching.

Systemic tacrolimus may interact with a number of other medications.

- These drugs may increase tacrolimus levels: bromocriptine, cimetidine, clarithromycin, clotrimazole, cyclosporine, danazol, diltiazem, erythromycin, fluconazole, itraconazole, ketoconazole, methylprednisolone, metoclopramide, nicardipine, and verapamil.
- Carbamazepine, phenobarbital, phenytoin, rifabutin, and rifampin may decrease levels of tacrolimus.
- Taking cyclosporine or other nephrotoxic drugs with tacrolimus may increase the risk of toxicity in the kidney.
- Tacrolimus should be used cautiously with other immunosuppressants, because the combination may suppress the immune system too much.
- Drugs that induce or inhibit the CYP450 enzyme system may increase the body's metabolism of tacrolimus.

Taking tacrolimus can result in adverse reactions in addition to those for all immunosuppressants, such as:

- constipation
- tremor

- hypertension
- leukopenia
- nephrotoxicity
- hepatotoxicity

URICOSURICS AND OTHER ANTIGOUT DRUGS

Gout is a type of arthritis that occurs when too much uric acid builds up in the body. Uric acid is a waste product of the kidneys. It's normally flushed out of the body in urine. An excess of uric acid can result when the body produces too much uric acid or when the body can't eliminate enough of it. Excess uric acid forms crystals, which are deposited in different areas of the body, such as:

- in joints (especially the big toe)
- under the skin
- in soft tissues
- in the kidney and urinary tract

These deposits of uric acid crystals cause inflammation and swelling. **Uricosurics** and other antigout drugs have anti-inflammatory actions that act to relieve gout.

Uricosurics

Uricosurics are typically used to treat two conditions:

- chronic gouty arthritis
- tophaceous gout (the deposit of tophi or urate crystals under the skin and in the joints)

The main goal in using uricosurics is to prevent or control the frequency of gouty arthritis attacks. Uricosurics work by increasing uric acid excretion in urine. They reduce the reabsorption of uric acid at the proximal convoluted tubules of the kidneys. This results in increased excretion of uric acid in urine, reducing the levels of uric acid in the blood.

Uricosurics shouldn't be given during an acute gouty attack because they can prolong inflammation. These drugs may increase the change of an acute gouty attack when therapy begins and whenever serum urate levels change rapidly. As a result, colchicine is given during the first three to six months of therapy with uricosuric drugs.

One uricosuric drug, probenecid, is used to treat hyperuricemia associated with gout and gouty arthritis. This prescription medication is sold in tablet form. It's also available in combination with colchicine as tablets. Probenecid may interact with many other drugs.

- Probenecid significantly increases or prolongs the effects of cephalosporins, penicillins, and sulfonamides.
- Serum urate levels may increase when probenecid is taken with antineoplastic drugs.
- Probenecid increases the blood serum concentration of dapsone, aminosalicylic acid, and methotrexate, causing toxic reactions.

PROCEED WITH CAUTION

Adverse Reactions to Probenecid

Adverse reactions to probenecid include:

■ headache
■ anorexia
■ vomiting
■ hypersensitivity reactions

Other Antigout Drugs

Other antigout drugs are used to prevent and relieve gouty attacks. These drugs act in different ways on the body.

Allopurinol

Allopurinol (Zyloprim, Aloprim) is used to treat primary gout, with the aim of preventing acute gouty attacks. It can be prescribed with uricosurics when smaller doses of each drug are directed. It's used:

■ to treat gout or hyperuricemia (buildup of uric acid in the blood) that may occur with blood abnormalities and during treatment of tumors or leukemia
■ to treat primary or secondary uric acid nephropathy (kidney disease), with or without the associated symptoms of gout
■ to prevent recurrent uric acid stone formation
■ to treat patients who respond poorly to maximum dosages of uricosurics or who have allergic reactions or intolerance to uricosuric drugs

Allopurinol and its metabolite oxypurinol work by blocking the action of xanthine oxidase, the enzyme responsible for making uric acid. By stopping the body from making uric acid, allopurinol eliminates the problems related to hyperuricosuria (abnormally high levels of uric acid in the urine).

Allopurinol is manufactured as tablets and as powder for injection. Injectable forms are used for patients with leukemia or tumors who are receiving cancer therapy and can't tolerate oral therapy.

Allopurinol interacts with several other drugs.

■ Allopurinol may increase the effects of oral anticoagulants.

PROCEED WITH CAUTION

Adverse Reactions to Other Antigout Drugs

The most common adverse reactions to these drugs include:

■ vomiting
■ diarrhea
■ intermittent abdominal pain

Other reactions vary with the specific antigout medication.

■ Allopurinol increases the blood serum concentration of mercaptopurine and azathioprine, increasing the risk of toxicity.
■ Angiotensin-converting enzyme inhibitors increase the risk of hypersensitivity reactions to allopurinol.
■ Allopurinol increases the levels of theophylline in the blood, leading to possible toxicity.
■ The risk of bone marrow depression increases when cyclophosphamide is taken with allopurinol.
■ Allopurinol increases the likelihood of skin rash when taken with ampicillin or amoxicillin.

Along with the adverse reactions noted for all other antigout medications, the most common adverse reaction to allopurinol is skin rash.

Colchicine

Colchicine is used to relieve the inflammation of acute gouty arthritis attacks. It's especially effective in relieving pain if given promptly. When colchicine is given during the first several months of therapy with other antigout medications, it may prevent the gouty attacks that sometimes occur with these drugs.

Colchicine acts to reduce the inflammatory response to urate crystals that are deposited in joint tissues. It may produce its effects by blocking the migration of white blood cells to the inflamed joint. This reduces phagocytosis and lactic acid production by white blood cells. The result is a decrease in uric acid deposits and reduced inflammation.

Colchicine is available by prescription only. It's manufactured as tablets. Colchicine is absorbed by the GI tract and is partially metabolized in the liver. The drug and its metabolites then re-enter the intestinal tract through biliary secretions. After readsorption from the intestines, colchicine is distributed to various tissues.

Prolonged administration of colchicine may cause bone marrow suppression.

QUICK QUIZ

Answer the following multiple-choice questions.

1. Which of the following drugs would *not* be used to treat a respiratory allergy?
   a. brompheniramine maleate
   b. clemastine fumarate
   c. folic acid
   d. loratadine
2. What key process do glucocorticoids disrupt?
   a. histamine synthesis
   b. capillary dilation
   c. capillary permeability
   d. all of the above
3. Which effect does taking hydrocortisone cause?
   a. decreased blood pressure
   b. salt and water retention
   c. allergic conjunctivitis
   d. all of the above

4. Which of the following would most likely *not* require treatment with an immunosuppressant drug?
   a. allograft rejection
   b. severe rheumatoid arthritis
   c. an allergic reaction to blood or plasma
   d. severe psoriasis
5. Which of the following drugs acts as an antihistamine, but is not chemically related to antihistamines?
   a. hydroxyzine
   b. diphenhydramine
   c. fexofenadine
   d. cyproheptadine

Please answer each of the following questions in one to three sentences.

1. How do sedating and nonsedating antihistamines differ in terms of their action on the body?

_____

_____

2. How do glucocorticoids work?

_____

_____

3. How do immunosuppressants work in transplant patients?

_____

_____

4. How are uricosurics different from other antigout drugs?

_____

_____

5. Explain how antihistamines and mast cell stabilizers differ in how they act on the body.

_____

_____

Answer the following questions as either true or false.

1. ___ Antihistamines can reverse the symptoms of an allergic response.
2. ___ Cromolyn sodium reduces smooth muscle contractions in the airways by blocking the action of leukotrienes.
3. ___ Because glucocorticoids block the immune response, they can cover up symptoms of serious infections.
4. ___ Chronic use of glucocorticoids can suppress the action of the adrenal gland.
5. ___ Uricosurics can prolong inflammation if given during acute attacks of gout.

Match the generic name of each drug in the left column with the correct trade name from the right column.

1. montelukast	a. Allegra
2. daclizumab	b. Medrol
3. fexofenadine	c. Zenapax
4. methylprednisolone	d. Prograf
5. tacrolimus	e. Singulair

DRUG CLASSIFICATION TABLE

Classification	Generic Name	Trade Name(s)
Sedating antihistamines	brompheniramine *brome-fen-ir'-a-meen*	*chewable tablets:* Brovex CT *extended-release tablets:* Bidhist, BPM, Lo-Hist 12, *extended-release capsules:* Lodrane 12 *oral suspension:* J-Tan, B-Vex, Brovex, TanaCof-XR oral solution: J-Tan PD, Vazol
	chlorpheniramine *klor-fen-eer'-a-meen*	*extended-release capsules (Rx):* CPM 12 mg *extended-release tablets (OTC):* Chlor-Trimeton Allergy *extended-release tablets (Rx):* ED-Chlor, Tan *oral suspension (Rx):* ED-Chlor Ped, TanaHist-PD, ChlorTan, P-Tann, PediaTan *tablets (OTC):* Aller-Chlor, Chlor-Trimeton Allergy *oral solution (OTC):* Aller-Chlor, Diabetic Tussin Allergy Relief
	cetirizine *se-tear'-i-zeen*	*chewable tablets:* Children's Zyrtec Allergy, *tablets:* Zyrtec Hives Relief, Zyrtec Allergy *syrup:* Zyrtec, Children's Zyrtec Allergy, Children's Zyrtec Hives Relief

continued

DRUG CLASSIFICATION TABLE (continued)

Classification	Generic Name	Trade Name(s)
Sedating antihistamines (continued)	cetirizine and pseudoephedrine *se-tear'-i-zeen soo-dow-e-fed'-rin*	*extended release tablets:* Zyrtec-D
	levocetirizine	*tablets:* Xyzal
	cyproheptadine *seye-proh-hep'-tuh-deen*	*tablets:* (no longer marketed under trade name) *oral solution:* (no longer marketed under trade name)
	clemastine *klem'-as-teen*	*tablets (OTC):* Tavist Allergy *tablets (Rx):* (no longer marketed under trade name) *syrup (Rx):* (no longer marketed under trade name)
	dimenhydrinate *dye-men-hye'-dri-nate*	*chewable tablets (OTC):* Dramamine *tablets (OTC):* Dramamine *injection (Rx):* (no longer marketed under trade name)
	diphenhydramine *dye-fen-hye'-dra-meen*	*capsules (OTC):* Benadryl Allergy *chewable tablets (OTC):* Benadryl Allergy *elixir (OTC):* (no longer marketed under trade name) *injection (Rx):* (no longer marketed under trade name) *orally disintegrating strips (OTC):* Benadryl Children's Allergy Quick Dissolve, Benadryl Allergy *orally disintegrating tablets (OTC):* Benadryl Children's Allergy Fastmelt *oral solution (OTC):* Benadryl Allergy, PediaCare Nighttime Cough *syrup (OTC):* (no longer marketed under trade name) *tablets (OTC):* Benadryl Allergy *topical cream (OTC):* Benadryl *topical gel (OTC):* Benadryl *topical solution (OTC):* Benadryl *topical spray (OTC):* Benadryl *tablet (OTC for treating insomnia):* Nytol, Simply Sleep, Sominex *capsule (OTC for treating insomnia):* Nytol, Unisom
	meclizine *mek'-li-zeen*	*chewable tablets (OTC):* Bonine *tablets (Rx):* Antivert *tablets (OTC):* Dramamine Less Drowsy
	promethazine *proe-meth'-a-zeen*	*injection:* Phenergan *tablets:* (no longer marketed under trade name) *oral solution:* (no longer marketed under trade name) *suppositories:* Phenadoz, Promethegan

continued

DRUG CLASSIFICATION TABLE (continued)

Classification	Generic Name	Trade Name(s)
Sedating antihistamines (continued)	promethazine and mepiridine *proe-meth'-a-zeen me-per'-i-deen*	*capsules (C-II):* (no longer marketed under trade name)
	promethazine and phenylephrine *proe-meth'-a-zeen fen-ill-ef'-rin*	*oral syrup:* Prometh VC Plain, Phen-Tuss AD
	promethazine, phenylephrine, and codeine *proe-meth'-a-zeen fen-ill-ef'-rin koe'-deen*	*oral syrup (C-V):* Prometh VC with Codeine
	promethazine and codeine *proe-meth'-a-zeen koe'-deen*	*oral syrup (C-V):* Prometh with Codeine
	promethazine with dextromethorphan	*oral syrup:* Phen Tuss DM, Prometh with Dextromethorphan
Nonsedating antihistamines	desloratadine *des-low-rah'-tah-deen*	*orally disintegrating tablets:* Clarinex RediTabs *syrup:* Clarinex *tablets:* Clarinex
	desloratadine and pseudoephedrine *des-low-rah'-tah-deen soo-dow-e-fed'-rin*	*extended-release tablets:* Clarinex-D 12-Hour, Clarinex-D 24-Hour
	fexofenadine *fecks-oh-fen'-a-deen*	*oral suspension:* Allegra *orally disintegrating tablets:* Allegra ODT *tablets:* Allegra
	fexofenadine and pseudoephedrine *fecks-oh-fen'-a-deen soo-dow-e-fed'-rin*	*extended-release tablets:* Allegra-D 12 Hour, Allegra-D 24 Hour
	loratadine *lor-a'-ta-dine*	*orally disintegrating tablets:* Alavert, Claritin RediTab, Dimetapp Children's Non-Drowsy Allergy *syrup:* Claritin Children's, Dimetapp Children's Non-Drowsy Allergy *tablets:* Claritin, Tavist ND *extended-release tablets:* Alavert, Claritin Hives Relief *oral solution:* Alavert, Claritin
	loratadine and pseudoephedrine *lor-a'-ta-dine soo-dow-e-fed'-rin*	*extended release tablets:* Claritin-D 12 Hour, Claritin-D 24 Hour, Alavert D-12 Hour
Leukotriene receptor antagonists	montelukast *mon-tell-oo'-kast*	*chewable tablets:* Singulair *oral granules:* Singulair *tablets:* Singulair
	zafirlukast *zah-fir'-luh-kast*	*tablets:* Accolate
Mast cell stabilizers	cromolyn sodium *kroe'-moe-lin*	*oral solution (Rx):* Gastrocrom *nasal solution (OTC):* Nasalcrom *oral inhalation (Rx):* Intal *nebulizer solution (Rx):* Intal *ophthalmic solution (Rx):* Crolom
Miscellaneous anti-allergy agents	epinephrine *ep-i-nef'-rin*	*inhalation solution (OTC):* Primatene Mist *injection (Rx):* Twinject, EpiPen, EpiPen Jr., Adrenalin *nasal spray (Rx):* Adrenalin

continued

DRUG CLASSIFICATION TABLE (continued)

Classification	Generic Name	Trade Name(s)
Miscellaneous anti-allergy agents *(continued)*	hydroxyzine *hye-drox'-i-zeen*	*capsules:* Vistaril *oral suspension:* (no longer marketed under trade name) *tablets:* (no longer marketed under trade name) *injection:* (no longer marketed under trade name) *oral solution:* (no longer marketed under trade name)
Glucocorticoids	beclomethasone *be-kloe-meth'-a-sone*	*aerosol:* QVAR *nasal spray:* Beconase AQ
	betamethasone *bay-ta-meth'-a-zone* *betamethasone diproprionate*	*injection:* Celestone Soluspan *syrup:* Celestone *topical cream:* Betanate, Del-Beta *topical lotion:* Del-Beta *topical ointment:* (no longer marketed under trade name)
	betamethasone diproprionate (augmented) *bay-ta-meth'-a-zone*	*topical cream:* Diprolene AF *topical gel:* Diprolene *topical lotion:* Diprolene *topical ointment:* Diprolene
	betamethasone valerate *bay-ta-meth'-a-zone*	*topical cream:* BetaDerm, Beta-Val *topical foam:* Luxiq *topical lotion:* Beta-Val *topical ointment:* (no longer marketed under trade name)
	cortisone *kor'-ti-zone*	*tablets:* (no longer marketed under trade name)
	dexamethasone *dex-a-meth'-a-sone*	*oral solution:* (no longer marketed under trade name) *tablets:* Decadron, DexPak *injection:* (no longer marketed under trade name) *ophthalmic suspension:* Maxidex *ophthalmic solution:* (no longer marketed under trade name)
	hydrocortisone *hye-droe-kor'-ti-zone*	*tablets (Rx):* Cortef *cream (OTC):* Corticaine, Cortaid, Cortizone, Dermarest DriCort *gel (OTC):* Corticool *ointment (OTC):* Cortizone, Cortaid, Tucks HC-1 *lotion (OTC):* AlaCort, Cortaid, Dermarest Eczema, Sarnol-HC, AlaScalp *spray (OTC):* Cortaid, Cortizone *topical solution (OTC):* (no longer marketed under trade name) *rectal cream (Rx):* Anusol HC, Proctocream HC, Proctosol-HC, Proctozone-HC, Procto-Kit, Proctocort

continued

DRUG CLASSIFICATION TABLE (continued)

Classification	Generic Name	Trade Name(s)
Glucocorticoids (continued)	hydrocortisone acetate *hye-droe-kor'-ti-zone*	*cream (Rx):* Caldecort, Hytone, Instacort *gel (Rx):* Instacort-10, NuZon *lotion (Rx):* (no longer marketed under trade name) *rectal foam (Rx):* Cortifoam *rectal suppository (Rx):* Anucort HC, Anusol HC, Proctosol-HC, Rectasol-HC, Hemril, Proctocort, Proctosert-HC, Anumed-HC
	hydrocortisone butyrate *hye-droe-kor'-ti-zone*	*cream (Rx):* Locoid *lipocream (Rx):* Locoid Lipocream *ointment (Rx):* Locoid *topical solution (Rx):* Locoid
	hydrocortisone probutate *hye-droe-kor'-ti-zone*	*cream (Rx):* Pandel
	hydrocortisone sodium succinate *hye-droe-kor'-ti-zone*	*injection (Rx):* Solu-Cortef
	hydrocortisone valerate *hye-droe-kor'-ti-zone*	*cream (Rx):* Westcort *ointment (Rx):* Westcort
	methylprednisolone *meth-ill-pred-niss'-oh-lone*	*tablets:* Medrol *injection suspension:* Depo-Medrol *injection solution:* A-Methapred, Solu-Medrol
	prednisolone *pred-niss'-oh-lone*	*orally disintegrating tablets:* Orapred ODT *oral solution:* Orapred, Pediapred, Prelone, Millipred *ophthalmic suspension:* Pred Mild, Econopred, Econopred Plus, Omnipred, Pred-Forte *ophthalmic solution:* (no longer marketed under trade name) *tablets:* Prednoral
	prednisone *pred'-ni-sone*	*oral solution:* (no longer marketed under trade name) *tablets:* (no longer marketed under trade name) *tablets (dose paks):* Sterapred
	triamcinolone *trye-am-sin'-oh-lone*	*aerosol:* Azmacort *nasal spray:* Nasacort AQ *injection suspension:* Kenalog, Aristospan *injection solution:* Tac-3 *topical spray:* Kenalog *cream:* Cinalog, SP Rx, Triderm *lotion:* (no longer marketed under trade name) *ointment:* Triderm *dental paste:* Kenalog in Orabase, Oralone
Mineralocorticoids	fludrocortisone *floo-droe-kor'-te-sone*	*tablets:* (no longer marketed under trade name)

continued

DRUG CLASSIFICATION TABLE (continued)

Classification	Generic Name	Trade Name(s)
Noncorticoid immunosuppressants	anakinra *an-ah-kin'-rah*	*injection:* Kineret
	azathioprine *ay-za-thye'-oh-preen*	*injection:* (no longer marketed under trade name) *tablets:* Azasan, Imuran
	basiliximab *bass-ih-lix'-ih-mab*	*injection:* Simulect
	cyclosporine *sye'-kloe-spor-een*	*capsules:* Sandimmune, Gengraf, Neoral *oral solution:* Sandimmune, Gengraf, Neoral *injection:* Sandimmune *ophthalmic suspension:* Restasis
	cyclophosphamide *sye-klo-foss'-fam-ide*	*tablets:* Cytoxan *injection:* Cytoxan
	daclizumab *da-klye'-zue-mab*	*injection:* Zenapax
	antithymocyte globulin [equine] *an'-tye-thye'-moe-site glob'-yoo-lin*	*injection:* ATGAM
	antithymocyte globulin [rabbit] *an'-tye-thye'-moe-site glob'-yoo-lin*	*injection:* Thymoglobulin
	muromonab-CD3 *mue'-roe-moe'-nab*	*injection:* Orthoclone OKT
	mycophenolate *mye'-koe-fen'-oh-late*	*capsules:* CellCept *oral suspension:* CellCept *tablets:* CellCept *injection:* CellCept *gastro-resistant tablets:* Myfortic
	sirolimus *sir-oh'-li-mus*	*tablets:* Rapamune *oral solution:* Rapamune
	temsirolimus *tem'- sir-oh'-li-mus*	*injection:* Torisel
	tacrolimus *tak-roe'-li-mus*	*oral capsules:* Prograf *injection:* Prograf *ointment:* Protopic
Uricosurics	probenecid *proe-ben'-e-sid*	*tablets:* (no longer marketed under trade name)
	probenecid and colchicine *proe-ben'-e-sid kol'-chi-seen*	*tablets:* (no longer marketed under trade name)
Other antigout drugs	allopurinol *al-oh-pure'-i-nole*	*tablets:* Zyloprim *injection:* Aloprim
	colchicine *kol'-chi-seen*	*tablets:* (no longer marketed under trade name)

CHAPTER 11

Psychotropic Drugs

CHAPTER OBJECTIVES

- Match brand and generic names of commonly used psychotropic drugs
- Identify the classification of commonly used psychotropic drugs
- Identify the uses of commonly used psychotropic drugs
- Match the brand or generic names of commonly used psychotropic drugs to the appropriate schedule
- Differentiate between a sedative and a hypnotic
- Compare and contrast the mechanism of action of antidepressants and mood stabilizers
- Identify drugs and foods that interact with monoamine oxidase inhibitors
- Compare and contrast the use of oral and parenteral routes of administration for antipsychotics
- List the extrapyramidal effects seen with typical antipsychotics
- Describe common dosing regimens for stimulants in treating attention deficit hyperactivity disorder

KEY TERMS

antianxiety drugs (anxiolytics)—a group of drugs that are mainly used to treat anxiety disorders

antidepressants—drugs that are used to treat depression

antipsychotic drug—a type of drug that controls psychotic symptoms and thought disorders that can occur with schizophrenia, mania, and other psychoses

anxiety— a feeling of apprehension, worry, or uneasiness that may or may not be based on reality

atypical antipsychotics—a group of drugs designed to treat schizophrenia

barbiturates—a class of drugs that reduce overall CNS alertness and are used for sedation, sleep inducement, anxiety relief, and to relieve the effects of seizures and convulsions

benzodiazepines—a class of drugs used for sedation, sleep inducement, relief of anxiety and tension, skeletal muscle relaxation, and relief of the effects of seizures and convulsions

bipolar disorder—a psychiatric disorder characterized by severe mood swings from extreme hyperactivity to clinical depression

central nervous system (CNS)—one of two main divisions of the nervous system consisting of the brain and spinal cord

depression—a psychiatric disorder that impairs functioning and is characterized by feelings of intense sadness, helplessness, and worthlessness

extrapyramidal effects—adverse reactions that occur in the extrapyramidal portion of the nervous system, causing abnormal muscle movements

hypnotic—a drug that induces sleep

neuroleptic malignant syndrome—a rare reaction to antipsychotic drugs characterized by a combination of extrapyramidal effects, hyperthermia, and autonomic disturbance

psychotic disorders—disorders that are characterized by personality disorganization and loss of grip on reality

sedatives—drugs that reduce anxiety, tension, or excitement

selective serotonin reuptake inhibitors (SSRIs)—a group of drugs that treat depression with fewer adverse reactions than other antidepressant drugs

tardive dyskinesia—a syndrome consisting of potentially irreversible, involuntary dyskinetic movements of the tongue, face, mouth, jaw, and sometimes the extremities

tricyclic antidepressants (TCAs)—a group of drugs used to treat major depression

typical antipsychotics—a group of older drugs that once were commonly used for treating psychotic disorders, but which today have been largely replaced by drugs with fewer and less severe side effects

This chapter presents the classes of drugs that are used to treat various sleep and psychogenic disorders, such as anxiety, depression, and psychotic disorders. You'll learn about the uses and various actions of drugs that alter psychogenic behavior and promote sleep. You'll also learn about drug interactions and adverse reactions to these drugs.

THE CENTRAL NERVOUS SYSTEM

The nervous system is the body's communication network. Although all parts of the nervous system work in coordination, portions may be grouped together on the basis of structure or function. The drugs discussed in this chapter affect the structural division of the nervous system known as the **central nervous system (CNS)**, which includes the brain and spinal cord.

The functional cells of the nervous system are highly specialized cells called neurons. As you can see in figure 11-1, each neuron is made up of a soma (the body of the neuron), dendrites, and an axon. Terminals called synapses link these structures. Different types of neurons carry out one of three functions:

- conduct electrical impulses to the spinal cord and brain
- carry impulses from the CNS to the body's muscles and glands
- relay information within the CNS

The nervous system works by means of electrical impulses sent along neuron fibers and transmitted from cell to cell. Information passes from one cell to another at the synapse across a tiny gap between the cells. Information usually crosses this gap in the form of a chemical known as a neurotransmitter.

You've learned about several neurotransmitters in previous chapters, including epinephrine (adrenaline), norepinephrine, and acetylcholine. Cells have special sites, or receptors, that are ready to pick up and respond to specific neurotransmitters. These receptors influence how or if that cell will respond to a given neurotransmitter.

SEDATIVE AND HYPNOTIC DRUGS

Sedatives reduce **anxiety**—a feeling of apprehension, worry, or uneasiness that may or may not be based on reality, tension, or excitement. Sedatives commonly cause some degree of drowsiness. When given in large doses, sedatives are considered **hypnotics**—drugs that induce a state resembling natural sleep.

The three main classes of synthetic dugs used as sedatives and hypnotics include:

- benzodiazepines
- barbiturates
- nonbenzodiazepine-nonbarbiturate drugs

Other sedatives may include sedating **antidepressants**, such as trazodone hydrochloride, and OTC sleep aids. Antidepressants are drugs that are used to treat **depression**, a psychiatric disorder that impairs functioning and is characterized by feelings of intense sadness, helplessness, and worthlessness.

Benzodiazepines

Benzodiazepines produce many therapeutic effects, including:

- inducing sedation and sleep
- relieving anxiety and tension
- relaxing skeletal muscle tension
- relieving convulsions

NEURON

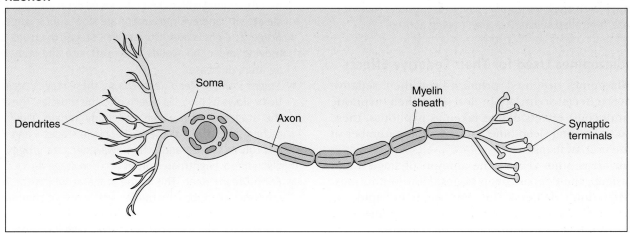

FIGURE 11-1 Neurons are the communication channels of the nervous system. (From Willis M. *Medical Terminology: The Language of Health Care.* 2nd Ed. Baltimore, MD: Lippincott Williams & Wilkins; 2006.)

As a result of their effects, these drugs are used in a variety of ways. These include:

- treating insomnia
- treating anxiety and seizure disorders
- treating alcohol-withdrawal symptoms
- producing skeletal muscle relaxation
- IV anesthesia
- relaxing patients before surgery

Benzodiazepines work by stimulating gamma-aminobutyric acid (GABA) receptors in a portion of the brain called the ascending reticular activating system (RAS). The RAS is associated with wakefulness and attention.

Low doses of benzodiazepines decrease anxiety. At low dosage levels, these drugs can usually calm or sedate a patient without causing drowsiness. At higher dosages, they induce sleep. Some benzodiazepines have active metabolites, which may give these drugs longer periods of action.

Few drugs interact with benzodiazepines, except for other CNS depressants and alcohol. When alcohol and other CNS depressants (such as anticonvulsants) are taken with benzodiazepines, the results are increased sedation and CNS depressant effects. These effects can include:

- reduced muscle coordination
- reduced level of consciousness
- respiratory depression
- death

Benzodiazepines also have a potential for abuse, tolerance, and physical dependence. For this reason, they are classified as Schedule IV controlled substances. In addition, benzodiazepines with active metabolites or a long half-life (the period of retention in the body) may accumulate and cause adverse effects in older adult patients. In general, lower starting doses with gradual dosage increases should be used with older adult patients.

TIP As a pharmacy technician, you will refill medications. It's very important that you help the pharmacist monitor patients' compliance with their benzodiazepine prescriptions to ensure that these controlled substances aren't being abused.

Benzodiazepines Used for Their Sedative Effects

Benzodiazepines are used primarily for their sedative (calming) effects or in larger doses for their hypnotic (sleep-inducing) effects. When taken as hypnotics, these drugs increase total sleep time and reduce the number of times the user awakens.

Benzodiazepines reduce the amount of stage 3 and stage 4 sleep, the deepest sleep stages. However, in most cases, they don't decrease the time spent in rapid-eye-movement (REM) sleep. This gives benzodiazepines a significant advantage as hypnotics over barbiturates.

Estazolam

Estazolam is prescribed as oral tablets. It is used for the short-term treatment of insomnia. It can work to improve

---

PROCEED WITH CAUTION

Adverse Reactions to Benzodiazepines

Benzodiazepines may cause:

- amnesia
- fatigue
- unintentional daytime sedation
- muscle weakness
- dry mouth
- nausea and vomiting
- dizziness
- ataxia (impaired ability to coordinate movement)
- rebound insomnia

These drugs may also have a hangover effect, or residual drowsiness and impaired reaction time upon awakening.

---

the quality and length of disrupted patient sleep cycles for up to 12 weeks.

This drug is not fast acting. On average, it requires two hours to reach peak concentrations in the bloodstream. However, its metabolites can remain in the body for up to 24 hours.

Flurazepam

Flurazepam (Dalmane) is available as oral capsules. This is another drug that is used to treat insomnia. It's one of the

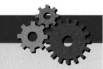

HOW IT WORKS

Sleep Cycles

People cycle between stages while they sleep. Each cycle lasts about 90 minutes. The average person has about three to five sleep cycles per night.

- *Stage 1: Drowsiness.* This is a short stage lasting five to ten minutes during which the person is easily awakened. Muscle activity and eye movement are slow during stage 1.
- *Stage 2: Light sleep.* During this stage, the eyes stop moving under the eyelids, and heart rate and body temperature decrease.
- *Stages 3 and 4: Deep sleep.* During these stages, brain activity slows as blood is diverted to the muscles. These are the stages during which the body repairs itself and recharges its physical energy. People in stages 3 and 4 are difficult to arouse and, when awakened, are groggy and disoriented. Nightmares often occur in stage 4.
- *REM: Dream sleep.* This is the stage at which the brain processes emotions, memories, and stress in the form of dreams. The person's eyes jerk rapidly back and forth under the eyelids, which is what gives this stage its name.

If the sleeper awakens during the REM stage, she returns to stage 1 to start the next cycle. Otherwise, REM sleep is followed by the light sleep of stage 2.

fastest-acting benzodiazepines. Flurazepam reaches peak concentration in the blood about 30 to 60 minutes after it is taken. However, hormonal contraceptives may reduce the body's metabolism of this drug, increasing the risk of toxicity.

Lorazepam

Lorazepam (Ativan) is produced as tablets and as a concentrated solution for oral administration. It's also available in prefilled syringes for IV or IM injection. The injection forms are usually used to reduce anxiety and sedate patients before surgical procedures. Intravenous lorazepam is also used to treat epileptic seizures. Oral forms of this drug are used to manage anxiety disorders and for short-term treatment of anxiety symptoms or anxiety associated with depression.

Quazepam

Quazepam (Doral) is prescribed as oral tablets for patients who have difficulty falling asleep or who awaken frequently during sleep. Peak concentrations in the blood are reached after about two hours, and metabolites of the drug remain in the body for up to 39 hours.

Temazepam

Temazepam (Restoril) is an oral capsule that has the same uses as quazepam. However, this drug is slower acting and more quickly eliminated than quazepam. Temazepam reaches peak levels in the blood two to three hours after taking it, and, on average, its metabolites remain in the body for about ten hours.

T I P The generic names of most benzodiazepines end with the letters -*pam*, which makes it easy to identify them.

Triazolam

Triazolam (Halcion) is prescribed as oral tablets for the short-term treatment of insomnia. Prescriptions are usually written for a seven- to ten-day supply only. You should question any prescription for quantities or refills that provide more than a one-month supply.

Like flurazepam, this drug is fast acting. However, its action may be affected by inhibitors of the cytochrome P-450 system, such as erythromycin or ketoconazole.

Benzodiazepines Used for the Treatment of Anxiety

Some benzodiazepines are primarily used to reduce tension, anxiety, and excitement. They include the drugs discussed below.

Alprazolam

Alprazolam is available for oral administration as immediate-release tablets, extended-release tablets, and in a concentrated oral solution. The oral solution must be mixed in water, juice, or some other liquid before being consumed.

An orally disintegrating tablet is also available for sublingual administration, meaning it is placed on the tongue where it dissolves.

The various forms of alprazolam have different therapeutic uses. The immediate-release tablets and oral solution are used in treating anxiety disorders, whereas the brand name drugs Xanax (tablets), Xanax XR (extended-release tablets), and Niravam (orally disintegrating tablets) are used to treat panic disorder.

Chlordiazepoxide

Chlordiazepoxide (Librium) is produced as capsules. The drug is used to:

- reduce apprehension and anxiety before surgery
- provide short-term relief of anxiety symptoms
- manage anxiety disorders
- treat the symptoms of acute alcohol withdrawal

The main use of chlordiazepoxide is in treating seizure disorders.

Chlordiazepoxide is also found in combination with clidinium (Librax). This combination drug, which comes in capsule form, is used to treat stomach or bowel problems such as ulcers, bowel irritability, or inflammation. Another combination drug, chlordiazepoxide and amitriptyline (Limbitrol), is used to treat moderate to severe depression with moderate to severe anxiety. This drug is available in tablet form.

Clonazepam

Clonazepam (Klonopin) is manufactured as oral tablets and as orally disintegrating tablets for sublingual administration. The main use of this drug is in treating seizure disorders.

Clorazepate

Clorazepate is prescribed as immediate-release tablets (Tranxene) and as extended-release tablets (Tranxene SD). This drug is used in the following ways:

- to manage anxiety disorders
- for short-term relief of anxiety symptoms
- as adjunct therapy in managing partial seizures
- to relieve the symptoms of acute alcohol withdrawal

Diazepam

Diazepam (Valium) is available for oral administration as tablets and as an oral solution. It may also be administered by injection or in the form of a rectal gel (Diastat).

This drug is used in treating convulsive disorders as well as anxiety disorders and short-term relief of anxiety symptoms. In addition, diazepam is used to relieve agitation, tremors, and other symptoms associated with acute alcohol withdrawal. The rectal gel is generally used during seizures or in other instances when patients can't take the oral forms.

How It Works

Benzodiazepines

Figure 11-2 shows how benzodiazepines work at the cellular level.

1. The number of chloride ions in the postsynaptic neuron influences the speed of impulses from a presynaptic neuron across a synapse—low chloride, more speed. The passage of chloride ions into the postsynaptic neuron is aided by the action of GABA.

2. When GABA is released from the presynaptic neuron, it travels across the synapse and binds to the GABA receptors on the postsynaptic neuron. This binding opens the chloride channels, which allows chloride ions to flow into the post-synaptic neuron and causes the nerve impulses to slow down.

3. Benzodiazepines bind to receptors on or near the GABA receptor. This action enhances the effect of GABA and allows more chlorine ions to flow into the postsynaptic neuron. This depresses the nerve impulses, causing them to slow down or stop.

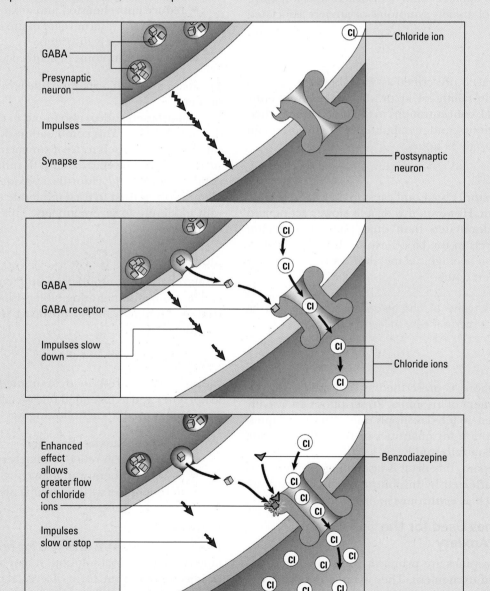

FIGURE 11-2   How benzodiazepines work. (From *Clinical Pharmacology Made Incredibly Easy.* 2nd Ed. Philadelphia, PA: Lippincott Williams & Wilkins; 2005.)

Oxazepam

Oxazepam is administered orally as capsules. This drug is used for the short-term relief of anxiety symptoms, management of anxiety disorders, and treatment of the symptoms of alcohol withdrawal. It has been found to be especially effective in treating older adult patients.

Barbiturates

The major pharmacological action of **barbiturates** is to reduce overall CNS alertness. They appear to act throughout the CNS.

These drugs have many clinical uses. These uses include:

- daytime sedation for short periods of time (typically less than two weeks)
- aiding sleep in patients with insomnia
- preoperative sedation and anesthesia
- relief of anxiety
- anticonvulsant effects

Barbiturates depress the sensory cortex of the brain, decrease motor activity, alter cerebral function, and produce drowsiness, sedation, and hypnosis. Low doses of these drugs depress the sensory and motor cortex, causing drowsiness. However, high doses may cause respiratory depression and death because of their ability to depress all levels of the CNS.

Barbiturates may interact with many other drugs.

- They may reduce the effects of beta blockers (such as metoprolol and propranolol), chloramphenicol, corticosteroids, doxycycline, oral anticoagulants, hormonal contraceptives, quinidine, tricyclic antidepressants, metronidazole, theophylline, and cyclosporine.
- Their use with methoxyflurane may stimulate the production of metabolites that are toxic to the kidneys.
- Their use with other CNS depressants may cause excessive CNS depression.
- Valproic acid may increase barbiturate levels.
- Monoamine oxidase inhibitors (MAOIs) inhibit the metabolism of barbiturates, increasing their sedative effects.
- When barbiturates are taken with acetaminophen, the risk of liver toxicity increases.

Barbiturates are classified as Schedule II, Schedule III, or Schedule IV controlled substances. Patients develop tolerance to barbiturates more quickly than they do to benzodiazepines. Physical dependence on barbiturates can occur, even with a small daily dose. In comparison, benzodiazepines are relatively safe and effective. For these reasons, benzodiazepines have replaced barbiturates as the sedatives and hypnotics of choice.

 T I P Since benzodiazepines are safer and just as effective as barbiturates, these drugs are the sedatives and hypnotics of choice.

Amobarbital

Amobarbital (Amytal), a Schedule II controlled substance, is available as a powder that must be made into a solution and then administered by IM or IV injection. This drug is used as a sedative and as a preliminary drug before administering anesthesia. It's also used for short-term relief of insomnia. However, amobarbital loses its effectiveness for that purpose after about two weeks of use.

Butabarbital

Butabarbital (Butisol) is administered orally as tablets or as an oral solution. This drug is a Schedule III controlled substance. Its main use is as a sedative or hypnotic. But like amobarbital, it loses effectiveness after about two weeks of use.

Mephobarbital

Mephobarbital (Mebaral) is a Schedule IV controlled substance. This drug is prescribed as tablets for oral administration. It's used as a sedative for relieving anxiety, tension, and apprehension. Mephobarbital is also used as an anticonvulsant in treating grand mal and petit mal epileptic seizures.

! PROCEED WITH CAUTION

Adverse Reactions to Barbiturates

Barbiturates may have widespread adverse effects. Possible central nervous system reactions include:

- drowsiness
- lethargy
- headache
- depression

Adverse cardiovascular and respiratory effects may include:

- hypotension
- hypoventilation, resulting in a low oxygen content and/ or high carbon dioxide content in the bloodstream
- spasm of the larynx (voice box) and bronchi
- reduced rate of breathing
- severe respiratory depression

Other reactions include:

- vertigo
- nausea and vomiting
- diarrhea
- epigastric pain
- allergic reactions

TIP Most barbiturates have the letters *-barbital* in the generic name, which makes them easy to identify.

Pentobarbital

Pentobarbital (Nembutal) is available as a solution for IM injection. This drug is classified as a Schedule II controlled substance. Its main uses are for the short-term treatment of insomnia and for treatment of convulsions resulting from seizure activity or other causes.

Phenobarbital

Phenobarbital (Luminal) is a Schedule IV controlled substance. It's manufactured in several oral forms, including tablets and oral solution. Phenobarbital is also available as a solution for IV infusion. Like most other barbiturates, this drug is used as a sedative, a short-term hypnotic, and an anticonvulsant in treating epilepsy.

Hydantoins, such as phenytoin, reduce the metabolism of phenobarbital. This may produce increased toxic effects.

Secobarbital

Secobarbital (Seconal), a Schedule II controlled substance, is administered orally as capsules. Its main use is as a short-term hypnotic. But like many other barbiturates, it loses its effectiveness for this purpose after about two weeks of use.

Nonbenzodiazepine-Nonbarbiturates

Nonbenzodiazepine-nonbarbiturates act as hypnotics and are used for short-term treatment of simple insomnia. Their depressant effects are similar to those of barbiturates, but their mechanism of action isn't known.

These drugs offer no special advantages over other sedatives, and with the exception of zolpidem, they lose their effectiveness by the end of the second week of use. Other uses include sedation before surgery or before electroencephalographic studies.

Some serious drug interactions can result from the use of nonbenzodiazepine-nonbarbiturates.

- When used with other CNS depressants, additive CNS depression occurs. Drowsiness, respiratory depression, stupor, coma, or death can result.
- Use with IV furosemide may produce sweating, flushing, variable blood pressure, and uneasiness.

Chloral Hydrate

Chloral hydrate is available as capsules (Somnote) and solution for oral administration and as rectal suppositories (Aquachloral). It's classified as a Schedule IV controlled substance. In addition to its uses as a sedative and hypnotic, oral chloral hydrate is used as adjunct therapy in postoperative pain control.

The rectal form of chloral hydrate is used in older adult patients, young patients, or patients who might not

PROCEED WITH CAUTION

Adverse Reactions to Nonbenzodiazepine-Nonbarbiturates

The most common adverse reactions to these drugs include:

- nausea and vomiting
- gastric irritation
- hangover effects (possibly leading to respiratory depression or even respiratory failure)

tolerate oral administration. This form of the drug is also used to prevent or control the symptoms of acute alcohol withdrawal.

Older adult patients seem to tolerate chloral hydrate better than barbiturates. However, chloral hydrate may increase the risk of bleeding in patients who are taking oral anticoagulants.

Zaleplon

Zaleplon (Sonata), a Schedule IV controlled substance, is prescribed as capsules for the short-term treatment of insomnia. It is most effective in reducing the length of time it takes the patient to fall sleep. However, zaleplon does not seem to be effective in increasing the length of sleep or in decreasing the number of awakenings.

Zolpidem

Zolpidem is also a Schedule IV controlled substance. This drug is available as immediate-release tablets (Ambien) and extended-release tablets (Ambien CR). Unlike other nonbenzodiazepine-nonbarbiturates, which lose their effectiveness after two weeks of use, zolpidem can be effective for up to 35 days.

Eszopiclone

Eszopiclone (Lunesta) is available in tablet form. It is classified as a Schedule IV controlled substance.

ANTIANXIETY DRUGS

Antianxiety drugs, which are also called **anxiolytics**, are some of the most commonly prescribed drugs in the United States. They are used mainly to treat anxiety disorders.

You've already read about benzodiazepines and barbiturates—two of the three main types of antianxiety drugs. The third type is a class of drugs known as azaspirodecanedione derivatives. The main drug in this class is buspirone (BuSpar).

Orally administered as tablets, buspirone's structure and mechanism of action differ from those of other antianxiety drugs. Although buspirone's exact mechanism of action is unknown, it's known that the drug doesn't affect

GABA receptors like benzodiazepines do. In fact, patients who haven't received benzodiazepines seem to respond better to buspirone.

Buspirone seems to produce various effects in the midbrain and acts as a midbrain modulator. This may be due to the drug's chemical attraction to serotonin receptors.

Buspirone is used to treat generalized anxiety states. But because it has a slow onset of action, it is not effective when quick relief from anxiety is needed, such as during a panic attack. Except for this drawback, buspirone has several advantages over other antianxiety drugs. These advantages include:

- less sedation
- no increase in depressant effects when mixed with alcohol or other CNS depressants, such as sedatives and hypnotics
- a lower potential for abuse

Dosing Control

A unique preparation of buspirone hydrochloride is packaged under the brand name BuSpar DIVIDOSE. Because adjusting the dosage of buspirone takes time and a wait-and-see approach to determine the effectiveness from patient to patient, the DIVIDOSE is an attractive prescribing option for physicians.

The tablets are available in two strengths, 15 mg and 30 mg, and they are scored so that they can be either bisected or trisected. Thus, a single 15-mg tablet can provide the following doses: 15 mg (entire tablet), 10 mg (two thirds of a tablet), 7.5 mg (one half of a tablet), or 5 mg (one third of a tablet). A single 30-mg tablet can provide the following doses: 30 mg (entire tablet), 20 mg (two thirds of a tablet), 15 mg (one half of a tablet), or 10 mg (one third of a tablet). A typical initial dose is 15 mg daily divided into two doses, but the maximum daily dose could increase to 60 mg.

Because of the flexibility provided by the tablet's formulation, physicians can adjust a patient's medication without having to prescribe multiple doses. Instead, they can use the convenient scored tablets to increase or decrease a patient's dose gradually.

Adverse Reactions to Busiprone

Because of its low potential for abuse, buspirone is not classified as a controlled substance by the Drug Enforcement Administration (DEA).

The most common adverse reactions to buspirone include:

- dizziness
- light-headedness
- insomnia
- rapid heart rate
- heart palpitations
- headache

ANTIDEPRESSANT AND MOOD STABILIZER DRUGS

Antidepressant and mood stabilizer drugs are used to treat affective disorders—that is, mood disturbances characterized by depression or elation. Unipolar disorders are characterized by periods of clinical depression. These disorders are treated with:

- tricyclic antidepressants
- MAOIs
- selective serotonin reuptake inhibitors
- miscellaneous antidepressants

Bipolar disorders are characterized by alternating periods of manic behavior and clinical depression. These disorders are usually treated with lithium and anticonvulsant drugs. Other mood stabilizers include divalproex sodium, carbamazepine, and olanzapine.

TIP Because antidepressant and mood stabilizer drugs may cause suicidal thoughts in young adults, all must include a black box warning in their product labeling. As you learned in Chapter 4, a black box warning is a warning required by the FDA for certain drugs that list any serious or life-threatening adverse reactions.

Tricyclic Antidepressants

Tricyclic antidepressants (TCAs) are used to treat major depression. They're especially effective in treating depression made manifest by weight loss, anorexia, or insomnia. Physical signs and symptoms may lessen after one to two weeks of therapy; psychological symptoms abate after two to four weeks of treatment.

TCAs are less effective in treating atypical depression, depression accompanied by delusions, or hypochondriasis (abnormal concern about health). When given with a mood stabilizer, these drugs may be helpful in treating acute episodes of depression in bipolar disorder.

It's believed that TCAs increase the amount of norepinephrine, serotonin, or both in the CNS by preventing reuptake of these neurotransmitters. Reuptake occurs when a neurotransmitter rapidly reenters the neuron from which it was released. Preventing reuptake increases the levels of these neurotransmitters in the synapses, which relieves depression. TCAs also block acetylcholine and histamine receptors.

TCAs are also used for preventing migraine headaches and in treating:

- phobias (panic disorder with agoraphobia)
- attention deficit disorder (ADD)

- obsessive-compulsive disorder (OCD)
- neuropathic pain (chronic pain that can occur with nerve damage from a number of causes)
- diabetic neuropathy (nerve degeneration caused by diabetes)
- enuresis (urinary incontinence)

TCAs interact with several commonly used drugs.

- They increase the effects of amphetamines and sympathomimetics, leading to hypertension.
- Barbiturates increase the body's metabolism of TCAs, which decreases TCA levels in the blood.
- Cimetidine impairs metabolism of TCAs by the liver, which increases the risk of toxicity.
- Using TCAs with MAOIs may cause very high body temperatures, excitability, and seizures.
- When anticholinergic drugs are taken with TCAs, increased anticholinergic effects such as dry mouth, urine retention, and constipation may result.
- TCAs reduce the antihypertensive effects of clonidine and guanethidine.

Amitriptyline

Amitriptyline is prescribed as tablets to relieve the symptoms of depression. An off-label use is for pain manage-

PROCEED WITH CAUTION

Adverse Reactions to Tricyclic Antidepressants

Adverse reactions to TCAs include:

- orthostatic hypotension
- sedation
- jaundice
- rashes
- photosensitivity reactions
- a fine resting tremor
- decreased sexual desire
- inhibited ejaculations
- transient eosinophilia (abnormal increase in the number of eosinophils in the blood)
- reduced white blood cell count
- manic episodes (in patients with or without bipolar disorder)
- exacerbation of psychotic symptoms in susceptible patients

In rare instances, TCA therapy may also lead to:

- granulocytopenia (a deficiency of granulocytes in the blood)
- heart palpitations
- heart conduction delays
- rapid heartbeat
- cardiovascular adverse reactions (in older adult patients)
- impaired cognition (in older adult patients)

ment therapy. This drug can also cause sedation, which may occur before its therapeutic effect takes place. Patients may need to take this drug for as long as 30 days for a therapeutic benefit to occur.

Amoxapine

Amoxapine is taken orally as tablets to relieve the symptoms of certain types of depression. These include:

- neurotic depressive disorders
- reactive depressive disorders
- psychotic depression
- depression accompanied by anxiety or agitation

Clomipramine

Clomipramine (Anafranil) is available in capsules for oral administration. It is mainly used in the treatment of OCD.

Desipramine

Desipramine (Norpramin) is prescribed as tablets. Its main use is in treating depression. Off-label uses include treatment of patients with alcohol dependence, as well as:

- attention deficit hyperactivity disorder (ADHD)
- anxiety
- bulimia nervosa
- diabetic neuropathy
- Tourette syndrome
- urinary incontinence

Sudden death has occurred in children and adolescents taking desipramine. For this reason, a baseline electrocardiogram is recommended before TCAs are prescribed to patients in this age group.

TIP TCAs can be used to treat many ailments besides depression. Don't assume the patient receiving the drug is being treated for depression.

Doxepin

Doxepin is manufactured as capsules and as an oral solution that patients must dilute in water, milk, or juice. It is also available in the form of a topical cream (Prudoxin, Zonalon). This drug is prescribed to treat depression or anxiety associated with bipolar disorders, alcoholism, and other causes. The following symptoms respond especially well to doxepin:

- sleep disturbances and other somatic symptoms
- lack of energy
- tension
- guilt, fear, apprehension, and worry

Imipramine

Imipramine hydrochloride (Tofranil) is manufactured in tablet form. It is primarily used to treat depression. However, this drug may also be used as temporary adjunctive therapy in treating urinary incontinence in children six years of age and older.

A similar compound, imipramine pamoate (Tofranil PM), comes in the form of capsules. This drug is also used to treat depression.

With both imipramine hydrochloride and imipramine pamoate, one to three weeks of treatment may be needed before these drugs have their maximum effect.

Nortriptyline

Nortriptyline (Pamelor) is available as capsules and as an oral solution. This drug is used to treat depression.

Protriptyline

Protriptyline (Vivactil) is manufactured as tablets. It is generally used only to treat depressed patients who are under close medical supervision. This drug is especially suitable for patients who are introverted and who fail to react to an injected antigen or allergen.

Trimipramine

Trimipramine (Surmontil) is prescribed as capsules. It is most effective in treating moderately depressed patients. However, trimipramine is less effective than some other TCAs in treating certain types of severe depression.

Monoamine Oxidase Inhibitors

MAOIs are believed to work by inhibiting MAO. MAO is an enzyme that occurs throughout the body and metabolizes many neurotransmitters, including norepinephrine, dopamine, and serotonin. Blocking the metabolism of these neurotransmitters leaves more of them available to the receptors. This blocking relieves the symptoms of depression.

MAOIs may be more effective than other antidepressants in treating atypical depression. Atypical depression produces signs opposite to those of typical depression. For example, a patient may gain weight, sleep more, and have a higher susceptibility to feel rejected by others.

MAOIs may also be used to treat typical depression that is resistant to other therapies or when other therapies are contraindicated. Other uses for MAOIs include treatment for:

- panic disorder with agoraphobia
- hypochondriasis and other phobic anxieties
- post-traumatic stress disorder (PTSD)
- neurodermatitis (an itchy skin disorder seen in nervous, anxious people)
- refractory narcolepsy (sudden sleep attacks)
- eating disorders
- pain disorders

MAOIs interact with a wide variety of drugs:

- Taking MAOIs with amphetamines, methylphenidate, levodopa, sympathomimetics, and nonamphetamine appetite suppressants may cause a hypertensive crisis.

- Taking MAOIs with TCAs, fluoxetine, citalopram, clomipramine, trazodone, sertraline, paroxetine, or fluvoxamine may result in elevated body temperature, excitability, and seizures.
- Taking MAOIs with doxapram may cause hypertension and arrhythmias. MAOIs may also increase the adverse reactions to doxapram.
- MAOIs may enhance the hypoglycemic effects of antidiabetic drugs.
- Taking MAOIs with meperidine may lead to excitability, hypertension or hypotension, extremely high body temperatures, and coma.
- MAOIs should be discontinued two weeks before starting another antidepressant. Patients should also wait two weeks (five weeks for fluoxetine) after discontinuing an antidepressant before they begin taking an MAOI.

TIP Before a patient begins taking an MAOI, he should have a "washout" period of at least two weeks during which he receives no medication. A washout period is also necessary for patients discontinuing MAOIs.

Certain foods also can interact with MAOIs and produce severe reactions. The most serious reactions involve

PROCEED WITH CAUTION

Adverse Reactions to Monoamine Oxidase Inhibitors

Adverse reactions to MAOIs include:

- hypertensive crisis (when taken with tyramine-rich foods)
- orthostatic hypotension
- restlessness
- drowsiness
- dizziness
- headache
- insomnia
- constipation
- anorexia
- nausea and vomiting
- weakness
- joint pain
- dry mouth
- blurred vision
- peripheral edema
- urine retention
- transient impotence
- rash
- skin and mucous membrane hemorrhage

Adverse reactions may be avoided by giving the drug in small, divided doses.

tyramine-rich foods such as red wine, aged cheese, and fava beans. Foods with moderate tyramine content, such as yogurt and ripe bananas, can be eaten occasionally but with care.

Phenelzine

Phenelzine (Nardil) is prescribed as tablets to treat patients with depression who have anxiety and phobias or hypochondriasis.

Tranylcypromine

Tranylcypromine (Parnate) is available in the form of tablets. This drug is used to treat major depressive episodes in patients who have failed to respond to more common antidepressants.

Selective Serotonin Reuptake Inhibitors

Selective serotonin reuptake inhibitors (SSRIs) were developed to treat depression with fewer adverse reactions than those caused by TCAs and MAOIs. Although they inhibit the reuptake of the neurotransmitter serotonin, SSRIs are chemically different from TCAs and MAOIs.

SSRIs are used to treat the same major depressive episodes as TCAs, and they have the same degree of effectiveness. They may also be useful in treating:

- panic disorders
- eating disorders
- personality disorders
- impulse-control disorders
- anxiety disorders

Drug interactions with SSRIs involve their ability to inhibit a liver enzyme that's responsible for the oxidation of many drugs, including TCAs and some antipsychotics. The use of SSRIs with MAOIs can cause serious and possibly fatal reactions. Individual SSRIs also have their own interactions. These are included with the discussion of each drug that follows.

Citalopram

Citalopram (Celexa) is available as tablets and as a solution for oral administration. It should not be taken with war-

farin, however, due to the potential for increased bleeding. In addition, carbamazepine may increase the clearance of citalopram. Using citalopram may also cause orthostatic hypotension.

Escitalopram

Escitalopram (Lexapro) is prescribed as tablets or an oral suspension for the treatment of generalized anxiety disorder (GAD) and major depressive disorder (MDD). A diagnosis of MDD requires that at least five of the following symptoms be present:

- depressed mood that interferes with daily functioning
- loss of interest in usual activities
- significant change in weight and/or appetite
- increased fatigue
- insomnia or hypersomnia (excessive sleep)
- psychomotor agitation or retardation
- slowed thinking or impaired concentration
- feelings of guilt or worthlessness
- a suicide attempt or suicidal ideation

Fluoxetine

Fluoxetine (Prozac, Prozac Weekly) is available as tablets, immediate-release capsules, extended-release capsules, and oral solution. It's used in the treatment of bulimia nervosa (a disorder characterized by binge eating and vomiting), MDD, OCD, and panic disorder.

Another fluoxetine drug, Sarafem and Selfemra, is prescribed for the treatment of premenstrual dysphoric

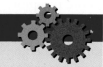

HOW IT WORKS

Selective Serotonin Reuptake Inhibitors

Serotonin (along with other neurotransmitters) carries messages in the form of electrical impulses between cells in the brain. It is released (transmitted) from the neuron of one brain cell and passes through a space or gap called a synapse to receptors on the neuron of another brain cell. However, not all serotonin that is released reaches the receptors. Some of it is reabsorbed into the neuron that released it to be used again to transmit another message. This reabsorption process is called "reuptake."

If too little serotonin is released, the brain's communication about sleep, emotions, and other messages carried by serotonin becomes slower and less efficient. Depression is the result.

SSRIs block the reuptake process and prevent serotonin from being reabsorbed by the transmitting neuron. This makes more serotonin available to the receiving neuron, even if serotonin levels remain low. As the amount of serotonin reaching the receiving neuron increases, better communication is restored, and depression is alleviated.

PROCEED WITH CAUTION

Adverse Reactions to Selective Serotonin Reuptake Inhibitors

Adverse reactions to SSRIs include:

- anxiety
- insomnia
- somnolence (drowsiness)
- heart palpitations
- various rashes
- sexual dysfunction

disorder (PMDD). PMDD is marked by mood swings, anxiety, anger or irritability, appetite and sleep changes, lack of energy, and difficulty concentrating that some women experience a few days before a menstrual period.

Fluoxetine increases the half-life of diazepam and displaces highly protein-bound drugs, leading to toxicity. In addition, decreased plasma levels can occur with fluoxetine.

Fluvoxamine

Fluvoxamine is prescribed as tablets and extended-release capsules (Luvox CR) for the treatment of OCD. It's also used in treating bulimia nervosa, depression, panic disorder, and social phobia.

Fluvoxamine should not be used with diltiazem hydrochloride. This combination may cause bradycardia (an abnormally slow heartbeat).

Paroxetine

Paroxetine (Paxil, Paxil CR, Pexeva) is available as immediate-release tablets, controlled-release tablets, and an oral suspension. It's used to treat GAD, MDD, OCD, panic disorder, PTSD, PMDD, and social anxiety disorder.

A number of other drugs interact with paroxetine:

- The use of paroxetine with warfarin may lead to increased bleeding.
- Paroxetine shouldn't be used with tryptophan because this combination may cause headache, sweating, nausea, and dizziness.
- Paroxetine may increase procyclidine levels, causing increased anticholinergic effects.
- Cimetidine, phenobarbital, and phenytoin may reduce the metabolism of paroxetine by the liver, increasing the risk of toxicity.
- Paroxetine may interact with other highly protein-bound drugs, causing adverse reactions to either drug.

In addition to the adverse reactions that may occur with other SSRIs, paroxetine may cause orthostatic hypotension.

T I P The Food and Drug Administration has approved paroxetine (Paxil) and sertraline (Zoloft) as the drugs of choice for treating post-traumatic stress disorder (PTSD). For these drugs to be prescribed, the patient must have symptoms such as intense fear, helplessness, and horror that last for a month or more and that significantly impair the patient's functioning.

Sertraline

Sertraline (Zoloft) is produced as tablets and as an oral solution. It's used to treat the same conditions as paroxetine. Like paroxetine, sertraline may interact with other highly protein-bound drugs to cause adverse reactions.

 PROCEED WITH CAUTION

Tapering Selective Serotonin Reuptake Inhibitors

Patients who are taking SSRIs need to be aware that abruptly stopping the drug may cause the following physical symptoms to occur:

- dizziness and vertigo
- headache
- fatigue
- nausea and vomiting
- ataxia (inability to coordinate voluntary muscle movements)
- tremor
- muscle pain

The psychological side effects of abruptly stopping an SSRI include:

- anxiety
- irritability
- crying spells and feelings of sadness
- memory problems
- vivid dreams

Tapering the dosage of the drug slowly over several weeks can prevent discontinuation symptoms. Patients should be advised to consult with their physician before discontinuing any SSRI.

Selective Serotonin and Norepinephrine Reuptake Inhibitors

Selective serotonin and norepinephrine reuptake inhibitors (SSNRIs) are another class of antidepressants. These drugs affect both mood and feelings of pain.

Venlafaxine

Venlafaxine (Effexor, Effexor XR) is produced as immediate-release tablets and extended-release capsules. The tablets are used in treating MDD. The extended-release capsules are usually prescribed for GAD or social anxiety disorder.

Adverse reactions to this drug include headache, somnolence, dizziness, and nausea.

Duloxetine

Duloxetine (Cymbalta) is FDA approved to treat major depressive disorder, diabetic nerve pain, and general anxiety disorder. Duloxetine is available in delayed-release capsule form.

Dizziness, fatigue, somnolence, constipation, and decreased appetite are potential adverse reactions for this drug. Patients should not take duloxetine with MAOIs or thioridazine, an antipsychotic drug.

T I P The prescribing physician should be consulted if an MAOI is prescribed in conjunction with some antidepressants.

Miscellaneous Antidepressants

Other drugs are used to treat depression as well. These miscellaneous antidepressants may all have serious and possibly fatal effects if they're combined with MAOIs.

Maprotiline

Maprotiline is prescribed as tablets for the treatment of depression, depression-related anxiety, and bipolar disorder. It is a tetracyclic antidepressant that's believed to work by increasing the amount of norepinephrine, serotonin, or both in the CNS by blocking their reuptake by presynaptic neurons (nerve terminals).

This drug interacts with CNS depressants to cause an additive effect. Common adverse reactions include seizures, orthostatic hypotension, tachycardia, and electrocardiographic changes.

Mirtazapine

Mirtazapine is manufactured as tablets (Remeron) and orally disintegrating tablets (Remeron Soltab). Like maprotiline, it's a tetracyclic antidepressant and is believed to work in the same way as maprotiline.

This drug's main use is the treatment of MDD. Like maprotiline, it may interact with CNS depressants to cause an additive effect. Adverse reactions include tremors, confusion, nausea, and constipation.

Bupropion

Bupropion is prescribed as immediate-release tablets (Wellbutrin) and extended-release tablets (Wellbutrin SR, Wellbutrin XL). All forms are used to treat MDD. Off-label uses include weight loss and treatment of neuropathic pain and ADHD. One brand of this drug, Zyban, is used to help people to stop smoking.

Bupropion is classified as a dopamine reuptake-blocking agent. However, it is no longer believed to work in that manner. It more likely acts on nonadrenergic receptors instead.

Adverse reactions to bupropion include:

- headache
- confusion
- tremors
- agitation
- tachycardia
- anorexia
- nausea and vomiting

The risk of these adverse reactions—as well as the risk of seizures—increases when bupropion is combined with levodopa, TCAs, or phenothiazines.

Trazodone

Trazodone is prescribed as tablets to treat depression with or without anxiety. It is also used off-label in treating cocaine withdrawal and insomnia. Although its mechanism of action is unknown, trazodone is believed to lessen depression by inhibiting the reuptake of serotonin and norepinephrine in the presynaptic neurons.

Adverse reactions to trazodone include dizziness and drowsiness. This drug may increase serum levels of digoxin and phenytoin. Its use with antihypertensive agents may increase hypotensive effects. CNS depression may be enhanced if trazodone is administered with other CNS depressants.

Nefazodone

Nefazodone is administered orally as tablets. This drug works by inhibiting the uptake of serotonin and norepinephrine by the neurons. It's also a serotonin antagonist, which explains its effectiveness in treating anxiety.

Nefazodone may increase digoxin levels if it is administered with digoxin. It also increases CNS depression when combined with CNS depressants. Adverse reactions include headache, somnolence, dizziness, and nausea.

Lithium

The discovery of lithium was a milestone in treating mania and bipolar disorders. It's believed that in mania, the patient experiences excessive catecholamine stimulation. (Catecholamines include epinephrine, norepinephrine, dopamine, and similar amines that function as hormones, neurotransmitters, or both.) In bipolar disorder, the patient is affected by swings between excessive catecholamine stimulation during mania and the diminished catecholamine stimulation of depression. Lithium is used to treat the manic phases of bipolar disorder. Other uses being researched for lithium include:

- preventing unipolar depression and migraine headaches
- treating depression, alcohol dependence, anorexia nervosa, syndrome of inappropriate antidiuretic hormone, and neutropenia

Lithium's exact mechanism of action is unknown. It may regulate catecholamine release by:

- increasing norepinephrine and serotonin uptake
- reducing the release of norepinephrine from the presynaptic neurons
- inhibiting norepinephrine's action in the postsynaptic neurons

Lithium carbonate is available as immediate-release capsules and tablets. It's also manufactured as extended-release tablets (Lithobid). Another lithium compound, lithium citrate, is administered in the form of an oral solution.

Lithium has a narrow margin of safety. A blood level that is even slightly higher than the therapeutic level can be dangerous. Patients who are taking this drug must be monitored closely. Blood samples must be drawn twice a week to determine serum lithium levels when the patient

AT THE COUNTER

Lithium Logistics

A patient is admitted to the hospital and diagnosed with bipolar disorder. What two types of medications would you expect to see an order for?

An antidepressant and lithium would most likely be prescribed.

What labs would you expect to see ordered with the lithium?

Lithium blood levels should be monitored routinely. Lithium has a narrow therapeutic margin of safety. High levels of lithium can be dangerous and may cause confusion, lethargy, slurred speech, increased reflex reactions, and seizures.

starts taking this drug. Blood draws should continue until serum lithium levels and the patient's clinical condition stabilize. Serious interactions with other drugs can occur because of lithium's narrow therapeutic range.

- The risk of lithium toxicity increases when lithium is taken with thiazide and loop diuretics and nonsteroidal anti-inflammatory drugs.
- Patients on a severe salt-restricted diet are susceptible to lithium toxicity. On the other hand, increased sodium intake may reduce lithium's therapeutic effects.
- The administration of lithium with haloperidol, phenothiazines, or carbamazepine may increase the risk of neurotoxicity.
- Lithium's effects are reduced when taken with theophylline.
- Sodium bicarbonate may increase the body's excretion of lithium, reducing the drug's effects.
- Lithium may increase the hypothyroid effects of potassium iodide.

Common adverse reactions to lithium include:

- thirst
- elevated white blood cell count
- polyuria (excessive urination)
- reversible electrocardiogram changes

ANTIPSYCHOTIC DRUGS

Antipsychotic drugs can control psychotic symptoms such as delusions and hallucinations. They are also used to treat thought disorders that can occur with schizophrenia, mania, and other psychoses. These drugs have several different names, including:

- *Antipsychotic.* These can eliminate signs and symptoms of psychoses.
- *Major tranquilizer.* These can calm an agitated patient.
- *Neuroleptic.* These have an adverse neurobiological effect that causes abnormal body movements.

All antipsychotic drugs belong to one of two major groups: atypical antipsychotics and typical antipsychotics.

Atypical Antipsychotics

Atypical antipsychotics are drugs designed to treat schizophrenia. They block the dopamine receptors, but they do so to a lesser extent than typical antipsychotics. This results in far fewer unwanted neurological effects than with typical antipsychotics. Atypical antipsychotics also block serotonin receptor activity.

These combined actions account for their effectiveness and, along with their improved tolerability, make atypical antipsychotics the first line of treatment for patients with schizophrenia. In lower doses, they are commonly used to treat behavioral and psychotic symptoms in patients with dementia.

Except for clozapine, these drugs also carry only a small risk for seizures. However, atypical antipsychotics counteract the effects of levodopa and other dopamine agonists. Also, drugs that alter the cytochrome P-450 enzyme system affect the metabolism of some atypical antipsychotics.

TIP Antipsychotics with anticholinergic properties should not be prescribed to older adult patients.

Aripiprazole

Aripiprazole (Abilify) is available as oral tablets and disintegrating oral tablets (Abilify Discmelt), as an oral solution, and as a solution for IM injection. Aripiprazole injections are indicated only for treating agitation in patients with schizophrenia or bipolar disorder. Therapy for schizophrenia or bipolar disorder itself is accomplished with oral aripiprazole. This drug is a fairly new atypical antipsychotic and may produce mild sedation.

AT THE COUNTER

Clozapine Considerations

A patient comes into the pharmacy with a prescription for clozapine. What do you need to know before you can fill the prescription?

Is the patient registered through a national registry for clozapine? All patients who are taking clozapine must be registered. Registration must be completed by the physician specifically for the patient prior to a prescription being dispensed. The medication has very specific monitoring parameters that the physician must follow. Not all pharmacies stock and dispense clozapine.

Why does clozapine require such specific monitoring?

Clozapine may cause agranulocytosis, which is a condition characterized by a severe decrease in white blood cell count (WBC). The patient's WBC and absolute neutrophil count must be closely monitored while he is receiving clozapine therapy.

Clozapine

Clozapine is prescribed as tablets (Clozaril) and orally disintegrating tablets (Fazaclo). It's used to treat patients with severe schizophrenia who have not responded to other therapies. The standard tablets are also used to control recurrent suicidal behavior in patients with schizophrenia and certain other psychiatric disorders.

This drug is associated with agranulocytosis (an abnormal decrease in white blood cells). Weight gain is common with this drug, and seizures may also occur.

Olanzapine

Olanzapine (Zyprexa) is available as tablets, orally disintegrating tablets (Zyprexa Zydis), and a powder that is mixed with sterile water for IM injection. The uses of each form of this drug are the same as for aripiprazole. Like aripiprazole, this drug should not be administered by IV infusion.

Olanzapine is also available in a combination product with fluoxetine (Symbyax). This drug, which is available in capsule form, is used in treating depressive episodes associated with bipolar disorder.

Weight gain is a common side effect of olanzapine. This drug also places the patient at risk for extrapyramidal effects, although the risk is minimal. (**Extrapyramidal effects** are a group of adverse reactions in the nervous system that cause abnormal muscle movements.)

Quetiapine

Quetiapine is prescribed as immediate-release tablets (Seroquel) and extended-release tablets (Seroquel XR) for the treatment of schizophrenia. The immediate-release form is also used to treat bipolar disorder. The most common adverse reaction to this drug is sedation.

Risperidone

Risperidone (Risperdal) is available as tablets, orally disintegrating tablets (Risperdal M-Tab), and oral solution. It's also manufactured as a powder that must be mixed with the liquid in the dose pack and administered by IM injection (Risperdal Consta). Injected risperidone is an extended-release drug that is given once every two weeks. Daily oral administration usually begins with the first risperidone injection.

Risperidone has a higher risk of extrapyramidal effects than other atypical antipsychotics, especially if it's prescribed at higher doses than six milligrams per day. Risperidone is used to treat bipolar mania and irritability associated with autism. In addition, it's used in treating schizophrenia. Off-label uses include treatment of OCD and treatment of tics associated with Tourette syndrome.

Ziprasidone

Ziprasidone (Geodon) is prescribed as capsules for oral administration and as a powder that is mixed with sterile water for IM injection. Ziprasidone injections are used to relieve acute agitation in patients with schizophrenia. The oral form is used to treat bipolar mania and schizophrenia.

This drug may cause electrocardiogram changes. For this reason, it's usually recommended only after the patient has failed to respond to other atypical antipsychotics.

Typical Antipsychotics

As their name suggests, **typical antipsychotics** are generally older drugs that once were "typical" therapies for **psychotic disorders**—disorders that are characterized by personality disorganization and a loss of grip on reality in the patient. Although typical antipsychotics remain effective, their serious long-term adverse effects now limit their use. Instead, clinicians now prefer the newer, less potentially harmful atypical antipsychotics.

The major typical antipsychotics include:

- chlorpromazine
- fluphenazine decanoate
- fluphenazine
- haloperidol (Haldol)
- haloperidol decanoate (Haldol Decanoate)
- loxapine (Loxitane)
- molindone (Moban)
- perphenazine
- perphenazine and amitriptyline
- pimozide (Orap)
- thioridazine
- thiothixene (Navane)
- trifluoperazine

STIMULANTS

Stimulants are used to treat ADHD, a condition marked by inattention, impulsiveness, and hyperactivity. They're believed to work by increasing the patient's levels of dopamine and norepinephrine in one of three ways:

- by blocking the reuptake of dopamine and norepinephrine

PROCEED WITH CAUTION

Adverse Reactions to Typical Antipsychotics

Neurological reactions are the most common and serious adverse reactions to these drugs.

- Extrapyramidal effects may appear after the first few days of therapy. **Tardive dyskinesia**, or a number of potentially irreversible involuntary muscle movements, may occur after several years of treatment.
- **Neuroleptic malignant syndrome** may occur. This is a potentially fatal condition that produces muscle rigidity, extreme extrapyramidal effects, severely elevated body temperature, hypertension, and rapid heart rate. If left untreated, it can result in respiratory failure and cardiovascular collapse.

- by enhancing the presynaptic release
- by inhibiting MAO

Stimulants are the treatment of choice for ADHD. They help improve attention, which can lead to improved performance at work or school. They also decrease impulsivity and hyperactivity, if those symptoms are troublesome.

Here are a few important considerations about this class of drugs that you should keep in mind:

- Stimulants should not be used within 14 days of discontinuing therapy with an MAOI.
- Stimulants are easy to abuse. (All stimulants discussed in this chapter are classified as Schedule II controlled substances.) Close monitoring of their use is required.

In addition, drug holidays are recommended every year to assess whether the need for the drug still exists. Many parents with children who have ADHD suspend use of the drug during summer vacations from school to see if the child still needs the medication.

TIP Most, but not all, of the stimulants used to treat ADHD are Schedule II controlled substances. It's important to know how each medication is classified because the laws for Schedule II substances are much stricter than for the other schedules.

Dextroamphetamine

Dextroamphetamine, a Schedule II controlled substance, is prescribed as immediate-release tablets (Dextrostat) or as sustained-release capsules (Dexedrine). The capsules are taken once a day at the same time every day. Patients who are taking tablets should take the first dose on awaking each morning and then one or two more doses during the day at four- to six-hour intervals.

Tablets can be taken with or without food, but should not be taken with fruit juice. Foods and drinks that contain large amounts of caffeine—such as chocolate, coffee, and cola drinks—should be avoided at all times because they can increase this drug's adverse effects.

Adverse reactions to dextroamphetamine include:

- restlessness
- tremors
- insomnia
- tachycardia
- heart palpitations
- cardiac arrhythmias
- dry mouth
- unpleasant taste
- diarrhea

Methylphenidate and Dexmethylphenidate

Methylphenidate and dexmethylphenidate are two similar drug compounds used to treat ADHD. Both are classified as Schedule II controlled substances.

Methylphenidate may be prescribed in one of several different forms, including:

- immediate-release tablets (Ritalin)
- chewable tablets (Methylin)
- extended-release tablets (Metadate ER, Concerta, Ritalin SR)
- extended-release capsules (Ritalin LA, Metadate CD)
- oral solution (Methylin)
- transdermal patch (Daytrana)

In children, the oral solution or the immediate-release or chewable tablets should be taken twice daily, before breakfast and lunch. The adult dose is two to three times daily. In patients who develop sleep difficulties while taking methylphenidate, the final dose should be taken before 6:00 P.M. The extended-release tablets and capsules remain effective for about eight hours. The patch is applied to the hip two hours before its effect is needed. It must be removed nine hours after application.

Dexmethylphenidate is available in the form of tablets (Focalin) and extended-release capsules (Focalin XR). The immediate-release form of dexmethylphenidate should be taken twice daily, at least four hours apart, with or without food. The extended-release capsules, however, should be taken once daily, in the morning. Capsules may be swallowed whole or administered by opening the capsules and sprinkling the contents on a small amount of applesauce. The applesauce mixture should be taken immediately and may not be stored for future use.

Adverse reactions to methylphenidate and dexmethylphenidate may include:

- dizziness
- headache
- insomnia
- heart palpitations
- cardiac arrhythmias
- tachycardia
- abdominal pain
- anorexia
- nausea
- hypersensitivity reactions (such as skin rash, urticaria, and fever)

Methylphenidate and dexmethylphenidate may also decrease the effects of guanethidine and may increase the effects of TCAs, warfarin, and some anticonvulsant drugs.

Mixed Amphetamine Salts

Mixed amphetamine and dextroamphetamine salts are combinations of amphetamines in a single compound. They are available in immediate-release tablets (Adderall) and extended-release capsules (Adderall XR) and have been found to be very effective in the treatment of ADHD. These drugs are also used in treating narcolepsy (a chronic disorder that results in recurrent attacks of drowsiness and sleep during daytime).

Adverse reactions to mixed amphetamine salts include:

- restlessness
- insomnia
- hyperexcitability
- heart palpitations
- cardiac arrhythmias
- tremors
- abdominal pain
- dry mouth
- unpleasant taste

QUICK QUIZ

Answer the following multiple-choice questions.

1. Patient education about taking an SSRI should include which of the following instructions?
   a. Slowly increase your dosage until your depression is relieved.
   b. Be sure to drink plenty of water while you are taking this drug.
   c. Avoid exercise for an hour after taking this medication.
   d. Don't discontinue this drug without consulting your physician.
2. If a patient is taking chloral hydrate, what adverse reactions is she most likely to experience?
   a. cardiac irregularities
   b. blood pressure changes
   c. GI symptoms and hangover effects
   d. dizziness and light-headedness
3. What adverse reactions are common with the drugs that are used to treat anxiety?
   a. light-headedness, dizziness, and vertigo
   b. skin rash and other hypersensitivity reactions
   c. anger, irritability, and combativeness
   d. extrapyramidal effects
4. What medications should a patient who is being treated with lithium avoid?
   a. antihypertensive drugs
   b. hormonal contraceptives
   c. antidiabetic drugs
   d. loop diuretics
5. Drugs used to treat ADHD in children are usually withheld at all of the following times *except:*
   a. before breakfast
   b. within 14 days of discontinuing an MAOI
   c. before bedtime
   d. during school vacations

Please answer each of the following questions in one to three sentences.

1. What is the difference between a sedative and a hypnotic?

   _____

   _____

2. In what circumstances would the use of an injectable antipsychotic be indicated over oral administration of the drug?

   _____

   _____

3. What similarities and differences exist in how TCAs, MAOIs, and SSRIs work?

   _____

   _____

4. How does the reason for prescribing an antipsychotic differ from the reason for prescribing an antidepressant?

   _____

   _____

5. What extrapyramidal effect may appear in patients after long-term treatment with typical antipsychotics?

   _____

   _____

Answer the following questions as either true or false.

1. ___ A person taking an MAOI should avoid eating foods that are high in tyramine.
2. ___ Fluoxetine (Prozac) is one of the most commonly prescribed drugs for treating depression.
3. ___ Stimulants such as dextroamphetamine (Dexedrine) are the frontline drugs for treating ADHD.
4. ___ Antipsychotic drugs are used to treat delusions and other thought disorders that accompany schizophrenia and mania.
5. ___ Typical antipsychotics are generally safer for patients to use than atypical antipsychotics.

Match each psychotropic drug in the left column with its classification in the right column.

1. buspirone	a. antianxiety drugs
2. clozapine	b. antidepressants and mood stabilizers
3. dextroamphetamine	c. antipsychotics
4. diazepam	d. sedatives and hypnotics
5. lithium	e. stimulants

DRUG CLASSIFICATION TABLE

Classification	Generic Name	Trade Name(s)
Benzodiazepines	estazolam *es-taz'-e-lam*	*tablets:* (no longer marketed under trade name)
	flurazepam *flur-az'-e-pam*	*capsules:* Dalmane
	lorazepam *lor-a'-ze-pam*	*tablets:* Ativan *oral solution:* (no longer marketed under trade name) *injection:* Ativan
	quazepam *kwa'-ze-pam*	*tablets:* Doral
	temazepam *te-maz'-e-pam*	*capsules:* Restoril
	triazolam *trye-ay'-zoe-lam*	*tablets:* Halcion
	alprazolam *al-prah'-zoe-lam*	*tablets:* Xanax *extended-release tablets:* Xanax XR *orally disintegrating tablets:* Niravam *solution:* (no longer marketed under trade name)
	chlordiazepoxide *klor-dye-az-e-pox'-ide*	*capsules:* Librium
	chlordiazepoxide and clidinium *klor-dye-az-e-pox'-ide klih'-dih-nee-uhm*	*capsules:* Librax
	chlordiazepoxide and amitriptyline *klor-dye-az-e-pox'-ide am-ee-trip'-ti-leen*	*tablets:* Limbitrol
	clonazepam *clo-nay'-zeh-pam*	*tablets:* Klonopin *orally disintegrating tablets:* Klonopin
	clorazepate *klor-az'-e-pate*	*tablets:* Tranxene *extended-release tablets:* Tranxene SD
	diazepam *dye-az'-e-pam*	*tablets:* Valium *oral solution:* (no longer marketed under trade name) *rectal gel:* Diastat *injection:* (no longer marketed under trade name)
	oxazepam *ox-a'-ze-pam*	*capsules:* (no longer marketed under trade name)
Barbiturates	amobarbital *am-oh-bar'-bi-tal*	*injection:* Amytal
	butabarbital *byoo-ta-bar'-bi-tal*	*tablets:* Butisol *oral solution:* Butisol
	mephobarbital *me-foe-bar'-bi-tal*	*tablets:* Mebaral
	pentobarbital *pen-toe-bar'-bi-tal*	*injection:* Nembutal
	phenobarbital *fee-noe-bar'-bi-tal*	*tablets:* (no longer marketed under trade name) *injection:* Luminal *oral solution:* (no longer marketed under trade name)
	secobarbital *see-koe-bar'-bi-tal*	*capsules:* Seconal
Nonbenzodiazepine-nonbarbiturates	chloral hydrate *klor-al hye'-drate*	*capsules:* Somnote *rectal suppositories:* Aquachloral *oral solution:* (no longer marketed under trade name)

continued

DRUG CLASSIFICATION TABLE (continued)

Classification	Generic Name	Trade Name(s)
Nonbenzodiazepine-nonbarbiturates (continued)	zaleplon zal'-ah-plahn	capsules: Sonata
	zolpidem zol'-pih-dem	tablets: Ambien extended-release tablets: Ambien CR
	eszopiclone e-zo'-pic-clone	tablets: Lunesta
Antianxiety drugs	buspirone byoo-spye'-rone	tablets: BuSpar
Tricyclic antidepressants	amitriptyline am-ee-trip'-ti-leen	tablets: (no longer marketed under trade name)
	amoxapine a-mox'-a-peen	tablets: (no longer marketed under trade name)
	clomipramine kloe-mi'-pra-meen	capsules: Anafranil
	desipramine dess-ip'-ra-meen	tablets: Norpramin
	doxepin dox'-e-pin	capsules: (no longer marketed under trade name) oral solution: (no longer marketed under trade name) topical cream: Prudoxin, Zonalon
	imipramine hydrochloride im-ip'-ra-meen	tablets: Tofranil
	imipramine pamoate im-ip'-ra-meen	capsules: Tofranil PM
	nortriptyline nor-trip'-ti-leen	capsules: Pamelor oral solution: Pamelor
	protriptyline proe-trip'-ti-leen	tablets: Vivactil
	trimipramine trye-mi'-pra-meen	capsules: Surmontil
Monoamine oxidase inhibitors	phenelzine fen'-el-zeen	tablets: Nardil
	tranylcypromine tran-ill-sip'-roe-meen	tablets: Parnate
Selective serotonin reuptake inhibitors	citalopram si-tal'-oh-pram	tablets: Celexa oral solution: Celexa
	escitalopram es-sye-tal'-oh-pram	tablets: Lexapro oral suspension: Lexapro
	fluoxetine floo-ox'-e-teen	tablets: (no longer marketed under trade name) capsules: Prozac extended-release capsules: Prozac Weekly oral solution: Prozac tablets (PMDD): Sarafem capsules (PMDD): Selfemra
	fluoxetine and olanzapine floo-ox'-e-teen oh-lan'-za-peen	capsules: Symbyax
	fluvoxamine floo-voks'-a-meen	tablets: (no longer marketed under trade name) extended-release capsules: Luvox CR
	paroxetine par-ox'-e-teen	tablets: Paxil, Pexeva controlled-release tablets: Paxil CR oral suspension: Paxil
	sertraline sir'-trah-leen	tablets: Zoloft oral solution: Zoloft

continued

DRUG CLASSIFICATION TABLE (continued)

Classification	Generic Name	Trade Name(s)
Selective serotonin and norepinephrine reuptake inhibitors	venlafaxine *ven-la-fax'-een*	*tablets:* Effexor *extended-release capsules:* Effexor XR
	duloxetine *du-lox'-e-teen*	*delayed release capsules:* Cymbalta
Miscellaneous antidepressants	maprotiline *map-roe'-ti-leen*	*tablets:* (no longer marketed under trade name)
	mirtazapine *mer-tah'-zah-peen*	*tablets:* Remeron *orally disintegrating tablets:* Remeron Soltab
	bupropion *byoo-proe'-pee-on*	*tablets:* Wellbutrin *extended-release tablets:* Wellbutrin XL, Wellbutrin SR *extended-release tablets (smoking cessation):* Zyban
	trazodone *traz'-oh-done*	*tablets:* (no longer marketed under trade name)
	nefazodone *ne-faz'-oh-done*	*tablets:* (no longer marketed under trade name)
Mood stabilizer drugs	lithium carbonate *lith'-ee-um*	*capsules:* (no longer marketed under trade name) *tablets:* (no longer marketed under trade name) *extended-release tablets:* Lithobid
	lithium citrate *lith'-ee-um*	*oral solution:* (no longer marketed under trade name)
Atypical antipsychotic drugs	aripiprazole *ar-i-pip'-ra-zole*	*tablets:* Abilify *orally disintegrating tablets:* Abilify Discmelt *oral solution:* Abilify *injection:* Abilify
	clozapine *kloe'-za-peen*	*tablets:* Clozaril *orally disintegrating tablets:* Fazaclo
	olanzapine *oh-lan'-za-peen*	*tablets:* Zyprexa *orally disintegrating tablets:* Zyprexa Zydis *injection:* Zyprexa
	olanzapine and fluoxetine *oh-lan'-za-peen floo-ox'-e-teen*	*capsules:* Symbyax
	quetiapine *kwe-tie'-ah-pine*	*tablets:* Seroquel *extended-release tablets:* Seroquel XR
	risperidone *ris-per'-i-done*	*tablets:* Risperdal *orally disintegrating tablets:* Risperdal M-Tab *oral solution:* Risperdal *injection:* Risperdal Consta
	ziprasidone *zih-pray'-sih-dohn*	*capsules:* Geodon *injection:* Geodon
Typical antipsychotic drugs	chlorpromazine *klor-proe'-ma-zeen*	*tablets:* (no longer marketed under trade name) *injection:* (no longer marketed under trade name)
	fluphenazine decanoate *floo-fen'-a-zeen*	*injection:* (no longer marketed under trade name)

continued

DRUG CLASSIFICATION TABLE (continued)

Classification	Generic Name	Trade Name(s)
Typical antipsychotic drugs (continued)	fluphenazine *floo-fen'-a-zeen*	*tablets:* (no longer marketed under trade name) *elixir:* (no longer marketed under trade name) *solution:* (no longer marketed under trade name) *injection:* (no longer marketed under trade name)
	haloperidol *ha-loe-per'-i-dole*	*tablets:* (no longer marketed under trade name) *oral solution:* (no longer marketed under trade name) *injection:* Haldol
	haloperidol decanoate *ha-loe-per'-i-dole*	*injection:* Haldol Decanoate
	loxapine *lox'-a-peen*	*capsules:* Loxitane
	molindone *moe-lin'-done*	*tablets:* Moban
	perphenazine *per-fen'-a-zeen*	*tablets:* (no longer marketed under trade name)
	perphenazine and amitriptyline *per-fen'-a-zeen am-ee-trip'-ti-leen*	*tablets:* (no longer marketed under trade name)
	pimozide *pi'-moe-zide*	*tablets:* Orap
	thioridazine *thye-oh-rid'-a-zeen*	*tablets:* (no longer marketed under trade name)
	thiothixene *thye-oh-thix'-een*	*capsules:* Navane
	trifluoperazine *try-floo-oh-per'-a-zeen*	*tablets:* (no longer marketed under trade name)
Stimulants	dextroamphetamine *dex-troe-am-fet'-a-meen*	*tablets:* Dextrostat *sustained-release capsules:* Dexedrine
	methylphenidate *meh-thyl-fen'-ih-date*	*tablets:* Ritalin *chewable tablets:* Methylin *extended-release tablets:* Metadate ER, Concerta, Ritalin SR *oral solution:* Methylin *transdermal patch:* Daytrana *extended-release capsules:* Ritalin LA, Metadate CD
	dexmethylphenidate *dex-meh-thyl-fen'-ih-date*	*extended-release capsules:* Focalin XR *tablets:* Focalin
	mixed amphetamine salts *am-fet'-a-meen*	*extended-release capsules:* Adderall XR *tablets:* Adderall

CHAPTER 12

Endocrine Drugs

- Match brand and generic names of commonly used endocrine drugs
- Identify the classification of commonly used endocrine drugs
- Identify the uses of common endocrine drugs
- Compare and contrast type 1 and type 2 diabetes, including the medications used for each type
- Describe a sliding scale dosing for insulin
- Explain the advantages and disadvantages of hormone-replacement therapy
- Explain the mechanism of action for oral contraceptives and emergency contraception
- Discuss when a progestin-only oral contraceptive would be used instead of a combination estrogen-progestin oral contraceptive
- Describe the strengths of thyroid drugs found for various brand and generic names, and explain the unique nature of some of the strengths

KEY TERMS

anterior pituitary drugs—drugs that mimic the effects of hormones produced in the anterior pituitary gland

antithyroid drugs—drugs that act as antagonists to thyroid hormones; also known as *thyroid antagonists*

emergency contraceptives—drugs used to prevent pregnancy only after unprotected intercourse or in situations in which contraceptives are known or suspected to have failed

estrogens—substances that mimic the effects of a natural female hormone

glands—specialized clusters of cells that release substances into the blood or into cavities inside the body or its outer surface

glucagon—a hyperglycemic agent used to increase blood glucose levels

hormonal contraceptives—drugs used regularly to prevent pregnancy; also known as oral contraceptives or birth control pills

hormones— the chemical transmitters secreted by glands in response to stimulation

hyperglycemic drugs—drugs that increase blood glucose levels

hyperthyroidism—a condition in which the thyroid gland produces too much thyroid hormone

hypoglycemic drugs—drugs that decrease blood glucose levels

insulin—a hormone produced by the pancreas that helps maintain blood glucose levels within normal limits

oral antidiabetic drugs—drugs used to treat type 2 diabetes that are administered by mouth

pituitary drugs—natural or synthetic hormones that mimic the action of hormones produced by the pituitary gland

progestins—substances that mimic the effects of a naturally occurring female hormone (progesterone)

thyroid antagonists—see *antithyroid drugs*

thyroid drugs—natural or synthetic substances that replace or substitute for thyroid hormones

type 1 diabetes—a chronic condition, usually diagnosed during childhood, in which the body does not produce enough insulin

type 2 diabetes—a chronic condition in which either too little insulin is produced or the cells can't properly use the insulin that is produced

The endocrine system consists of **glands**, which are specialized cell clusters, and **hormones**, the chemical transmitters secreted by the glands in response to stimulation. Together with the central nervous system, the endocrine system regulates and integrates the body's metabolic activities. The aim is to maintain homeostasis (the body's internal balance or equilibrium). Situations that might require drugs that affect the endocrine system include:

- diabetes
- diagnostic tests
- **hyperthyroidism** (a condition in which the thyroid gland produces too much thyroid hormone)
- contraception

Drugs from three general classes are used to treat endocrine system disorders:

- natural hormones and their synthetic analogs
- hormonelike substances
- drugs that stimulate or suppress hormone secretion

ANTIDIABETIC DRUGS AND GLUCAGON

Antidiabetic drugs and **glucagon** help the body control levels of glucose, a type of sugar, in the body. Normally, the body controls blood glucose levels by releasing a hormone called **insulin**. Insulin is released in small amounts throughout the day as blood glucose levels change. Insulin is needed for cells to convert glucose, starches, and other foods into energy.

Diabetes mellitus, or just diabetes, is a chronic disease in which the body can't properly regulate glucose. It's characterized by disturbances in carbohydrate, protein, and fat metabolism. This leads to elevated levels of glucose in the body. The disease appears in two main forms.

- In **type 1 diabetes** (formerly called insulin-dependent diabetes mellitus), the body doesn't produce enough insulin. Patients must take insulin to control blood glucose levels. Type 1 diabetes is usually diagnosed during childhood.
- In **type 2 diabetes** (formerly called non-insulin-dependent diabetes mellitus), the body can produce insulin but has insulin resistance. Either too little insulin is produced or the cells can't properly use the insulin that is produced. Type 2 diabetes is the more common type of diabetes.

Substances used to regulate glucose and control diabetes may either increase or decrease blood glucose levels.

- **Hypoglycemic drugs** decrease blood glucose levels. Insulin, a pancreatic hormone, and oral antidiabetic drugs are hypoglycemic drugs.
- **Hyperglycemic drugs** increase blood glucose levels. Glucagon, another pancreatic hormone, is classified as a hyperglycemic drug.

Insulin

The hormone insulin is normally produced by beta cells in the pancreas. It's needed for the body to use glucose and to store amino acids and fatty acids. Patients may need to receive a form of insulin to control blood glucose levels for type 1 diabetes. Insulin is also used to treat type 2 diabetes in the following situations:

- when other methods of controlling glucose levels have failed or are contraindicated
- when blood glucose levels are elevated during periods of emotional or physical stress (such as infection or surgery)
- when oral antidiabetic drugs are contraindicated because of pregnancy or hypersensitivity

Insulin is also used to treat several complications of diabetes.

- Diabetic ketoacidosis is a serious condition in which the blood becomes acidic due to a buildup of toxic substances called ketones. This condition is more common with type 1 diabetes.
- Hyperosmolar hyperglycemic nonketotic syndrome occurs when blood glucose levels increase and the body tries to eliminate the excess sugar in the urine. It's most common in patients with type 2 diabetes.
- Hyperkalemia (elevated serum potassium levels) in patients without diabetes can also be treated with insulin. Potassium moves with glucose from the bloodstream into the cell, lowering serum potassium levels.

Insulin can't be taken orally because the GI tract breaks down the protein molecule before it reaches the bloodstream. However, insulin may be given by SubQ injection. The absorption of injected insulin varies according to several factors including:

- the injection site
- the blood supply
- the degree of tissue hypertrophy (enlargement) at the injection site

Insulin may also be given by IV infusion and in dialysate fluid (a fluid that cleanses the blood) infused into the peritoneal cavity for patients on peritoneal dialysis therapy.

Insulin is referred to as an anabolic, or building, hormone. It helps by doing the following:

- promoting storage of glucose as glycogen
- increasing protein and fat synthesis
- slowing the breakdown of glycogen, protein, and fat
- balancing fluids and electrolytes

Although it has no antidiuretic effect, insulin can correct polyuria (excessive urination) and polydipsia (excessive thirst). These symptoms often occur with osmotic diuresis (increased pressure in the kidney tubules) that occurs in hypoglycemia as a result of the decreased blood glucose level. Insulin also aids the movement of potassium from the extracellular fluid into the cell.

Patients need to monitor their blood glucose levels using a glucometer several times a day. Physicians may prescribe insulin on a sliding scale basis. The prescription shows the amount of insulin required for different blood glucose levels. Patients check their blood glucose levels to determine the exact dose required. This allows good control of blood glucose, to ensure that the amount of insulin taken matches what the body needs.

It's important to store insulin properly. Preparations can be stored at room temperature for one month. Prefilled glass or plastic syringes are stable for 28 days under refrigeration.

Some drugs interact with insulin, changing its ability to decrease the blood glucose level. Other substances may directly affect glucose levels.

- Anabolic steroids, salicylates, alcohol, and MAOIs may increase the hypoglycemic effect of insulin.
- Corticosteroids, sympathomimetic drugs, thiazide diuretics, and dextrothyroxine sodium may reduce the effects of insulin, resulting in hyperglycemia.
- Beta-adrenergic blockers may prolong the hypoglycemic effect of insulin and may mask signs and symptoms of hypoglycemia.

Insulins are divided into four groups, depending on their duration of action after administration. The following table shows the onset and duration of action for each group. However, the specific onset and duration depend on the brand (see table 12-1).

Insulin Lispro

Insulin lispro (Humalog) is a rapid-acting insulin that is available by prescription only. It has a faster onset and a shorter duration of action than regular insulin. When patients use this drug to treat type 1 diabetes, a longer-acting insulin is also needed to maintain glycemic control. The amount of longer-acting insulin may need to be adjusted. For type 2 diabetes, it may be used without a longer-acting insulin as part of a therapy regimen with sulfonylurea drugs.

Insulin lispro is manufactured in vials, cartridges, and disposable pen delivery devices. It may be injected within 15 minutes before or after a meal. Insulin lispro should be stored in a refrigerator. It may be diluted with sterile

TABLE 12-1 Insulin: Onset and Duration of Action

Insulin Preparations	Onset of Action	Duration of Action
Rapid-acting	15 minutes	2 to 5 hours
Short-acting	30 to 60 minutes	8 to 16 hours
Intermediate-acting	1 to 2 hours, 30 minutes	24 hours
Long-acting	4 to 8 hours	20 to 36 hours

PROCEED WITH CAUTION

Adverse Reactions to Insulin

Adverse reactions to insulin include:

- hypoglycemia (below normal blood glucose levels)
- Somogyi effect (hypoglycemia followed by rebound hyperglycemia)
- hypersensitivity reactions
- lipodystrophy (disturbance in fat deposition)
- insulin resistance

In insulin resistance, the body no longer responds well to insulin. High levels of insulin are needed to maintain normal blood sugar.

diluent or certain other insulins. Diluted insulin lispro must be used within 28 days if refrigerated and 14 days if at room temperature.

TIP As a pharmacy technician, you should know which insulins require a prescription and which do not. If a prescription is not required, always double-check that you have the correct product before selling it to the patient.

Insulin Aspart

Insulin aspart (Novolog) is a rapid-acting insulin. It is available by prescription only and is used to control hyperglycemia in patients with diabetes. Insulin aspart is given by injection and should normally be used in treatment regimens together with an intermediate- or long-acting insulin.

Insulin Glulisine

Insulin glulisine (Apidra) is a rapid-acting insulin used to control hyperglycemia in adults with diabetes. Administered by injection, this drug has a more rapid onset of action and a shorter duration of action than regular human insulin. It should normally be used in treatment regimens together with a longer-acting insulin. Insulin glulisine is available by prescription only.

Regular Insulin

Regular insulin (Humulin R, Novolin R) is short acting. It's used to treat types 1 and 2 diabetes that can't be controlled by diet and exercise. Regular insulin is manufactured in vials for injection as synthetic human insulin. This type of insulin is available with or without a prescription.

Regular human insulin should be clear and colorless. It doesn't need to be shaken before use. Shaking may lead to air bubbles. Regular insulin is usually given 30 to 60 minutes before a meal. Peak effects last from two to five hours.

Insulin Isophane

Insulin isophane (Humulin N, Novolin N), abbreviated NPH, is an intermediate-acting insulin. Intermediate-acting insulin is developed as synthetic human insulin.

HOW IT WORKS

How Insulin Aids Glucose Uptake

Insulin is normally produced by the beta cells of the pancreas. It allows body cells to use glucose for energy. Figure 12-1 shows the following process:

1. Glucose can't enter the cell without the aid of insulin.
2. Insulin binds to the receptors on the surface of the target cell. Insulin and its receptor first move inside the cell. This

activates glucose transporter channels to move to the surface of the cell.

3. These channels allow glucose to enter the cell. The cell can then use the glucose for metabolism.

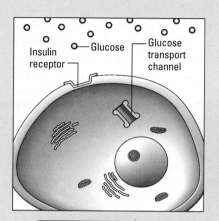
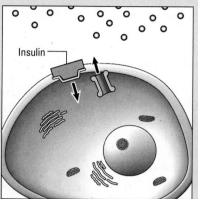
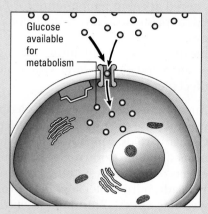

FIGURE 12-1 How insulin aids glucose uptake. (From *Clinical Pharmacology Made Incredibly Easy.* 2nd Ed. Philadelphia, PA: Lippincott Williams & Wilkins; 2005.)

NPH insulin is available without a prescription. This type of insulin is manufactured as a suspension for injection and as cartridges for use with an injection pen. NPH insulin is administered once or twice a day within 60 minutes of a meal.

Insulin Detemir

Insulin detemir (Levemir) is an intermediate- to long-acting insulin. It is a prescription drug used to treat adults and children with type 1 diabetes or adult patients with type 2 diabetes who require long-acting insulin for the control of hyperglycemia. Insulin detemir is available in the form of prefilled cartridges and syringes or in vials for injection.

TIP Insulin is typically stored in the refrigerator in the pharmacy. Most pharmacies do not place the insulin bag on the shelf waiting for the customer to pick it up, but instead leave it labeled in the refrigerator. Make sure when retrieving the product from the refrigerator that you have not only the correct patient, but also the correct product. This provides you with the perfect opportunity to make sure that the correct insulin is being dispensed.

Insulin Glargine

Insulin glargine (Lantus) is a long-acting insulin. Like insulin detemir, it is used to treat adults and children with type 1 diabetes or adult patients with type 2 diabetes who require long-acting insulin for the control of hyperglycemia.

It is a prescription drug available as vials and cartridges for injection.

Combination Insulin Products

Combination drugs are also used to control hyperglycemia in patients with diabetes.

- Insulin aspart protamine and insulin aspart (Novolog Mix 70/30) is only available by prescription and is administered by injection. However, this drug should not be given intravenously.
- Insulin lispro protamine and insulin lispro (Humalog Mix 75/25, Humalog Mix 50/50) is available by prescription in the form of vials and disposable pen delivery devices for injection.

Another combination drug, insulin NPH suspension and regular insulin (Novolin 70/30, Humulin 70/30, Humulin 50/50), is used to treat type 1 diabetes, certain cases of type 2 diabetes, and gestational diabetes (a temporary condition that may occur during pregnancy). This drug is available over the counter in the form of vials for injection.

TIP Insulin requirements change during pregnancy. Patients who are pregnant should monitor their glucose levels more often.

Oral Antidiabetic Drugs

Many types of **oral antidiabetic drugs** have been approved for use in the United States. These drugs are used to treat

AT THE COUNTER

The Proper Tools for Insulin

A patient drops off a prescription for insulin. When the patient picks the prescription up, he asks for syringes to go with his insulin. How do you know which syringes the patient needs?

First, you will need to determine how many units of insulin the patient will take for each dose. Insulin syringes are different from others in that they are calibrated in units instead of milliliters. Insulin syringes are available in 30 units (3/10 mL), 50 units (1/2 mL), or 100 units (1 mL). Once you know how many units per dose, then choose the largest number and find the smallest syringe in which that number of units will fit. For example, if the patient is to take 30 units at breakfast, 40 units at lunch, and 35 units at dinner, then choose a 50-unit (1/2 mL) syringe.

When you are looking at the patient's prescription to determine which syringes he'll need, the patient tells you that he needs enough for 30 days because he is going on vacation. How many boxes of syringes will he need?

If the patient injects himself three times a day, then he would need 90 syringes for 30 days. So a box of 100 syringes will be enough.

Also, the patient asks you to make sure that he has enough insulin for 30 days. How many vials of insulin will he need?

Insulin comes in 100 units per 1 mL. So if the patient's prescription is for a 10 mL vial, then it would contain 1000 units. The patient is taking 30 units at breakfast, 40 units at lunch, and 35 units at dinner. Therefore, each day he'll need 105 units. So for 30 days the patient will use 3150 units, which is three vials and part of a fourth vial. So you should make sure that he has four vials in his prescription.

patients with type 2 diabetes if diet and exercise can't control blood glucose levels. Oral antibiotic drugs aren't effective in patients with type 1 diabetes, however, because these patients' pancreatic cells are functioning at a level lower than the minimum.

Combinations of multiple oral antidiabetic drugs or an oral antidiabetic drug with insulin therapy may be needed for some patients who don't respond to either therapy alone. These combination therapies aren't recommended for children or pregnant women. When using these combination therapies, it's important to monitor kidney function to help prevent lactic acidosis associated with using metformin.

Oral antidiabetic drugs are believed to act both within and outside the pancreas to regulate blood glucose. They probably stimulate pancreatic beta cells to release insulin in a patient with a minimally functioning pancreas. Within a few weeks to a few months of starting treatment, pancreatic insulin secretions will decrease to pretreatment levels. However, the blood glucose levels will remain normal or near

normal. Most likely, the oral antidiabetic agents are acting outside the pancreas to maintain this control.

Extrapancreatic actions (actions outside the pancreas) of antidiabetic drugs may decrease and control blood glucose. These drugs work in the following ways.

- They can go to work in the liver and decrease glucose production there.
- They can increase the number of insulin receptors in peripheral tissues. This provides more opportunities for the cells to bind with insulin and start the process of glucose metabolism.

Guidelines from the American Diabetes Association suggest that glucose levels should be maintained within normal ranges for good health. They recommend that beginning steps to control diabetes may include diet, exercise, and the use of an oral antidiabetic drug called metformin or an insulin. If blood glucose levels are still higher than normal ranges, alternative approaches may be used, including taking other oral antidiabetic drugs.

Hypoglycemia is a major adverse reaction to oral antidiabetic drugs, especially when combination therapy is used.

TIP Older adult patients may have reduced kidney function. They shouldn't take oral antidiabetic combination drugs without being tested to show that their kidneys are working adequately.

Incretin Enhancers

Incretin enhancers, also called DPP-4 inhibitors, work to inactivate dipeptidyl peptidase-4, an enzyme that limits the effectiveness of certain hormones helpful in the treatment of type 2 diabetes. Incretin enhancers can limit the degradation of these hormones.

Sitagliptin (Januvia) is an incretin enhancer used as an adjunct to diet and exercise to improve glycemic control in patients with type 2 diabetes. Sitagliptin is available by prescription in tablet form. It can be taken with or without food.

Sitagliptin is also available in combination with metformin (Janumet). This drug treats type 2 diabetes in adults as an adjunct to diet and exercise to improve glycemic control. It is available in the form of prescription tablets and should be taken twice daily with food.

Metformin

Metformin is manufactured as tablets (Glucophage), extended-release tablets (Fortamet, Glucophage XR, Glumetza), and oral solution (Riomet). Children older than 10 years may take the immediate-release tablets or oral solution. The extended-release tablets are indicated for adults older than 17 years of age. The extended-release tablets are usually taken once a day with the evening meal. Other forms of metformin are typically taken twice a day with meals. Metformin may be used in combination with a sulfonylurea drug or with insulin in adults older than 17 to control blood sugar levels. It's manufactured in several combination tablets.

Metformin works differently than other antidiabetic drugs. It decreases the production of glucose by the liver and the intestinal absorption of glucose. It also improves insulin sensitivity.

Hypoglycemia may occur when metformin is combined with any of the following drugs:

- cimetidine
- nifedipine
- procainamide
- ranitidine
- vancomycin

Hypoglycemia is less likely to occur when metformin is used as a single agent.

Because metformin given with iodinated contrast dyes can cause acute renal failure, metformin doses shouldn't be given to patients undergoing procedures that require IV contrast dye. Metformin should not be given to patients with heart failure, kidney disease, and acute or chronic metabolic acidosis. It shouldn't be used during pregnancy or by patients older than 80 years.

In addition to hypoglycemia, metformin may cause the following adverse reactions:

- metallic taste in the mouth
- nausea and vomiting
- abdominal discomfort

Sulfonylureas

Sulfonylureas are used along with diet and exercise to lower blood glucose levels in patients with type 2 diabetes. While a patient is taking sulfonylureas, blood glucose levels must be monitored to make sure the patient is taking the smallest dose that is effective. Sulfonylureas may also be used along with insulin in patients with difficult-to-control glucose levels.

Sulfonylureas may be grouped as first- or second-generation sulfonylureas. Second-generation sulfonylureas were developed later. They typically have fewer adverse effects than first-generation sulfonylureas.

Sulfonylureas may interact with other drugs and substances. Hypoglycemia may occur when sulfonylureas are combined with any of the following:

- alcohol
- anabolic steroids
- chloramphenicol
- cimetidine
- clofibrate
- fluconazole
- gemfibrozil
- MAOIs
- NSAIDs
- probenecid
- ranitidine
- salicylates

- sulfonamides
- warfarin

Hyperglycemia may occur when sulfonylureas are taken with any of the following:

- corticosteroids
- dextrothyroxine
- rifampin
- sympathomimetics
- thiazide diuretics

Sulfonylureas may cause the following adverse reactions:

- anorexia
- epigastric fullness
- blood abnormalities
- water retention
- rash
- hyponatremia (low blood sodium level)
- photosensitivity (abnormally heightened reactivity of the skin to sunlight)

Chlorpropamide

Chlorpropamide is a first-generation sulfonylurea drug. It's available by prescription as tablets. This drug is usually taken once a day with breakfast. If patients are transferred from insulin to chlorpropamide, there is a risk of hypoglycemia during the transition period.

Chlorpropamide is rapidly absorbed. Its effects last for at least 24 hours. Because of these long-lasting effects, adverse reactions to this drug may be more prolonged or severe than those of other sulfonylureas.

Glimepiride

Glimepiride (Amaryl) is a prescription medication available as tablets. This second-generation drug may be used on its own or in combination with metformin or insulin to lower blood glucose levels. It's typically taken once per day with breakfast.

T **I** **P** Patients who are taking certain sulfonylureas, such as chlorpropamide and glimepiride, shouldn't drink alcohol. It can interact with these drugs and cause a facial flushing reaction.

Glipizide

Glipizide is a second-generation sulfonylurea drug. It's manufactured as tablets (Glucotrol) and extended-release tablets (Glucotrol XL). Unlike other sulfonylureas, the body's absorption of glipizide is delayed when taken with food. The standard tablets are most effective when taken about 30 minutes before a meal.

The combination drug glipizide and metformin (Metaglip) is manufactured as oral tablets. It's taken once or twice a day with meals. To begin, a low dose is given. Doses are gradually increased to avoid hypoglycemia and adverse GI reactions, and to determine the minimum effective dose.

Glipizide and metformin may interact with many other substances.

- Alcohol increases the risk of lactic acidosis.
- Cationic drugs (for example, digoxin, morphine, ranitidine) may interact with metformin and require careful monitoring.

When given with glipizide and metformin, some drugs may increase the risk of hypoglycemia, including:

- ACE inhibitors (such as benazepril)
- azole antifungals (such as miconazole)
- beta-blockers
- chloramphenicol
- cimetidine
- clofibrate
- fenfluramine
- MAOIs (such as isocarboxazid)
- NSAIDs
- probenecid
- warfarin

Drugs that may lead to hyperglycemia include the following:

- calcium channel blockers (such as amlodipine)
- corticosteroids
- diazoxide
- estrogens
- isoniazid
- nicotinic acid
- oral contraceptives
- phenothiazines
- phenytoin
- rifamycins
- sympathomimetics
- thyroid replacement drugs

Glyburide

Glyburide is a second-generation sulfonylurea drug manufactured as tablets (Diabeta, Micronase) and micronized tablets (Glynase) of varying strengths. It's typically taken in a single dose at breakfast.

Glyburide also comes in a combination tablet with metformin (Glucovance) for use in situations when glyburide and diet don't provide enough control over blood sugar levels. This combination drug is given as oral tablets once or twice daily with meals. Dosage is gradually increased over a two-week period to reach the minimum effective dose to control blood glucose. This drug should be stored in light-resistant containers. A thiazolidinedione may also be used with this combination therapy for patients who need more glycemic control.

Tolazamide

Tolazamide is a first-generation sulfonylurea drug. It's prescribed as tablets to control mild to moderately severe type 2 diabetes. Like other sulfonylureas, it's usually taken as a single dose with breakfast.

Tolbutamide

Tolbutamide is another first-generation sulfonylurea drug. It's manufactured as oral tablets. Oral tolbutamide may be taken as a single dose with breakfast or in divided doses throughout the day.

Alpha-Glucosidase Inhibitors

Alpha-glucosidase inhibitors slow down the digestion of carbohydrates. This results in a smaller increase in glucose levels in the body after meals. As with other antidiabetic drugs, it's important to individualize dosages and monitor blood glucose levels when taking these drugs.

Alpha-glucosidase inhibitors block the action of alpha-glucosidases, enzymes that convert carbohydrates to glucose in the small intestine. By blocking these enzymes, the breakdown of carbohydrates into glucose and other sugars is slowed down. This reduces blood glucose level after meals.

Because alpha-glucosidase inhibitors work differently than sulfonylureas, insulin, or metformin, the effects of alpha-glucosidase inhibitors are additive when taken with these drugs. Alpha-glucosidase inhibitors may also interact with other drugs.

- Taking these drugs with digoxin may reduce the body's digoxin level.
- Digestive enzyme preparations (such as those containing amylase or pancreatin) or intestinal adsorbents (charcoal) may reduce the effects of alpha-glucosidase inhibitors.

Taking alpha-glucosidase inhibitors with some drugs may result in hypoglycemia. These drugs include:

- calcium channel blockers
- corticosteroids
- estrogens
- hormonal contraceptives
- isoniazid
- nicotinic acid
- phenothiazine
- phenytoin
- sympathomimetics
- thyroid products
- thiazides

Alpha-glucosidase inhibitors are not recommended for patients with cirrhosis, inflammatory bowel disease, or chronic intestinal diseases.

Acarbose

Acarbose (Precose) is available by prescription as tablets. It's used to lower blood glucose levels as an adjunct to diet in treating type 2 diabetes. It may be used in combination with sulfonylureas, insulin, or metformin therapy. In these combinations, acarbose produces an additive effect. This can increase the risk of hypoglycemia.

Dosages of acarbose must be individualized for each patient. It's usually taken three times a day at the start of each meal.

Miglitol

Miglitol (Glyset) is sold by prescription as tablets. It may be used as an adjunct to diet or in combination with a sulfonylurea when diet alone hasn't been effective. This drug is usually taken three times a day, at the beginning of each meal.

Meglinitides

Meglinitides are amino acid derivatives. These drugs act to increase insulin secretion from the pancreas. They stimulate beta cells in the pancreatic islets to produce insulin. The amount of insulin released depends on the glucose levels in the body, and it decreases if glucose levels are low.

These drugs may interact with other medications. The following medications may reduce hypoglycemic effects:

- calcium channel blockers
- corticosteroids
- estrogens
- sympathomimetics
- thiazides
- thyroid products

Some drugs taken with meglinitides may increase hypoglycemic effects, including:

- coumarins
- MAOIs
- nonselective beta-blockers
- NSAIDs
- salicylates

Meglinitides shouldn't be taken during pregnancy. They should be carefully monitored in patients with liver or kidney disease. Adverse reactions to meglinitides that are different from those of other oral antidiabetic drugs include:

- bronchitis
- back pain
- headache
- rhinitis
- upper respiratory tract infection

Nateglinide

Nateglinide (Starlix) is manufactured as tablets to be used alone or in combination with metformin or a thiazolidinedione. This drug is normally taken three times a day, up to 30 minutes before meals.

Repaglinide

Repaglinide (Prandin) is prescribed as tablets. It may be used alone or in combination therapy with metformin or thiazolidinediones if necessary. Therapy must be individualized for each patient. Depending on the patient's meal pattern, this drug may be taken two, three, or four times a day. Tablets are taken within 15 minutes of a meal.

Taking repaglinide with CYP450 inhibitors (such as ketoconazole or clarithromycin) may increase levels of repaglinide in the body.

Thiazolidinediones

Thiazolidinediones act to improve insulin sensitivity. For thiazolidinediones to work, insulin must be present in the body. These drugs improve insulin sensitivity in muscle and adipose tissue cells. They are used as an adjunct to diet and exercise in treating type 2 diabetes. Thiazolidinediones may also be used in combination with metformin, insulin, or a sulfonylurea drug if diet and exercise don't provide enough control over blood glucose levels.

Patients taking thiazolidinediones should have their liver enzyme levels monitored from time to time. These drugs must be used with caution in patients who have experienced jaundice while taking troglitazone. Because of the potential for fluid retention when taking these drugs, they are not recommended for patients with severe heart failure.

Thiazolidinediones may interact with other medications.

- Thiazolidinedione levels may be decreased when taken with atorvastatin for seven or more days.
- Ketoconazole may increase blood levels of thiazolidinediones.

Adverse reactions to thiazolidinediones that differ from those for other oral antidiabetic drugs include:

- headache
- back pain
- diarrhea
- swelling
- sinusitis
- upper respiratory tract infections
- weight gain

Patients taking thiazolidinediones should be watched carefully for signs and symptoms of heart failure. Thiazolidinediones can cause or worsen congestive heart failure.

Pioglitazone

Pioglitazone (Actos) is manufactured as an oral tablet for prescription use. It's taken once a day with or without meals. It's also manufactured as tablets in combination with metformin (Actoplus Met) or glimepiride (Duetact).

Rosiglitazone

Rosiglitazone (Avandia) is available by prescription as tablets. It may be taken as a single dose or twice a day, with or without food.

Rosiglitazone is also manufactured as tablets in combination with glimepiride (Avandaryl) or as a combination with metformin (Avandamet). Rosiglitazone and metformin is taken once or twice a day. A low dose is given to start, and the dose is gradually increased to the minimum effective dose. This reduces adverse GI reactions. Patients taking this drug combination have increased risks for congestive heart failure and lactic acidosis.

Exenatide

Exenatide (Byetta) is used to treat patients with type 2 diabetes who are taking metformin, a sulfonylurea, or both. This drug shouldn't be given to patients with type 1 diabetes.

Exenatide is manufactured as an injection solution in a prefilled pen. It's given by SubQ injection in the thigh, abdomen, or upper arm. The injection is given twice a day within one hour before the morning and evening meals. This drug should be stored in the refrigerator.

Exenatide has several actions on the body, including:

■ stimulating insulin production
■ blocking the release of glucagon after meals
■ slowing gastric emptying

Exenatide may interact with other drugs.

■ Because of its effects on gastric emptying, exenatide may affect the absorption of some oral drugs, such as

---

HOW IT WORKS

How Glucagon Increases Glucose Levels

When the body has enough stored glycogen, glucagon can increase glucose levels in patients with severe hypoglycemia. What happens is easy to follow (see figure 12-2).

1. First, glucagon stimulates the formation of the enzyme adenylate cyclase in the liver cell.
2. Adenylate cyclase then converts adenosine triphosphate (ATP) to cyclic adenosine monophosphate (cAMP).

3. This product starts a series of reactions that result in an active phosphorylated glucose molecule.
4. In this phosphorylated form, the large glucose molecule can't pass through the cell membrane.
5. Through glycogenolysis (the breakdown of glycogen, the stored form of glucose), the liver removes the phosphate group. This allows the glucose to enter the bloodstream, increasing blood glucose levels for short-term energy needs.

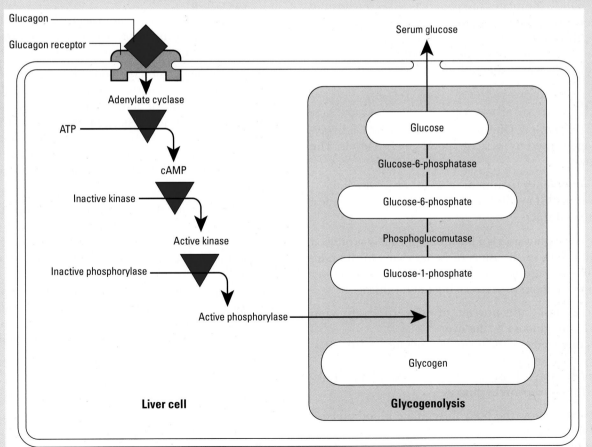

FIGURE 12-2 How glucagon raises glucose levels. (From *Clinical Pharmacology Made Incredibly Easy*. 2nd Ed. Philadelphia, PA: Lippincott Williams & Wilkins; 2005.)

acetaminophen, antibiotics, or hormonal contraceptives. These drugs should be taken at least an hour before exenatide.

- Taking exenatide with sulfonylureas may increase the risk of hypoglycemia.

The most common adverse reactions to exenatide include:

- diarrhea
- dizziness
- headache
- jittery feeling
- nausea
- vomiting

Exenatide (Byetta) is a new synthetic medication for treating type 2 diabetes. Scientists studying hormones found that the peptide exendin-4 found in the Gila monster's saliva was able to lower blood sugar. Based on their research, synthetic exendin-4 has been produced and is used to achieve the same effect.

- It's the first of a new class of drugs called incretin mimetics that help the body make the right amount of insulin at the right time.
- It's used with metformin and/or medications in the sulfonylurea family, such as glyburide and glipizide.
- Exenatide stimulates the pancreas to secrete insulin when blood sugar is high.
- The drug also slows down how fast the stomach empties and can decrease a patient's appetite.
- Exenatide is available only as an injectable.

Glucagon

Glucagon (GlucaGen, Glucagon Emergency Kit), a hyperglycemic agent used to increase blood glucose levels. The drug is used:

- for emergency treatment of severe hypoglycemia
- to reduce GI motility during radiologic examination of the GI tract

In the body, glucagon is a hormone normally produced by the alpha cells of the islets of Langerhans in the pancreas. It acts to regulate the rate of glucose production. There are three main processes affected by glucagon:

- glycogenesis, the process of converting glycogen back into glucose by the liver
- gluconeogenesis, the formation of glucose from free fatty acids and proteins
- lipolysis, the release of fatty acids from adipose tissue for conversion to glucose

These processes allow the body to regulate blood glucose levels and metabolism.

Glucagon is administered by SubQ, IM, or IV injection. It's manufactured as powder for injection in single-use vials or disposable syringes with diluent. Glucagon must be reconstituted before use. The reconstituted solution must be used immediately.

Glucagon may interact with oral anticoagulants, increasing the tendency to bleed.

ESTROGENS

The body naturally produces two female hormones: estrogen and progesterone. These hormones develop and maintain the female reproductive system. **Estrogens** and **progestins** are substances that mimic the physiological effects of these naturally occurring hormones.

Estrogens are used therapeutically to correct estrogen-deficient states and to prevent pregnancy, along with progestin, in hormonal contraceptives. They may be synthetic or produced from natural sources. Estrogens are prescribed in several different situations:

- for hormone-replacement therapy in postmenopausal women to relieve symptoms caused by loss of ovarian function
- for hormone-replacement therapy in women with primary ovarian failure or female hypogonadism (a condition in which hormone secretion is reduced)
- for hormone-replacement therapy in women who have had their ovaries surgically removed (female castration)
- palliatively to treat advanced, inoperable breast cancer in postmenopausal women and prostate cancer in men

How estrogen acts on the body isn't clearly understood. It's believed to increase the synthesis of DNA, RNA, and protein in tissues in the female breast, urinary tract, and genital organs. Synthetic estrogens are metabolized slowly in the liver and other tissues. As a result, they may have a higher potency than natural estrogens when taken orally.

There are relatively few drug interactions with estrogens.

- Estrogens may decrease the effects of anticoagulants, increasing the risk of blood clots.
- Antibiotics, barbiturates, carbamazepine, phenytoin, primidone, and rifampin reduce estrogen effectiveness.
- Estrogens interfere with the absorption of dietary folic acid, which can lead to a folic acid deficiency.
- Estrogens may interfere with the effectiveness of tamoxifen when these drugs are taken together.

Estrogens should be avoided by patients with the following conditions:

- known or suspected pregnancy
- abnormal genital bleeding
- breast cancer (except for palliative care)
- estrogen-dependent neoplasia (abnormal cell growth)
- thrombophlebitis or thromboembolic disorders

PROCEED WITH CAUTION

Adverse Reactions to Estrogens

Common adverse reactions to estrogens include:

- abdominal cramps and bloating
- breast pain or tenderness
- hair loss
- headache
- hypertension
- mild nausea or vomiting

Severe adverse reactions include:

- thromboembolism (blood vessel blockage caused by a blood clot)
- thrombophlebitis (vein inflammation associated with clot formation)

Conjugated Estrogenic Substances

Some conjugated estrogens (Premarin) contain a mixture of equine estrogens from natural sources. Other conjugated estrogens (Cenestin, Enjuvia) are synthetic. Both are available by prescription in tablets.

Conjugated estrogen is prescribed for hormone-replacement therapy and for palliative care of patients with metastatic breast or prostate cancer.

To treat symptoms of menopause and to prevent osteoporosis, patients should take the lowest oral dose possible that reduces symptoms. Tablets are usually taken once a day. They may be taken continuously without interruptions or in cycles (for example, 25 days on and 5 days off). For other conditions, tablets may be taken in cycles (three weeks on and one week off). The tablets should be stored at room temperature.

TIP Premarin tablets come in a variety of colors. You should learn which strength is which color because it will help you prevent mistakes when pulling the product from the shelf and counting. For example, Premarin 1.25-mg tablets are yellow, and 0.625-mg tablets are maroon. If you know the difference, you won't confuse them when preparing prescriptions.

Premarin is named after the source of its estrogen: pregnant mare's urine. When female horses are pregnant, their urine is collected in a rubber cup. The use of pregnant horses for this purpose has prompted concerns about their treatment due to the lack of mobility for the animals during the collection period.

Other sources of conjugated estrogen, such as plant-derived or synthetic estrogens, are also safe and effective. Mexican soybeans and yams are some plants that are used to produce conjugated estrogen products. Patients who are concerned about Premarin can discuss these alternative treatment options with their physicians.

Estradiol

This drug is sold by prescription in several different forms. Oral estradiol is taken as tablets (Estrace, Gynodiol, Femtrace) of varying strengths. It should be stored at room temperature in a light-resistant container.

Some formulations of estradiol are absorbed through the skin, including:

- transdermal patch (Alora, Vivelle, Climara, Menostar, Estraderm)
- gel (Elestrin, EstroGel, Divigel)
- emulsion (Estrasorb)
- spray (Evamist)

Transdermal estradiol is manufactured as a patch with varying release rates. It may be applied to the abdomen, upper inner thigh, upper arm, buttock, or outer hip. The patch is replaced once or twice a week, depending on the product. It shouldn't be exposed to sunlight. Swimming, bathing, or sauna use may affect the delivery of the medication.

The gel and emulsion forms of estradiol are both applied to clean, dry skin on the thighs. These forms come in a single-dose foil pouch. Patients should avoid washing the skin for at least one hour after application.

In addition to the adverse reactions for other estrogens, estradiol gel, spray, and emulsion may cause skin irritation or rash.

TIP Sunscreen might interfere with the action of estradiol gel or emulsion. These products shouldn't be used together.

Estradiol is also manufactured in several forms for vaginal use. These forms are used to treat vulval and vaginal atrophy, including symptoms such as dryness, burning, and itching.

- Estradiol acetate comes as a vaginal ring (Estring, Femring). It's used in the treatment of moderate to severe symptoms of menopause, including vasomotor symptoms and vulvar and vaginal atrophy. The ring remains in place for three months after insertion.
- Estradiol vaginal cream (Estrace) may be used daily initially. However, its use should be reduced to one to three times a week as symptoms improve.
- Estradiol vaginal tablets (Vagifem) are inserted using an applicator. At first, they are inserted once a day for two weeks. Later, they are used twice a week.
- Estradiol cypionate in oil (Depo-Estradiol) is manufactured in vials for injection. It must be given by IM injection. This drug is used to treat hypogonadism and moderate to severe vasomotor symptoms associated with menopause. For treatment of menopause, short-term cyclic use is recommended, with injections given every three to four weeks. Use of this drug should be reevaluated every three to six months.

■ Estradiol valerate in oil (Delestrogen) is given by injection. It's normally administered by deep IM injection into the upper, outer quadrant of the gluteal muscle. Every three to six months, the patient and physician should evaluate whether to continue or begin to taper this drug.

Estropipate

Estropipate (Ogen) is derived from natural substances. It's used to treat moderate to severe symptoms associated with menopause. This drug is sold by prescription as tablets of several different strengths. One tablet is taken daily in a cycle (three weeks on and one week off). After three to six months, the patient should try to taper or stop using the medication.

Esterified Estrogens

Esterified estrogens (Menest) are available by prescription as film-coated tablets. As with other estrogens, patients should take the lowest dose that will control symptoms. The drug is usually taken in cycles of three weeks on and one week off.

Taking esterified estrogens with dantrolene or hepatotoxic drugs may increase the risk of hepatotoxicity.

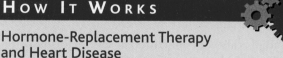

HOW IT WORKS

Hormone-Replacement Therapy and Heart Disease

Estrogen that is taken for hormone-replacement therapy in postmenopausal women has several advantages for the patient, including:

■ reducing moderate to severe hot flashes (flushing and sweating)
■ relieving moderate to severe dryness, itching, and burning around the vagina
■ lowering the risk of osteoporosis (loss of bone mass)

However, hormone-replacement therapy has several disadvantages as well. After a five-year study, the Women's Health Initiative reported increased risks of myocardial infarction, stroke, breast cancer, pulmonary embolism, deep vein thrombosis, and dementia in women being treated with conjugated equine estrogens and progesterone compared with those taking a placebo. In 2004, the U.S. Preventive Services Task Force recommended against the use of estrogen and progestin to prevent coronary heart disease in healthy women.

As a result, the Food and Drug Administration and American College of Obstetricians and Gynecologists recommend that women who choose to take hormone-replacement therapy for menopausal symptoms use these drugs for the shortest duration manageable and in the lowest possible dosages.

Hormonal Contraceptives

Many **hormonal contraceptives** are combinations of the hormones estrogen and progestin. Some contain only progestin. Hormonal contraceptives are used regularly to prevent pregnancy. These drugs have several actions on the body.

■ They block the release of eggs from the ovaries (ovulation).
■ They change the lining of the uterus to prevent implantation (attachment of the fertilized egg to the uterus wall).
■ They thicken cervical mucus (mucus at the opening of the uterus) to block sperm from entering.

Using hormonal contraceptives may provide health benefits that are not related to contraception. Some of these health benefits include:

■ regulating the menstrual cycle and decreasing blood loss
■ decreasing the chance of iron-deficiency anemia
■ reducing dysmenorrhea (painful menstruation)
■ decreasing the risk of developing ovarian cysts and ectopic pregnancies
■ reducing the likelihood of fibrocystic breast disease, pelvic inflammatory disease, endometrial cancer, and ovarian cancer
■ helping maintain bone density
■ reducing symptoms of endometriosis (a condition in which endometrial tissue grows outside the uterine cavity and may cause infertility, dysmenorrhea, and pelvic pain)

In addition, some oral contraceptives may also help reduce acne in women over 15 years old.

TIP Smoking increases the risk of serious cardiovascular adverse effects related to oral contraceptives. The risk increases especially for heavy smokers over age 35.

Many hormonal contraceptives are taken as oral tablets. The combination of estrogen and progestin in these oral contraceptives can lead to adverse reactions, depending on the balance of these hormones. Adjusting the balance of estrogen or progestin may minimize some of these effects.

There are many different brands of oral contraceptives that contain combinations of estrogens and progestins. They differ in the amount of estrogen they contain and how the doses of estrogen are given during the menstrual cycle.

Monophasic (one-phase) oral contraceptives provide a constant dose of estrogen and progestin for 21 days of the menstrual cycle. After 21 days, seven days are skipped. Some packages include a placebo or iron supplement on these days. Common monophasic drug combinations include:

- ethinyl estradiol and norethindrone (Brevicon, Modicon, Necon 0.5/35, Nortrel 0.5/35, Necon 1/35, Norinyl 1+35, Nortrel 1/35, Ortho-Novum 1/35, Ovcon 35, Zenchent, Ovcon 50, Balziva)
- ethinyl estradiol and norethindrone acetate (Junel 21 1/20, Loestrin 21 1/20, Microgestin 1/20, Junel 21 1.5/30, Loestrin 21 1.5/30, Microgestin 1.5/30)
- ethinyl estradiol and norethindrone acetate with iron days 25–28 (Loestrin 24 Fe 1/20, Junel Fe 1/20, Microgestin Fe 1/20)
- ethinyl estradiol and norethindrone with iron days 22–28 (Loestrin Fe 1/20, Loestrin Fe 1.5/30, Junel Fe 1.5/30, Microgestin Fe 1.5/30, Femcon Fe)
- ethinyl estradiol and ethynodiol diacetate (Kelnor 1/35, Zovia 1/35E, Zovia 1/50E)
- ethinyl estradiol and norgestrel (Lo/Ovral, Cryselle, Low-Ogestrel, Ogestrel 0.5/50, Ovral)
- ethinyl estradiol and norgestimate (Ortho-Cyclen, MonoNessa, Previfem Sprintec)
- ethinyl estradiol and desogestrel (Ortho-Cept, Apri, Desogen, Reclipsen, Solia)
- ethinyl estradiol and drospirenone (YAZ, Yasmin)
- ethinyl estradiol and levonorgestrel (Alesse, Aviane, Lessina, Levlite, Lutera, Sronyx, Levlen, Levora, Nordette, Portia, Lybrel); for extended cycle regimen (Jolessa, Quasense, Seasonale)
- mestranol and norethindrone (Necon 1/50, Norinyl 1+50, Ortho-Novum 1/50)

Biphasic (two-phase) oral contraceptives contain two different formulations during the menstrual cycle. During the first ten days, a smaller dose of progestin is given. The dose of progestin is increased for the rest of the cycle. The amount of estrogen remains constant, with a seven-day period without estrogen. The most common biphasic drug combination is ethinyl estradiol and norethindrone (Ortho-Novum 10/11, Necon 10/11). Ethinyl estradiol and levonorgestrel (Seasonique) is a biphasic drug combination for an extended cycle regimen. Ethinyl estradiol and desogestrel (Kariva, Mircette) make a unique combination tablet for days 1–21, followed by a placebo tablet on days 22–23, and estrogen tablet therapy for days 24–28.

Triphasic (three-phase) oral contraceptives contain varying amounts of progestin throughout the 21-day cycle. The amount of estrogen stays the same or changes, depending on the specific formulation. Packages usually include color-coded pills for each phase of the cycle. They may be packaged as 21-day or 28-day cycles. This depends on whether inactive or iron-containing pills are included for the seven-day break. The most common triphasic drug combinations include:

- ethinyl estradiol and norethindrone (Ortho-Novum 7/7/7, Necon 7/7/7, Nortrel 7/7/7, Aranelle, Leena, Tri-Norinyl)
- ethinyl estradiol and norethindrone acetate (Tri-Legest)

- ethinyl estradiol and norethindrone acetate with iron days 22-28 (Estrostep Fe, Tri-Legest Fe, Tilia Fe)
- ethinyl estradiol and norgestimate (Ortho Tri-Cyclen, TriNessa, Tri-Previfem, Tri-Sprintec, Ortho Tri-Cyclen Lo)
- ethinyl estradiol and desogestrel (Velivet, Cesia, Cyclessa)
- ethinyl estradiol and levonorgestrel (Triphasil, Enpresse, Trivora)

Norethindrone (Micronor, Camila, Errin, Jolivette, Nora-BE, Nor-QD) is a progestin-only contraceptive. It's sometimes referred to as the "mini-pill." This drug is safe for women who are breastfeeding because it doesn't affect milk production.

Norethindrone is manufactured as tablets in a 28-day package. Tablets are taken throughout the menstrual cycle, with no time off between packages. This product is most effective when patients take one tablet at the same time every day, without missing any doses. Pregnancy is more likely to occur when doses are taken late. Because this contraceptive doesn't contain estrogen, it causes fewer adverse reactions than other oral contraceptives.

Emergency Contraceptives

Some hormonal contraceptives are intended to prevent pregnancy only after unprotected intercourse or in situations where contraceptives are known or suspected to have failed. These drugs are sometimes referred to as **emergency contraceptives**. However, they are not effective if the patient is already pregnant. Emergency contraceptives are believed to work by preventing ovulation or fertilization of the egg. They may also prevent the process of implantation.

Levonorgestrel (Plan B) is used to prevent pregnancy after unprotected intercourse. It's manufactured as oral tablets. This drug has been approved for OTC sale to women 18 years of age and older. One tablet is taken within 72 hours of unprotected intercourse. A second tablet is normally taken 12 hours later. Treatment is more effective the sooner it is started.

PROGESTINS

Progestins are drugs that act on the body in the same way as the naturally occurring female hormone progesterone. Progesterone is produced in the ovaries, the placenta (during pregnancy), and the adrenal glands. It regulates the menstrual cycle and helps prepare the body for pregnancy.

- Progesterone levels change during the menstrual cycle. Increased levels of progesterone act to prepare the uterus for implantation of a fertilized egg. If pregnancy doesn't occur, progesterone levels decrease, leading to menstruation.

■ During pregnancy, progesterone acts with estrogen to suppress ovulation. It also encourages the growth of milk-producing glands in the breasts.

Progestins may be natural or synthetic. Synthetic progestins are used medically in the treatment of several conditions:

- amenorrhea (absence of menstrual periods)
- endometriosis
- uterine bleeding

They are also used alone or in combination with estrogen as oral contraceptives.

Progestins may interact with other drugs and substances.

- Aminoglutethimide or rifampin may decrease the effectiveness of progestins.
- Progestins may increase caffeine levels.
- Smoking while taking progestins may increase the risk of adverse cardiovascular effects.

Medroxyprogesterone

This drug is used in treating secondary amenorrhea and abnormal bleeding from the uterus. It may be used to reduce the chance of endometrial hyperplasia (an abnormal thickening of the lining of the uterus). Medroxyprogesterone is manufactured as tablets (Provera). It's also available as an injection for contraception (Depo-subQ Provera, Depo-Provera). The injection is given at three-month intervals.

Adverse reactions to medroxyprogesterone include:

- drowsiness
- fever
- rash
- weight gain or loss

These are in addition to the adverse reactions common to all progestins.

Megestrol

Megestrol tablets are used for palliative treatment of breast or endometrial cancer. This drug is also manufactured as

PROCEED WITH CAUTION

Adverse Reactions to Progestins

Adverse reactions to progestins may include:

- acne
- amenorrhea
- changes in menstrual flow
- chloasma or melasma (skin discoloration)
- edema
- mental depression

AT THE COUNTER

Similar-Sounding Trade Names

A patient is picking up her prescription for hormone-replacement therapy. In the past, she has received Premarin and Prempro, but this time her physician prescribed Premphase. She is curious about the differences in all the products since the names look so similar. What should you tell her?

Because this is a new prescription, the pharmacist should properly counsel the patient. You can tell her that Premarin, Prempro, and Premphase are all similar in that they all contain conjugated estrogen. Prempro and Premphase are similar in that they contain conjugated estrogen and medroxyprogesterone. However, Prempro and Premphase are different.

Is medroxyprogesterone available as a single-ingredient product?

Yes, as a single-ingredient product it is sold under the brand name Provera. So you will notice that Prempro comes from the two brand names of Premarin and Provera. Premphase, although it has the same two active ingredients, contains two different "phases" of treatment that involve one phase of Premarin only and a second phase of Premarin and Provera.

an oral suspension (Megace). Megestrol is used in the treatment of anorexia, cachexia (loss of body weight and muscle mass), and unexplained weight loss in patients with AIDS. This drug may interact with dofetilide, increasing the risk of cardiovascular toxicity.

Norethindrone

This medication (Aygestin) is available by prescription only. Tablets are taken daily, but doses vary according to the specific condition being treated and the patient's response to the drug.

In addition to the other adverse reactions common to progestins, norethindrone may cause nausea and, in rare cases, hematological reactions. This drug shouldn't be used for contraceptive purposes.

Progesterone

Progesterone is given to prevent endometrial hyperplasia in postmenopausal women who are taking conjugated estrogen. It may also be used to treat secondary amenorrhea. Progesterone is available by prescription only. It's manufactured as oral capsules (Prometrium) and in vials with oil for injection.

Oral capsules are taken once a day in the evening for ten or twelve days. The medication contained in these capsules is chemically identical with progesterone produced by the ovaries.

Progesterone injections are given for a period of six to eight days. The injection must be administered intramuscularly. The patient may experience irritation at the injection site.

Progesterone is also available as a vaginal gel (Prochieve, Crinone) or insert/suppository (Endometrin, First-Progesterone) to treat secondary amenorrhea. It's used on alternate days up to a total of six doses. This form of progesterone may also be used as part of a fertility treatment.

PITUITARY DRUGS

Pituitary drugs are natural or synthetic hormones that mimic the hormones produced by the pituitary gland. These drugs consist of two groups.

- **Anterior pituitary drugs** mimic the effects of hormones produced in the anterior pituitary gland. They may be used diagnostically or therapeutically to control the function of other endocrine glands, such as the thyroid gland, adrenals, ovaries, and testes.
- Posterior pituitary drugs may be used to regulate fluid volume and stimulate smooth muscle contraction in selected clinical situations.

The major adverse reactions to pituitary drugs are hypersensitivity reactions. Most other adverse reactions are drug specific.

Anterior Pituitary Drugs

The protein hormones produced in the anterior pituitary gland regulate growth, development, and sexual characteristics. They do this by stimulating the actions of other endocrine glands.

Anterior pituitary drugs have a significant effect on the body's growth and development. The hypothalamus controls secretions of the pituitary gland. In turn, the pituitary gland secretes hormones that regulate secretions or functions of other glands. The concentrations of hormones in the blood help determine how quickly or slowly these hormones are produced. Increased hormone levels stop hormone production; decreased levels increase production and secretion.

Adrenocorticotropic Drugs

Adrenocorticotropic drugs, or corticotropins, are used diagnostically to differentiate between primary and secondary failure of the adrenal cortex. They may also be used to treat adrenal insufficiency.

In the body, corticotropin stimulates the adrenal cortex to produce glucocorticoids. It acts on ACTH receptors on the adrenocortical cells. In turn, these cells begin the process of producing glucocorticoids.

Corticotropins may be derived from natural sources or produced synthetically. Natural corticotropins are derived from pork or pork products. Patients with allergies to pork or pork products shouldn't take corticotropins. Corticotropin can block skeletal growth, so it must be used with caution in children.

Corticotropins may interact with several other medications.

- Anticonvulsants, barbiturates, and rifampin increase the metabolism of corticotropin, reducing its effects.
- Corticotropin may increase the need for antidiabetic drugs, because it affects glycemic activity.
- Estrogens can increase the effect of corticotropin.
- Taking corticotropin with NSAIDs or salicylates may lead to GI bleeding. These drugs shouldn't be used together.
- Corticotropin may affect blood-clotting time. Careful monitoring is required when used with oral anticoagulants.
- Taking diuretics with corticotropin may increase potassium loss.
- Administering immunizations to a person taking corticotropin increases the risk of neurological complications and may reduce antibody response.

Long-term use of corticotropin can cause Cushing syndrome (a disease caused by overproduction of certain glucocorticoids). Other adverse reactions include:

- dizziness
- sodium and fluid retention

Repository Corticotropin

Repository corticotropin injections (H.P. Acthar Gel) are primarily used for diagnostic purposes for adrenocortical function. However, this drug may be used therapeutically as an anti-inflammatory or immunosuppressant for many disorders, such as:

- acute exacerbations of multiple sclerosis
- rheumatoid arthritis, ankylosing spondylitis, osteoarthritis, or bursitis (as adjunctive therapy)
- systemic lupus erythematosus (as maintenance therapy)
- allergic conditions that don't respond to standard treatment
- palliative management of leukemias

This prescription medication comes in the form of multidose vials. Repository corticotropin is administered by IM or SubQ injection every 24 to 72 hours. It shouldn't be given by IV administration, however. Repository corticotropin should be stored in the refrigerator and warmed to room temperature before use.

Cosyntropin

Cosyntropin (Cortrosyn) is a synthetic ACTH hormone. It's manufactured as powder for injection. It comes in vials with diluent and must be reconstituted before use. It's normally given by IM or direct IV injection when used as a rapid screening test for adrenal function. It may also be given as an IV infusion.

Taking estrogens, amphetamines, and lithium with cosyntropin can affect the results of adrenal function tests. Adverse reactions to cosyntropin are rare.

T I P Cosyntropin is less likely to cause an allergic reaction than ACTH preparations from natural sources.

Growth Hormone

Growth hormone is used to treat deficiencies of pituitary growth hormone. Growth is a complex process that involves bone growth, muscle growth, and changes in metabolism. In the body, growth hormone is normally secreted by the anterior pituitary gland. It regulates the process of growth up to early adulthood, when an individual stops growing in height. A deficiency of pituitary growth hormone can cause children to grow more slowly than normal.

The main growth hormone drug available in the United States is somatropin (Nutropin, Omnitrope, Saizen, Tev-Tropin, Genotropin, Norditropin, Humatrope, Serostim). It's used for long-term treatment of growth failure in children resulting from:

- inadequate secretion of growth hormone
- chronic kidney difficulties prior to kidney transplantation
- Turner syndrome
- Prader-Willi syndrome
- smaller size at birth (than the average for gestational age) without catching up by age two years
- short stature without a known cause when other known causes have been ruled out

It may also be used to treat adults with a growth hormone deficiency, as well as children and adults with AIDS-related lipoatrophy (the depletion of fat stores, especially in the limbs and cheeks). Children should only be treated with somatropin if their bones are still growing.

Somatropin is a synthetic product made using DNA technology. This makes it structurally identical with human growth hormone. Somatropin requires a prescription. It's normally given by SubQ injection. The drug is manufactured as a powder in multidose vials with a diluent, in a cartridge, or in a prefilled pen.

Gonadotropins

Gonadotropins are used in treating several different conditions:

- prepubertal cryptorchidism (failure of one or both testicles to descend into the scrotum) in boys aged four to nine years
- hypogonadism (underactive sex organs)
- anovulation (failure to ovulate) in women

These drugs work by mimicking the action of naturally occurring gonadotropins. In the body, gonadotropins have several actions.

- They influence the secretion of sex hormones, such as estrogen.
- They encourage the development of secondary sex characteristics.
- They influence the reproductive cycle in men and women by inducing sperm and egg production.

Gonadotropins are contraindicated in patients with uncontrolled thyroid or kidney dysfunction, abnormal uterine bleeding, and uterine fibromas or uterine cysts. They are also contraindicated in pregnant women and in men with normal pituitary function. These drugs have no known drug interactions. Adverse reactions to gonadotropins include:

- gynecomastia (development of male breasts)
- ovarian enlargement with pain and abdominal distention

Human Chorionic Gonadotropin

Human chorionic gonadotropin (HCG) (Pregnyl, Ovidrel, Novarel) is manufactured as powder for injection. It's given by IM injection only. Dosage depends on the patient's condition, age, and weight. This drug must be reconstituted before use.

This drug shouldn't be given during pregnancy. It should be used cautiously in patients with asthma, epilepsy, migraine headaches, and cardiac or renal disease.

Menotropins

Menotropins (Repronex, Menopur) is used to induce ovulation, alone or with human chorionic gonadotropin. This drug may also be used to treat hypogonadism in males. It comes as a lyophilized powder or pellet in vials with a diluent. It's administered by IM injection or SubQ injection to the lower abdomen. Doses must be individualized for each patient.

Thyrotropin Alfa

Thyrotropin alfa (Thyrogen) is used in testing levels of thyroglobulin (a thyroid hormone) in patients with thyroid cancer. It comes as a lyophilized powder for injection. The powder must be reconstituted immediately before use with the diluent provided.

This drug should be administered by IM injection only. It may be given in two doses every 24 hours or in three doses every 72 hours.

Thyrotropin alfa may cause hypersensitivity reactions that include urticaria, rash, itching, and flushing.

Posterior Pituitary Drugs

Posterior pituitary hormones are made in the hypothalamus. They are stored in the posterior pituitary gland, which, in turn, secretes all of the hormones into the blood.

Because enzymes in the GI tract can destroy all protein hormones, these drugs can't be given orally. Posterior pituitary drugs may be given by injection or intranasal spray. Posterior pituitary hormones affect:

- smooth muscle contraction in the uterus, bladder, and GI tract
- fluid balance through kidney reabsorption of water
- blood pressure through stimulation of the arterial wall muscles

Antidiuretic Hormone

Antidiuretic hormone (ADH) is prescribed for hormone-replacement therapy in patients with neurogenic diabetes insipidus (an excessive loss of urine caused by a brain injury or lesion that interferes with the production or release of ADH). Short-term ADH treatment is indicated for the following:

- patients with transient diabetes insipidus after head injury or surgery
- lifelong treatment for patients with idiopathic hormone deficiencies

This drug may also be used in the treatment of nighttime enuresis (bed-wetting).

ADH works to increase cyclic adenosine monophosphate (cAMP). This increases water reabsorption in the kidneys. High doses of ADH stimulate the contraction of blood vessels, increasing blood pressure. Caution should be taken when giving ADH to patients with coronary artery disease or kidney disease.

Several drugs can cause interactions with ADH.

- Alcohol, demeclocycline, and lithium may decrease ADH activity.
- Chlorpropamide, clofibrate, carbamazepine, and cyclophosphamide increase ADH activity.
- Synergistic effects may occur when barbiturates or cyclopropane anesthetics are used with ADH. This can result in coronary insufficiency or arrhythmias.

Two types of ADH are desmopressin acetate and vasopressin. Hypersensitivity reactions are the most common adverse reactions to ADH. With natural ADH, anaphylaxis may occur after injection. Natural ADH can also cause:

- ringing in the ears
- anxiety
- hyponatremia
- proteins in urine
- eclamptic attacks
- pupil dilation
- transient edema

Adverse reactions to synthetic ADH are rare.

Desmopressin Acetate

Desmopressin acetate is the drug of choice for long-term ADH deficiency. It's also used to treat primary nocturnal enuresis. This drug is available as oral tablets (DDAVP, Desmopressin), a nasal spray (DDAVP, Desmopressin, Minirin, Stimate), and as an injection (DDAVP).

Desmopressin acetate has a long duration of action and causes relatively few adverse reactions. It reduces diuresis and promotes blood clotting.

Vasopressin

This drug (Pitressin) is administered by SubQ or IM injection. For short-term therapy, vasopressin elevates blood pressure in patients with hypotension caused by lack of vascular tone. It also relieves gaseous distention after surgery. The antidiuretic effect of the drug lasts for two to six hours.

Temporary adverse reactions to vasopressin are blanching of the skin, abdominal cramps, and nausea. These reactions can be minimized by drinking one or two glasses of water when the drug is given.

Oxytocin

Oxytocin (Pitocin) is a hormone that stimulates the smooth muscle in the uterus and breast. It has several uses related to pregnancy and childbirth, such as:

- inducing labor and completing incomplete abortions
- treating preeclampsia, eclampsia, and premature rupture of membranes
- controlling bleeding and uterine relaxation after delivery
- speeding up the shrinking of the uterus after delivery
- stimulating lactation

Oxytocin is administered by injection. To induce labor, it must be administered using an IV infusion pump. A small dose is given initially, and the dose is gradually increased until labor contractions are regular. For postpartum therapy, oxytocin is given by IV infusion or by IM injection. This drug is absorbed quickly. Uterine effects last for two to three hours. Different brands of oxytocin require different methods of storage.

Some drugs may interact with oxytocin.

- Cyclophosphamide may increase the effect of oxytocin.
- Using vasopressors such as anesthetics, ephedrine, or methoxamine with oxytocin can increase the risk of hypertensive crisis and postpartum rupture of cerebral blood vessels.

Adverse reactions to oxytocin include:

- nausea
- vomiting
- intense or abrupt contractions of the uterus

THYROID AND ANTITHYROID DRUGS

Drugs that act on the thyroid have two main functions. They are used to correct the following conditions:

- thyroid hormone deficiency (hypothyroidism)
- thyroid hormone excess (hyperthyroidism)

Thyroid Drugs

Thyroid drugs act as replacement or substitute hormones. These drugs are used:

- to treat the many forms of hypothyroidism
- with antithyroid drugs to prevent goiter formation (an enlarged thyroid gland) and hypothyroidism
- to differentiate between primary and secondary hypothyroidism during diagnostic testing
- to treat papillary or follicular thyroid carcinoma

Thyroid drugs can be natural or synthetic hormones. They may contain triiodothyronine (T_3), thyroxine (T_4), or both. Natural thyroid drugs are made from animal thyroid. Synthetic thyroid drugs are actually the sodium salts of the L-isomers of the hormones.

Thyroid drugs increase the metabolic rate in body tissues. They act on the body in the following ways:

- affecting protein and carbohydrate metabolism
- stimulating protein synthesis
- promoting gluconeogenesis (the formation of glucose from free fatty acids and proteins)
- increasing the use of glycogen stores

Thyroid drugs also have several effects on the heart. These drugs:

- increase heart rate
- increase cardiac output (the amount of blood pumped by the heart each minute)
- may increase the heart's sensitivity to catecholamines
- increase the number of beta-adrenergic receptors in the heart (stimulation of beta receptors in the heart increases heart rate and contractility)

Not only do thyroid drugs affect the body's metabolism and the heart, they increase blood flow to the kidneys. These drugs increase the glomerular infiltration rate (the amount of plasma filtered through the kidney each minute) in hypothyroid patients, which produces diuresis.

Not surprisingly, thyroid drugs interact with several common medications.

- They increase the effects of oral anticoagulants, increasing the tendency to bleed.
- Cholestyramine and colestipol reduce the absorption of thyroid hormones.
- Taking thyroid drugs with digoxin may reduce serum digoxin levels, increasing the risk of arrhythmias or heart failure.
- Carbamazepine, phenytoin, phenobarbital, and rifampin increase metabolism of thyroid hormones, reducing their effectiveness.
- When theophylline is administered with thyroid drugs, serum theophylline levels may increase.
- Patients who are taking estrogen or oral contraceptives may need increased doses of thyroid drugs.

 PROCEED WITH CAUTION

Adverse Reactions to Thyroid Drugs

Most adverse reactions to thyroid drugs result from toxicity. They may affect the GI system, the cardiovascular system, or other areas of the body.

Adverse reactions in the GI system include:

- diarrhea
- abdominal cramps
- weight loss
- increased appetite

Adverse reactions in the cardiovascular system include:

- palpitations
- sweating
- rapid heart rate
- increased blood pressure
- angina
- arrhythmias

General signs and symptoms of toxic doses include:

- headache
- tremor
- insomnia
- nervousness
- fever
- heat intolerance
- menstrual irregularities

Thyroid USP (Desiccated)

Thyroid USP (desiccated) (Bio-Throid, Armour Thyroid, Nature Thyroid) is a natural hormone that contains both T_3 and T_4. This prescription medication is manufactured as tablets and capsules of different strengths. Low doses are given to start, with the dose increasing every two to three weeks. For diagnostic purposes, doses are given for seven to ten days. This drug is stored at room temperature.

T I P The brand name drug Synthroid comes in a variety of strengths. It's very important to double-check all prescriptions to make sure the correct strength is being dispensed. For convenience, the label has a color on it that matches the color of the tablet.

Levothyroxine

Levothyroxine (Levothroid, Levoxyl, Synthroid, Unithroid) is a synthetic hormone that contains T_4. It's the drug of choice for thyroid hormone-replacement therapy and for thyroid-stimulating hormone suppression therapy. This drug requires a prescription. It's manufactured as tablets of varying strengths and as powder for injection. The oral form of the drug is typically taken as a single daily dose. It should be taken on an empty stomach, at least 30 to 60 minutes before breakfast. It may take four to six weeks of regular treatment to achieve peak effects.

Levothyroxine can be used in newborns and children, with appropriate adjustments to the dosage. However, it must be used cautiously in older adult patients, patients with cardiovascular disease, and patients with adrenal insufficiency. Absorption of orally administered levothyroxine may be affected by foods containing dietary fiber, soybean flours, cottonseed meal, and walnuts.

TIP Synthroid may be prescribed in milligrams (mg) or micrograms (mcg). For example, prescriptions may be written for *Synthroid 0.125 mg* or *Synthroid 125 mcg*. Although the abbreviations may look similar, they represent very different dosages. When filling a prescription for Synthroid, always check to see if the drug has been prescribed in milligrams or micrograms.

Liothyronine

Liothyronine (Cytomel, Triostat) is a synthetic hormone that contains T_3. It's available by prescription as tablets or in vials for injection. Dosages must be individualized for each patient, according to the patient's response to the drug. Tablets are typically taken once a day. An IV preparation is sold for the treatment of myxedema coma (a serious condition related to hypothyroidism).

Liotrix

Liotrix (Thyrolar) is a synthetic hormone that contains both T_3 and T_4. It's sold as tablets of several different strengths and measured in micrograms. To start, this drug is given at a low dose. The dosage is increased every two to three weeks. Very low doses should be given to patients with angina pectoris and older adult patients. This drug should be refrigerated.

Antithyroid Drugs

A number of drugs act as **antithyroid drugs**, or **thyroid antagonists**. They are commonly used to treat hyperthyroidism (thyrotoxicosis). Graves disease (a form of hyperthyroidism) accounts for 85 percent of all cases.

Thioamides

Thioamides block iodine's ability to combine with tyrosine. This prevents the body from making thyroid hormone. Thioamides may interact with other substances.

- Thioamides may increase the effects of anticoagulants.
- Taking thioamides with cardiac glycosides may increase levels of glycosides.
- Potassium iodide may reduce the effectiveness of thioamides. Dosages may need to be adjusted.
- Foods containing iodine, such as iodized salt and shellfish, may change the effectiveness of thioamides.

Major adverse reactions to thioamide therapy include:

- granulocytopenia (low levels of granulocytes, a type of white blood cell)
- hypersensitivity reactions

Methimazole

Methimazole (Tapazole, Northyx) blocks thyroid hormone for long periods of time. Therefore, methimazole is well suited for once-daily administration to patients with mild to moderate hyperthyroidism. Therapy may continue for 12 to 24 months before remission occurs.

Methimazole is sold by prescription as oral tablets in several strengths. Doses vary depending on the severity of the condition. Usually, the daily amount is divided into three equal doses. These doses are given at eight-hour intervals.

Methimazole may cause hypoprothrombinemia (low levels of prothrombin) and bleeding. As a result, the patient's prothrombin time should be monitored carefully.

Propylthiouracil

This drug is usually used for rapid improvement of severe hyperthyroidism in adults and children. It may be used to reduce hyperthyroidism in preparation for surgery or radioactive iodine therapy. Propylthiouracil is sold by prescription as tablets. Three equal doses are taken each day, about eight hours apart. The drug should be taken with meals to avoid GI upset.

Iodides

Iodides act to decrease the amount of thyroid hormone in the body. They may be used in conjunction with surgery to remove the thyroid gland.

There are few drug interactions associated with iodides. However, they may interact with lithium, causing hypothyroidism.

Radioactive Iodine (Sodium Iodide)

Radioactive iodine is manufactured as therapeutic capsules and oral solution of varying strengths. Diagnostic capsules are also available. It's important to wear waterproof gloves when handling the drug. The appropriate dose should be measured by a radioactivity calibration system.

Radioactive iodine decreases hormone secretion by destroying thyroid tissue. This has two effects:

- acute radiation thyroiditis (inflammation of the thyroid gland)
- chronic gradual thyroid atrophy (shrinking of the thyroid over time)

! PROCEED WITH CAUTION

Adverse Reactions to Iodides

Iodides can cause several adverse reactions:

- unpleasant tastes
- increased salivation
- painful swelling of the parotid glands

In rare cases, IV iodine may cause an acute hypersensitivity reaction.

Acute radiation thyroiditis usually occurs three to ten days after administering radioactive iodine. Chronic thyroid atrophy may take several years to appear.

Stable Iodine (Potassium Iodide)

Stable iodine (SSKI) is used as an adjunct to antithyroid drugs to prepare for thyroid surgery. It's also used to treat thyrotoxic crisis, a condition related to overproduction of thyroid hormones. It's manufactured as a solution. To improve the taste of strong iodine solutions, they can be diluted with water or fruit juice.

Potassium iodide inhibits hormone synthesis through the Wolff-Chaikoff effect. In this effect, excess iodine decreases the amount of thyroid hormone produced. The amount of hormone released into the body is also decreased. Potassium iodide has an effect within 24 hours; however, it may take up to 15 days for the maximum effect.

Stable iodine may be used before surgical removal of the thyroid gland. This drug prepares the gland for surgery by firming it and decreasing its blood supply (vascularity). Stable iodine may also be used after radioactive iodine therapy to control symptoms of hyperthyroidism while the radiation takes effect.

QUICK QUIZ

Answer the following multiple-choice questions.

1. Which of the following drugs would most likely be used in the treatment of type 1 diabetes?
   a. exenatide
   b. miglitol
   c. insulin lispro
   d. nateglinide
2. Which of the following is *not* an anterior pituitary drug?
   a. cosyntropin
   b. thyrotropin alfa
   c. menotropins
   d. oxytocin
3. When would glucagon most likely be used?
   a. to lower blood glucose levels in a patient with type 1 diabetes
   b. for emergency treatment of severe hypoglycemia
   c. to improve insulin sensitivity in muscle cells
   d. to stimulate insulin production
4. Which of the following drugs is used to treat growth failure in children?
   a. somatropin
   b. liotrix
   c. cosyntropin
   d. methimazole

5. Which of the following is *not* an action of thyroid drugs?
   a. promoting the formation of glucose from free fatty acids and proteins
   b. increasing cardiac output
   c. decreasing the metabolic rate in body tissues
   d. increasing the amount of plasma filtered through the kidney each minute

Please answer each of the following questions in one to three sentences.

1. What is sliding-scale dosing for insulin, and how does it work?

_____

_____

2. What is the difference between type 1 and type 2 diabetes?

_____

_____

3. List three health benefits of taking contraceptive hormones that are unrelated to pregnancy prevention.

_____

_____

4. Give one advantage and one disadvantage of hormone-replacement therapy.

_____

_____

5. Explain the differences between monophasic, biphasic, and triphasic hormonal contraceptives.

_____

_____

Answer the following questions as either true or false.

1. ___ Gloves must be worn when handling stable iodine.
2. ___ Long-term use of corticotropin can cause Cushing syndrome.
3. ___ Levonorgestrel must be taken within 24 hours of unprotected intercourse to prevent pregnancy.
4. ___ Thyroid drugs can increase the effects of oral anticoagulants, leading to bleeding.
5. ___ Progestin-only oral contraceptives may be taken by women who are breastfeeding.

Match the generic name of each drug in the left column with the correct trade name from the right column.

1. levothyroxine	a. Femtrace
2. acarbose	b. Fortamet
3. estradiol	c. Precose
4. desmopressin	d. Stimate
5. metformin	e. Synthroid

DRUG CLASSIFICATION TABLE

Classification	Generic Name	Trade Name(s)
Insulins	insulin lispro *in'-su-lin lis'-pro*	*injection:* Humalog
	insulin aspart *in'-su-lin as'-part*	*injection:* Novolog
	insulin glulisine *in'-su-lin gloo'-lis-een*	*injection:* Apidra
	regular insulin *in'-su-lin*	*injection (OTC):* Humulin R, Novolin R
	insulin isophane (NPH) *in'-su-lin eye'-soe-fane*	*injection (OTC):* Humulin N, Novolin N
	insulin detemir *in'-su-lin de'-te-mir*	*injection:* Levemir
	insulin glargine *in'-su-lin glar'-jeen*	*injection:* Lantus
	insulin aspart and insulin aspart protamine *in'-su-lin as'-part in'-su-lin as'-part*	*injection:* Novolog Mix 70/30
	insulin lispro and insulin lispro protamine *in'-su-lin lis'-pro in'-su-lin lis'-pro*	*injection:* Humalog Mix 75/25, Humalog Mix 50/50
	insulin isophane (NPH) and regular insulin *in'-su-lin eye'-soe-fane in'-su-lin*	*injection (OTC):* Novolin 70/30, Humulin 70/30, Humulin 50/50
Oral antidiabetic drugs	sitagliptin *si-ta-glip'-tin*	*tablets:* Januvia
	sitagliptin and metformin *si-ta-glip'-tin met-for'-min*	*tablets:* Janumet
	metformin *met-for'-min*	*extended-release tablets:* Fortamet, Glucophage XR, Glumetza *tablets:* Glucophage *oral solution:* Riomet
	chlorpropamide *klor-proe'-pa-mide*	*tablets:* (no longer marketed under trade name)
	glimepiride *glye-meh'-per-ide*	*tablets:* Amaryl
	glipizide *glip'-i-zide*	*extended-release tablets:* Glucotrol XL *tablets:* Glucotrol
	glipizide and metformin *glip'-i-zide met-for'-min*	*tablets:* Metaglip
	glyburide *glye'-byoor-ide*	*micronized tablets:* Glynase *tablets:* Diabeta, Micronase
	glyburide and metformin *glye'-byoor-ide met-for'-min*	*tablets:* Glucovance
	tolazamide *tole-az'-a-mide*	*tablets:* (no longer marketed under trade name)
	tolbutamide *tole-byoo'-ta-mide*	*tablets:* (no longer marketed under trade name)
	acarbose *aye-kar'-bose*	*tablets:* Precose
	miglitol *mi'-gli-tole*	*tablets:* Glyset
	nateglinide *nah-teg'-lah-nyde*	*tablets:* Starlix
	repaglinide *re-pag'-lah-nyde*	*tablets:* Prandin
	pioglitazone *pie-oh-glit'-ah-zohn*	*tablets:* Actos
	pioglitazone and metformin *pie-oh-glit'-ah-zohn met-for'-min*	*tablets:* Actoplus Met

continued

DRUG CLASSIFICATION TABLE (continued)

Classification	Generic Name	Trade Name(s)
Oral antidiabetic drugs (continued)	pioglitazone and glimepiride *pie-oh-glit'-ah-zohn glye-meh'-per-ide*	*tablets:* Duetact
	rosiglitazone *roh-zee-glit'-ah-zohn*	*tablets:* Avandia
	rosiglitazone and glimepiride *roh-zee-glit'-ah-zohn glye-meh'-per-ide*	*tablets:* Avandaryl
	rosiglitazone and metformin *roh-zee-glit'-ah-zohn met-for'-min*	*tablets:* Avandamet
Other antidiabetic agents	exenatide *ex-en'-a-tide*	*injection pen:* Byetta
	glucagon *glue'-kuh-gahn*	*injection:* GlucaGen, Glucagon Emergency Kit
Estrogens	conjugated estrogen *ess'-troe-jen*	*tablets (equine):* Premarin *tablets (synthetic):* Cenestin, Enjuvia
	conjugated estrogen and medroxyprogesterone *ess'-troe-jen me-drox'-ee-pro-jess'-te-rone*	*tablets:* Prempro, Premphase
	estradiol *ess-troe-dye'-ole*	*tablets:* Estrace, Gynodiol, Femtrace *transdermal patch (biweekly):* Alora, Vivelle, Estraderm *transdermal patch (weekly):* Climara, Menostar *topical spray:* Evamist *topical emulsion:* Estrasorb *topical gel:* Elestrin, EstroGel, Divigel *vaginal cream:* Estrace *vaginal ring:* Estring, Femring *vaginal tablets:* Vagifem
	estradiol cypionate *ess-troe-dye'-ole sip-ee'-oh-nate*	*injection (in oil):* Depo-Estradiol
	estradiol valerate *ess'-truh-die'-ole val-eh-rate*	*injection (in oil):* Delestrogen
	estropipate *ess-troe-pi'-pate*	*tablets:* Ogen
	esterified estrogen *ess'-troe-jen*	*tablets:* Menest
Hormonal contraceptives	ethinyl estradiol and norethindrone *eth'-i-nil ess'-truh-die'-ole nor-eth-in'-drone*	*tablets (monophasic):* Brevicon, Modicon, Necon 0.5/35, Nortrel 0.5/35, Necon 1/35, Norinyl 1+35, Nortrel 1/35, Ortho-Novum 1/35, Ovcon 35, Zenchent, Ovcon 50, Balziva
	ethinyl estradiol and norethindrone *eth'-i-nil ess'-truh-die'-ole nor-eth-in'-drone*	*tablets (biphasic):* Ortho-Novum 10/11, Necon 10/11
	ethinyl estradiol and norethindrone *eth'-i-nil ess'-truh-die'-ole nor-eth-in'-drone*	*tablets (triphasic):* Ortho-Novum 7/7/7, Necon 7/7/7, Nortrel 7/7/7, Aranelle, Leena, Tri-Norinyl
	ethinyl estradiol and norethindrone acetate *eth'-i-nil ess'-truh-die'-ole nor-eth-in'-drone*	*tablets (monophasic):* Junel 21 1/20, Loestrin 21 1/20, Microgestin 1/20, Junel 21 1.5/30, Loestrin 21 1.5/30, Microgestin 1.5/30

continued

DRUG CLASSIFICATION TABLE (continued)

Classification	Generic Name	Trade Name(s)
Hormonal contraceptives (continued)	ethinyl estradiol and norethindrone acetate with iron days 25–28 eth'-i-nil ess'-truh-die'-ole nor-eth-in'-drone	tablets (monophasic): Loestrin 24 Fe 1/20, Junel Fe 1/20, Microgestin Fe 1/20
	ethinyl estradiol and norethindrone with iron days 22–28 eth'-i-nil ess'-truh-die'-ole nor-eth-in'-drone	tablets (monophasic): Loestrin Fe 1.5/30, Loestrin Fe 1/20, Junel Fe 1.5/30, Microgestin Fe 1.5/30, Femcon Fe
	ethinyl estradiol and norethindrone acetate eth'-i-nil ess'-truh-die'-ole nor-eth-in'-drone	tablets (triphasic): Tri-Legest
	ethinyl estradiol and norethindrone acetate with iron days 22–28 eth'-i-nil ess'-truh-die'-ole nor-eth-in'-drone	tablets (triphasic): Estrostep Fe, Tri-Legest Fe, Tilia Fe
	ethinyl estradiol and ethynodiol diacetate eth'-i-nil ess'-truh-die'-ole e-thye-noe-dye'-ole	tablets (monophasic): Kelnor 1/35, Zovia 1/35E, Zovia 1/50E
	ethinyl estradiol and norgestrel eth'-i-nil ess'-truh-die'-ole nor-jes'-trel	tablets (monophasic): Lo/Ovral, Cryselle, Low-Ogestrel, Ogestrel 0.5/50, Ovral
	ethinyl estradiol and norgestimate eth'-i-nil ess'-truh-die'-ole nor-jes'-ti-mate	tablets (monophasic): Ortho-Cyclen, MonoNessa, Previfem, Sprintec
	ethinyl estradiol and norgestimate eth'-i-nil ess'-truh-die'-ole nor-jes'-ti-mate	tablets (triphasic): Ortho Tri-Cyclen, TriNessa, Tri-Previfem, Tri-Sprintec, Ortho Tri-Cyclen Lo
	ethinyl estradiol and desogestrel eth'-i-nil ess'-truh-die'-ole des-oh-jes'-trel	tablets (monophasic): Ortho-Cept, Apri, Desogen, Reclipsen, Solia
	ethinyl estradiol and desogestrel eth'-i-nil ess'-truh-die'-ole des-oh-jes'-trel	tablets (biphasic): Kariva, Mircette
	ethinyl estradiol and desogestrel eth'-i-nil ess'-truh-die'-ole des-oh-jes'-trel	tablets (triphasic): Velivet, Cesia, Cyclessa
	ethinyl estradiol and drospirenone eth'-i-nil ess'-truh-die'-ole droe-spye'-re-none	tablets (monophasic): YAZ, Yasmin
	ethinyl estradiol and levonorgestrel eth'-i-nil ess'-truh-die'-ole lee'-voe-nor-jes'-trel	tablets (monophasic): Alesse, Aviane, Lessina, Levlite, Lutera, Sronyx, Levlen, Levora, Nordette, Portia, Lybrel tablets (monophasic extended cycle regimen): Jolessa, Quasense, Seasonale
	ethinyl estradiol and levonorgestrel eth'-i-nil ess'-truh-die'-ole lee'-voe-nor-jes'-trel	tablets (biphasic extended cycle regimen): Seasonique
	ethinyl estradiol and levonorgestrel eth'-i-nil ess'-truh-die'-ole lee'-voe-nor-jes'-trel	tablets (triphasic): Triphasil, Enpresse, Trivora
	mestranol and norethindrone mes'-tra-nole nor-eth-in'-drone	tablets (monophasic): Necon 1/50, Norinyl 1+50, Ortho-Novum 1/50
	norethindrone nor-eth-in'-drone	tablets (monophasic): Micronor, Camila, Errin, Jolivette, Nora-BE, Nor-QD
Emergency contraceptives	levonorgestrel lee'-voe-nor-jes'-trel	tablets: Plan B

continued

DRUG CLASSIFICATION TABLE *(continued)*

Classification	Generic Name	Trade Name(s)
Progestins	medroxyprogesterone acetate *me-drox'-ee-pro-jess'-te-rone*	*tablets:* Provera *injection:* Depo-subQ Provera, Depo-Provera
	megestrol acetate *me-jess'-troll*	*tablets:* (no longer marketed under trade name) *oral suspension:* Megace
	norethindrone *nor-eth-in'-drone*	*tablets:* Aygestin
	progesterone *proe-jess'-te-rone*	*capsules:* Prometrium *injection (in oil):* (no longer marketed under trade name) *vaginal inserts:* Endometrin *vaginal suppositories:* First-Progesterone *vaginal gel:* Prochieve, Crinone
Anterior pituitary drugs	repository corticotropin *kor-ti-ko-trop'-in*	*injection:* H.P. Acthar Gel
	cosyntropin *koe-sin-troe'-pin*	*injection:* Cortrosyn
	somatropin *soe-ma-tro'-pin*	*injection (vials):* Nutropin, Omnitrope, Saizen, Tev-Tropin, Genotropin, Norditropin, Humatrope, Serostim *injection (cartridges):* Saizen, Nutropin, Humatrope
	human chorionic gonadotropin (HCG) *go-nad'-oh-tro-pin*	*injection:* Pregnyl, Ovidrel, Novarel
	menotropins *men-oh-troe'-pins*	*injection:* Repronex, Menopur
	thyrotropin alfa *thigh'-row-trop-in*	*injection:* Thyrogen
Posterior pituitary drugs	desmopressin acetate *des-moe-pres'-in*	*tablets:* DDAVP, Desmopressin *nasal spray:* DDAVP, Desmopressin, Minirin, Stimate *injection:* DDAVP
	vasopressin *vay-soe-press'-in*	*injection:* Pitressin
	oxytocin *ox-i-toe'-sin*	*injection:* Pitocin
Thyroid drugs	thyroid USP (desiccated) *thye'-roid*	*capsules:* Bio-Throid *tablets:* Armour Thyroid, Nature Thyroid
	levothyroxine *lee-voe-thye-rox'-een*	*tablets:* Levothroid, Levoxyl, Synthroid, Unithroid *injection:* (no longer marketed under trade name)
	liothyronine *lye'-oh-thye'-roe-neen*	*tablets:* Cytomel *injection:* Triostat
	liotrix *lye'-oh-trix*	*tablets:* Thyrolar

continued

DRUG CLASSIFICATION TABLE (continued)

Classification	Generic Name	Trade Name(s)
Antithyroid drugs	methimazole *meth-im'-a-zole*	*tablets:* Tapazole, Northyx
	propylthiouracil *proe-pill-thye-oh-yoor'-a-sill*	*tablets:* (no longer marketed under trade name)
	radioactive iodine (sodium iodide) *eye'-oh-dine*	*capsules:* (product not marketed under a trade name) *oral solution:* (product not marketed under a trade name)
	stable iodine (potassium iodide) *eye'-oh-dine*	*oral solution:* SSKI

CHAPTER 13

Drugs for Fluid and Electrolyte Balance

CHAPTER OBJECTIVES

- List the four electrolyte replacement drugs, and identify whether they are typically found in intracellular or extracellular fluid
- Identify the uses of the four electrolyte replacement drugs
- Match the brands and generic names of commonly used electrolyte replacement drugs
- Identify situations that may cause a decrease in electrolyte stores or that may require electrolyte replacement
- Explain why the dosage strength for potassium is different from many other drugs commonly prescribed
- Describe the common dosage range for a calcium supplement being used to prevent osteoporosis
- List the functions of sodium in the body
- Identify alkalinizing and acidifying drugs by brand or generic name
- Describe the uses of alkalinizing and acidifying drugs
- Identify common drug interactions of alkalinizing and acidifying drugs

KEY TERMS

acidifying drugs—drugs that increase the blood's pH and are used in treating metabolic alkalosis

alkalinizing drugs—drugs that decrease the blood's pH and are used in treating metabolic acidosis

electrolyte—an electrically charged particle (ion) that's essential for normal cell function and is involved in various metabolic activities

electrolyte replacement drugs—organic or inorganic salts that increase depleted or deficient electrolyte levels

hypercalcemia—abnormally high calcium levels in the blood

hypernatremia—abnormally high sodium levels in the blood

hypocalcemia—low calcium levels in the blood

hypokalemia—low potassium levels in the blood

hyponatremia—low sodium levels in the blood

metabolic acidosis—a state of decreased serum pH caused by excess hydrogen in the extracellular fluid (ECF)

metabolic alkalosis—a state of increased serum pH caused by excess bicarbonate in the extracellular fluid (ECF)

Illness can easily disturb the mechanisms that help maintain the body's normal fluid and electrolyte balance. Loss of appetite, vomiting, surgery, diagnostic tests, and the administration of medication can also upset this delicate balance. Fortunately, numerous drugs can be used to correct these imbalances. In this chapter, you'll learn about the classes of drugs that affect fluid and electrolyte imbalances and the uses and varying actions of these drugs. You'll also learn about drug interactions and adverse reactions to these drugs.

ELECTROLYTE REPLACEMENT DRUGS

An **electrolyte** is an electrically charged particle (ion) that's essential for normal cell function and is involved in various metabolic activities. **Electrolyte replacement drugs** are organic or inorganic salts that increase depleted or deficient electrolyte levels by restoring the body's normal electrolyte balance, these drugs aid in maintaining homeostasis—a state of stability in the body's internal physiological conditions under changing environmental conditions.

The body's electrolytes include:

- potassium—the main electrolyte in intracellular fluid (ICF)
- calcium—a major electrolyte in extracellular fluid (ECF)
- magnesium—an electrolyte essential for homeostasis in ICF
- sodium—the principal electrolyte in ECF that is necessary for homeostasis

Potassium

Potassium is the major positively charged ion (cation) in ICF. Adequate potassium is needed for the proper functioning of all nerve and muscle cells, including the heart muscle, and it is important in nerve impulse transmission and muscle contraction. It's also essential for tissue growth and repair and for maintaining the body's acid-base balance.

Because the body can't store potassium, it must receive adequate amounts of this electrolyte daily. If potassium is depleted without being replaced, a condition called **hypokalemia** (low potassium levels in the blood) can result. Hypokalemia is common in conditions that increase potassium excretion or depletion. Some of these include:

- alcoholism
- clay ingestion
- starvation and anorexia nervosa
- vomiting or diarrhea
- laxative abuse
- excessive urination
- an excess of antidiuretic hormone
- some kidney diseases
- burns

- cystic fibrosis
- alkalosis (a dangerous decrease in the normal acidity of the blood)
- nasogastric suction (removing solids, liquids, or gases from the stomach or small intestine by a tube inserted through the nose)

The administration of the following drugs and other substances can also result in hypokalemia:

- potassium-depleting diuretics
- glucocorticoids
- intravenous amphotericin B
- vitamin B_{12}
- folic acid
- intravenous solutions that contain insufficient potassium

Potassium replacement therapy corrects hypokalemia. Replacement can be accomplished orally or intravenously with the potassium salts discussed in the following sections. Potassium also decreases the toxic effects of digoxin. Because potassium inhibits the excitability of the heart, normal potassium levels moderate the action of digoxin, therefore reducing the chances of digoxin toxicity.

Potassium should be used cautiously in patients who are taking:

- potassium-sparing diuretics such as amiloride, spironolactone, and triamterene
- ACE inhibitors such as captopril, enalapril, and lisinopril

PROCEED WITH CAUTION

Adverse Reactions to Potassium

Most adverse reactions to potassium are related to how it is administered. Common adverse reactions with oral administration include:

- nausea
- vomiting
- abdominal pain
- diarrhea

In addition, enteric-coated tablets may cause small-bowel ulceration, stenosis (narrowing or constriction of a blood vessel or valve), hemorrhage, or obstruction.

When administered by IV infusion, common adverse reactions to potassium include:

- pain at the injection site
- phlebitis (vein inflammation)
- increased risk of hyperkalemia (in patients with decreased urine production)

Given rapidly, IV potassium may also cause cardiac arrest.

Potassium Acetate

Potassium acetate is supplied as an injection. Potassium acetate is used when oral potassium replacement therapy is not practical.

TIP It's important to remember that potassium is usually dosed in milliequivalent units (mEq), not milligrams (mg).

Potassium Bicarbonate

Potassium bicarbonate (K-Lyte, K-Vescent, Klor-Con EF) is available in effervescent tablets, sometimes in combination with citric acid or potassium chloride. These tablets are dissolved in water to create an oral solution.

Potassium Chloride

Potassium chloride, often abbreviated KCl, is supplied in several forms for oral and IV administration. Oral forms include:

- controlled-release tablets (K-Tab, Klor-Con, Klotrix)
- controlled-release capsules (Micro-K)
- oral solution
- fruit-flavored powder (K-Lor, Klor-Con)

For IV infusion, potassium chloride is available in the following forms:

- IV bags
- concentrated solution that must be diluted before being infused

Dosage and rate of administration depend on the specific condition of each patient. Like potassium acetate, these forms of potassium are used when oral administration of potassium is not feasible.

Potassium Chloride can be used as a cardioplegic. Cardioplegia is the act of intentionally stopping cardiac activity, which is primarily used in cardiac surgery. The most common procedure for accomplishing this is infusing cardioplegia solution, typically consisting of potassium chloride, into the coronary circulation. This process is considered the most successful because it protects the heart muscle from damage. The heart remains stopped for a period of about 15 to 20 minutes with no electrical or mechanical activity. This is reversed over time by normal metabolic mechanisms.

TIP Potassium chloride is often used in intravenous products. The lid on potassium chloride injectable solution is black, which is different from all other injectable vial lids. When you see a black lid, this should remind you that it is potassium chloride and to double-check the dose before filling the order.

Other Potassium Salts

Other potassium salts include:

- potassium gluconate, which is available OTC in oral tablets
- potassium phosphate, which is available in tablets (K-Phos), powder for oral solution (Neutra-Phos-K), and as an injection

Calcium

Calcium is a major cation in ECF. Calcium has several important roles in the body:

- It's important for normal bone and tooth formation.
- It's important to normal functioning of the heart, kidneys, and lungs.
- It affects blood coagulation rate as well as cell membrane and capillary permeability.
- It's a factor in neurotransmitter and hormone activity, amino acid metabolism, vitamin B_{12} absorption, and gastrin secretion.

Pregnancy and breastfeeding increase calcium requirements. So do periods of bone growth in child-

---

HOW IT WORKS

How Potassium Works

Potassium works with sodium to regulate the amount of water that passes in and out of cells. We take in potassium from the foods we eat. Bananas, potatoes, and a number of other fruits and vegetables contain high amounts of potassium. When we eat these foods, the potassium in them is readily absorbed into the bloodstream from the GI tract.

As the blood circulates through the body, most of its potassium passes into the ICF. An enzyme maintains the concentration of potassium in the cells by pumping sodium out in exchange for potassium. Any excess potassium that is not absorbed into the cells is excreted in urine, stool, and sweat.

AT THE COUNTER

Working with Potassium Chloride

You receive an order for KCl 20 mEq in 1000 mL NS to be administered at a rate of 125 mL/hr. You retrieve the potassium chloride vial from the shelf. The label states that it contains 10 mL with a concentration of 2 mEq/mL. How much should you draw up into the syringe?

You should draw 10 mL into the syringe.

Why is it so important to make sure that the dose of potassium chloride is correct prior to injecting?

Potassium chloride can cause cardiac arrest if an incorrect dose is administered.

ren and adolescents. Calcium is useful in other ways as well:

- It's helpful in treating magnesium poisoning.
- It helps to strengthen myocardial tissue after defibrillation (electric shock to restore normal heart rhythm) or a poor response to epinephrine during resuscitation.
- It's used to supplement a calcium-deficient diet and to prevent osteoporosis.

Almost all of the body's calcium (99 percent) is stored in bone. When dietary intake of calcium isn't enough to meet the body's needs, these calcium stores are reduced. However, calcium moves quickly into ECF to restore calcium levels and reestablish balance.

Extracellular calcium exists in three forms:

- It's bound to plasma protein (mostly albumin).
- It's complexed with substances such as phosphate, citrate, or sulfate.
- It's ionized. Extracellular ionized calcium plays an essential role in normal nerve and muscle excitability.

Chronic insufficient calcium intake can result in bone demineralization. Calcium is replaced orally or intravenously with calcium salts such as those discussed in the following sections. These salts are readily absorbed and are eliminated in urine and stool.

Calcium has few significant interactions with other drugs. Here are some interactions that you should know:

- Administering calcium with digoxin may cause cardiac arrhythmias.
- Calcium replacement drugs may reduce the body's response to calcium channel blockers.
- Calcium supplements may inactivate tetracyclines.
- Calcium supplements may decrease the amount of atenolol available to the tissues, decreasing the effectiveness of the drug.
- When given in total parenteral nutrition, calcium may react with phosphorus present in the solution to form insoluble calcium phosphate granules. These may cause pulmonary embolism and possible death.

PROCEED WITH CAUTION

Adverse Reactions to Calcium

Calcium preparations may case **hypercalcemia** (abnormally high calcium levels in the blood). Early signs include:

- drowsiness and lethargy
- muscle weakness
- headache
- constipation
- metallic taste

Electrocardiographic changes also can occur with hypercalcemia. These changes include a shortened QT interval and heart block. Severe hypercalcemia can cause cardiac arrhythmias, coma, and cardiac arrest.

Oral Calcium

Oral calcium is commonly used to supplement a calcium-deficient diet, to prevent osteoporosis, and as an antacid for symptomatic relief of heartburn. It's also used to treat chronic **hypocalcemia** (low blood calcium levels) that can result from such conditions as:

- chronic hypoparathyroidism (a deficiency of parathyroid hormones)
- osteomalacia (softening of bones)
- long-term glucocorticoid therapy
- plicamycin and vitamin D deficiency

Calcium Carbonate

Calcium carbonate is supplied OTC as conventional tablets (Caltrate) and capsules. Some companies manufacture chewable tablets (Tums, Maalox Children's, Mylanta Children's, Pepto-Bismol Children's, Maalox, Alka-Mints) and soft chews (Rolaids). An oral suspension is also available.

Taken daily, this drug is used to prevent calcium deficiency. The usual daily dose is between 500 mg and 2 g, two to four times per day. It is recommended in doses of 1500 mg per day for men older than 65 years of age and for postmenopausal women not taking estrogen replacement therapy. Calcium carbonate can also be taken as needed for relief of aid indigestion, heartburn, and upset stomach.

HOW IT WORKS

Calcium: Building Strong Bones and Teeth

Calcium is one of the most vital minerals in the body. It works with other nutrients to build the hard structure that strengthens bones and teeth. Bones are a storage site for the body's calcium.

However, calcium is not only needed to form bones and teeth. It's also necessary for the following:

- proper functioning of organs and muscles
- blood clotting
- transmitting signals in nerve cells
- muscle contraction

These other functions of calcium are important for survival. When calcium intake is insufficient, the body will break down bone to maintain normal blood calcium levels. Calcium is continuously transported from bones into the bloodstream and replaced according to the body's daily calcium needs. The aging process also causes bone loss.

As you can see, adequate intake of calcium through dairy products and green leafy vegetables is an important step in maintaining the strong bones and teeth that were formed when you were young. It also aids in preventing the breakdown of bone in your body, known as osteoporosis.

Other Calcium Salts

The following are several other calcium salts.

- Calcium citrate (Citracal) is supplied OTC as tablets and caplets.
- Calcium glubionate (Calcionate) is available OTC as an oral solution. Calcium replacement therapy in pregnant women and woman who are breastfeeding is one tablespoon four times a day.
- Calcium lactate is available OTC in the form of tablets.
- Calcium acetate is a prescription product available in capsules (PhosLo) and tablets (Calphron).

Intravenous Calcium

The major clinical indication for IV calcium is acute hypocalcemia. This condition necessitates a rapid increase in serum calcium levels as found in:

- tetany (a nervous condition characterized by sharp flexion of the wrist and ankle joints, muscle twitching, cramps, and possible convulsions)

AT THE COUNTER

Calcium Supplements

A healthy 50-year-old patient comes to the pharmacy counter seeking a calcium supplement because she has heard it is good for the prevention of osteoporosis. The pharmacist makes a recommendation for Citracal and asks that you help the patient find the product. When you find the Citracal products, you notice that some contain vitamin D and others do not. Why is vitamin D included in some products?

Vitamin D promotes calcium absorption. Vitamin D can also be found in food and is made by the body after exposure to ultraviolet rays from the sun.

Would you expect that the patient's lifestyle and physical location would make a difference in whether the vitamin D is necessary or not?

Yes. If the patient is outside frequently, then her body is probably making enough vitamin D on its own. Also, if the patient lives in Miami, she is probably getting more sun exposure than a patient who lives in Seattle.

As you and the patient are looking at the different Citracal products, she notices that your pharmacy carries a lot of calcium supplements. She asks how they are different. What should you say?

There are a lot of calcium supplements on the market. The main difference among the different products is the salt attached to the calcium (for example, calcium carbonate, calcium citrate). Because the pharmacist recommended Citracal, you should encourage the patient to either purchase what the pharmacist recommended or speak to the pharmacist again.

- cardiac arrest
- parathyroid surgery
- vitamin D deficiency
- alkalosis

IV calcium is also used to prevent a hypocalcemic reaction during exchange transfusions.

Calcium salts used for these purposes include calcium chloride and calcium gluconate. Both drugs are available as injections. However, calcium chloride is not suitable for IM injection. It must be administered intravenously only. The typical adult dose is 5 to 10 mL infused slowly at a rate not to exceed 0.5 to 1.0 mL per minute, preferably into a central or deep vein.

Magnesium

Magnesium is the second most plentiful cation in ICF after potassium. About 65 percent of the body's magnesium is found in bone, and 20 percent is in muscle. The body uses magnesium in several ways:

- It is essential in transmitting nerve impulses to muscle.
- It stimulates parathyroid hormone secretion and thereby regulates ICF calcium levels.
- It aids in cell metabolism and in the movement of sodium and potassium across cell membranes.

The body's magnesium stores may be depleted in a number of ways. These include:

- malabsorption
- acute and chronic alcohol consumption
- chronic diarrhea
- prolonged treatment with diuretics
- prolonged therapy with parenteral fluids not containing magnesium
- nasogastric suctioning
- hyperaldosteronism
- hypoparathyroidism or hyperparathyroidism
- excessive release of adrenocortical hormones
- drugs such as cisplatin, aminoglycosides, cyclosporine, and amphotericin B

Magnesium replacement therapy is usually accomplished with magnesium oxide or magnesium sulfate, depending on how the drug is administered. Magnesium has few significant interactions with other drugs, although its use with digoxin may lead to heart attack.

Magnesium Oxide

Magnesium is provided orally as magnesium oxide. It is supplied OTC as tablets (MagOx, Phillips' Cramp-Free) and capsules (Uro-Mag, Mag Gel). Besides increasing the daily intake of magnesium, the tablets are also used to relieve acid indigestion and upset stomach.

A common adverse reaction to magnesium oxide is diarrhea. More serious adverse reactions may include:

- severe allergic reactions (such as rash, hives, difficulty breathing, and swelling of the mouth, face, lips, or tongue)

- black, tarry stools
- nausea
- slow reflexes
- vomit that looks like coffee grounds

Magnesium Sulfate

Magnesium is administered intravenously as magnesium sulfate. It is supplied in IV bags, and it is also available as a powder.

Magnesium sulfate is the drug of choice for replenishing and preventing magnesium deficiency. It also prevents or controls seizures by blocking neuromuscular transmission. It's widely used to treat or prevent eclamptic (convulsive) and preeclamptic seizure activity and to treat some ventricular arrhythmias. It's also used to treat seizures, severe toxemia (systemic bacterial infection), and acute nephritis (kidney inflammation) in children.

Magnesium sulfate is distributed widely throughout the body. Intravenous magnesium sulfate acts immediately, whereas the drug acts within 30 minutes after IM injection. Injections can also be painful, may induce sclerosis (hardening of tissue), and need to be repeated frequently.

Drug interactions with magnesium sulfate include the following:

- Increased CNS depressant effects may occur when magnesium sulfate is combined with alcohol, narcotics, antianxiety drugs, barbiturates, antidepressants, hypnotics, antipsychotic drugs, or general anesthetics.
- Magnesium sulfate combined with succinylcholine or tubocurarine increases and prolongs the neuromuscular blocking action of these drugs.

Adverse reactions to magnesium sulfate can be life threatening. They include:

- hypotension
- circulatory collapse
- flushing
- slow reflexes
- respiratory paralysis

Other Magnesium Salts

The following are several other magnesium salts:

- Magnesium gluconate (Mag-G, Magtrate) is available OTC as tablets.
- Magnesium chloride is a prescription drug available in the form of tablets (Mag-SR), injection, and delayed-release tablets (Mag-64).
- Magnesium lactate (Mag-Tab SR) is an OTC drug available as extended-release tablets.

Sodium

Sodium is the major cation in ECF. It performs many functions in the body:

- It maintains the osmotic pressure and concentration of ECF, acid-base balance, and water balance.
- It contributes to nerve conduction and neuromuscular function.
- It plays a role in glandular secretion.

Sodium replacement is necessary in conditions that cause rapid sodium loss. These conditions include:

- excessive perspiration
- anorexia
- excessive loss of GI fluids
- trauma or wound drainage
- adrenal gland insufficiency
- cirrhosis of the liver with ascites (abnormal secretion of fluid into the abdomen)
- syndrome of inappropriate antidiuretic hormone
- use of diuretics and tap water enemas
- prolonged IV infusion of dextrose in water (such as D5W) without other solutes

Sodium is typically replaced in the form of sodium chloride. It is available as in a variety of dosage forms including tablets and injection solutions. Sodium chloride is used for water and electrolyte replacement in patients with **hyponatremia** (low sodium levels in the blood) from electrolyte loss or severe sodium chloride depletion.

Severe sodium deficiency may be treated by IV infusion of a solution containing sodium chloride. In both its oral and parenteral forms, sodium chloride is quickly absorbed and distributed widely throughout the body. It replaces deficiencies of sodium and chloride ions in the blood plasma. It isn't significantly metabolized, however. Instead, it is eliminated primarily in urine, but also in sweat, tears, and saliva.

No significant drug interactions with sodium chloride have been reported.

ALKALINIZING AND ACIDIFYING DRUGS

Alkalinizing and acidifying drugs act to correct acid-base imbalances in the blood. The imbalances include:

- **metabolic acidosis**, a state of decreased serum pH caused by excess hydrogen in the extracellular fluid (ECF); treated with alkalinizing drugs
- **metabolic alkalosis**, a state of increased serum pH caused by excess bicarbonate in the extracellular fluid (ECF); treated with acidifying drugs

PROCEED WITH CAUTION

Adverse Reactions to Sodium

Adverse reactions to sodium include:
- pulmonary edema (if given too rapidly or in excess)
- **hypernatremia** (abnormally high sodium levels in the blood)
- potassium loss

Alkalinizing and acidifying drugs have opposite effects.

- An alkalinizing drug will increase the blood's pH and decrease the concentration of hydrogen ions.
- An acidifying drug will decrease blood pH and increase the concentration of hydrogen ions.

Some of these drugs also alter urine pH. This makes them useful in treating some urinary tract infections (UTIs) and drug overdoses.

Alkalinizing Drugs

Alkalinizing drugs are used to decrease the blood's pH and are used in treating metabolic acidosis. They are also used to raise urine pH to help remove certain substances, such as phenobarbital, after an overdose.

Most of the alkalinizing drugs can interact with a wide range of other drugs to increase or decrease the effects of those drugs.

- They may increase excretion and reduce the effects of ketoconazole, lithium, and salicylates.
- They may reduce the excretion and increase the effects of amphetamines, quinidine, and pseudoephedrine.
- They may reduce the antibacterial effects of methenamine.

Sodium Bicarbonate

Sodium bicarbonate is produced as tablets, effervescent tablets (Alka-Seltzer), effervescent granules for oral solution (Baros), and an injection (Neut). This drug separates into sodium and bicarbonate molecules in the blood buffer system to decrease the concentration of hydrogen ions and thereby increase blood pH. (Buffers prevent extreme changes in pH by taking or giving up hydrogen ions to neutralize acids or bases.)

Sodium bicarbonate is also used as an antacid to relieve acid indigestion, heartburn, and sour or upset stomach, and to increase urine pH.

Adverse reactions to sodium bicarbonate include:

- bicarbonate overdose
- cerebral dysfunction, tissue hypoxia, and lactic acidosis (with rapid administration for diabetic ketoacidosis)
- water retention and edema

Sodium Citrate

Sodium citrate (Oracit, Bicitra, Cytra-Z, Liqui-Dual Citra) is produced as an oral solution. It has the same mechanism of action as sodium bicarbonate. This drug is also used for the rapid relief of acid indigestion, heartburn, and sour stomach.

Adverse reactions to sodium citrate include:

- metabolic alkalosis, tetany, or aggravation of existing heart disease (with overdose)
- laxative effect (with oral administration)

Sodium Lactate

Sodium lactate is supplied as an injection for IV administration. It is used to prevent or control mild to moderate metabolic acidosis in patients with restricted oral intake. This drug acts similarly to sodium bicarbonate. It should be administered only by adding it to a larger volume of IV fluids.

Adverse reactions to sodium lactate include:

- metabolic alkalosis (with overdose)
- extravasation (escape of fluid from a blood vessel into surrounding tissue)
- water retention or edema (in patients with kidney disease or heart failure)

Tromethamine

Tromethamine, abbreviated THAM, is administered as an injection. It acts by combining with hydrogen ions to alkalinize the blood. The tromethamine-hydrogen ion complex that results is excreted in urine.

Adverse reactions to tromethamine include:

- hypoglycemia (low blood sugar)
- respiratory depression
- extravasation
- hyperkalemia
- toxic drug levels (if given for longer than 24 hours)

Acidifying Drugs

Acidifying drugs increase the blood's pH and are used in treating metabolic alkalosis. The action of most acidifying drugs is immediate, and they don't cause clinically significant drug interactions.

Adverse reactions to acidifying drugs are usually mild, such as GI distress. Overdose may lead to acidosis.

Acetazolamide

Acetazolamide (Diamox) is supplied as tablets, sustained-release capsules, and as an injection for parenteral administration. Its main use as an acidifying drug is in treating acute mountain sickness (adverse changes in the bodies of mountain climbers that result from the environmental conditions related to high altitudes). The drug increases the body's excretion of bicarbonate, which lowers blood and urine pH. Acetazolamide is also used to treat glaucoma and certain epilepsies. The injectable form is used to treat alkalosis.

Acetazolamide may produce metabolic acidosis. In addition, in patients with renal dysfunction, it may be ineffective and cause a loss of potassium in urine.

Adverse reactions to acetazolamide include:

- drowsiness
- nausea and vomiting
- diarrhea
- anorexia
- altered taste

- aplastic anemia
- seizures

T I P Acetazolamide can cause a number of side effects and may not be the best choice for patients with renal dysfunction.

Ammonium Chloride

Ammonium chloride is provided as an injection. Adverse reactions to ammonium chloride include metabolic acidosis and loss of electrolytes, especially potassium (with large doses).

Ascorbic Acid

Ascorbic acid is usually administered orally. It's available OTC in the following oral forms:

- tablets
- chewable tablets
- extended-release tablets
- extended-release capsules
- oral solution (Cecon)

When oral forms of the drug are absorbed poorly, or when oral administration is not practical, an injection solution (Ascor, Betac) may be used. This solution is usually administered by IM or SubQ injection.

Like ammonium chloride, ascorbic acid serves as a urinary acidifier. It directly acidifies urine, providing hydrogen ions and lowering urine pH.

Adverse reactions to ascorbic acid include:

- GI distress (with high doses)
- hemolytic anemia (in patients with glucose-6-phosphate dehydrogenase deficiency)

QUICK QUIZ

Answer the following multiple-choice questions.

1. What is the daily dose of calcium carbonate recommended for preventing osteoporosis in older adults?
   a. 100 mg
   b. 500 mg
   c. 1000 mg
   d. 1500 mg
2. How does sodium bicarbonate correct metabolic acidosis?
   a. It combines with hydrogen ions in the blood.
   b. It decreases hydrogen ion concentration.
   c. It increases hydrogen ion concentration.
   d. It lowers blood pH after being metabolized.
3. Which of these chemical elements is *not* an electrolyte?
   a. hydrogen
   b. magnesium
   c. potassium
   d. sodium

4. Severe loss of body fluid can deplete the body's supply of all of the following except:
   a. calcium.
   b. magnesium.
   c. potassium.
   d. sodium.
5. All these drugs can be used to treat heartburn and upset stomach except:
   a. calcium carbonate.
   b. sodium bicarbonate.
   c. sodium citrate.
   d. sodium chloride.

Please answer each of the following questions in one to three sentences.

1. How and why do the dosage strengths of some potassium replacement drugs differ from the dosage strengths of other electrolyte replacement drugs?

_____

_____

2. Why is it important that the body gets enough calcium?

_____

_____

3. What role does magnesium play in regulating the body's other electrolytes?

_____

_____

4. What functions does sodium perform in the body?

_____

_____

5. Why is it essential that the body has enough potassium?

_____

_____

Answer the following questions as either true or false.

1. ___ Most of the body's calcium is found in ECF.
2. ___ Most of the body's potassium is found in ECF.
3. ___ Most of the body's sodium is found in ECF.
4. ___ Most of the body's magnesium is found in ECF.
5. ___ An electrolyte replacement drug raises the blood's pH.

Match each drug in the left column with the condition it treats in the right column.

1. ascorbic acid	a. hypocalcemia
2. calcium citrate	b. hypokalemia
3. potassium chloride	c. hyponatremia
4. sodium citrate	d. metabolic acidosis
5. sodium chloride	e. metabolic alkalosis

DRUG CLASSIFICATION TABLE

Classification	Generic Name	Trade Name(s)
Electrolyte replacement drugs	potassium acetate *poe-tass'-ee-um*	*injection:* (no longer marketed under trade name)
	potassium bicarbonate *poe-tass'-ee-um*	*effervescent tablets:* K-Lyte, K-Vescent, Klor-Con EF
	potassium chloride *poe-tass'-ee-um*	*controlled-release tablets:* K-Tab, Klor-Con, Klotrix *controlled-release capsules:* Micro-K *oral solution:* (no longer marketed under trade name) *powder:* K-Lor, Klor-Con *injection:* (no longer marketed under trade name)
	potassium gluconate *poe-tass'-ee-um*	*tablets:* (no longer marketed under trade name)
	potassium phosphate *poe-tass'-ee-um*	*tablets:* K-Phos *injection:* (no longer marketed under trade name) *powder for oral solution:* Neutra-Phos-K
	calcium carbonate *kal'-see-um*	*tablets:* Caltrate *chewable tablets:* Tums, Maalox Children's, Mylanta Children's, Pepto-Bismol Children's, Maalox, Alka-Mints *oral suspension:* (no longer marketed under trade name) *soft chews:* Rolaids *capsules:* (no longer marketed under trade name)
	calcium citrate *kal'-see-um*	*tablets:* Citracal *caplets:* Citracal
	calcium glubionate *kal'-see-um*	*oral solution:* Calcionate
	calcium lactate *kal'-see-um*	*tablets:* (no longer marketed under trade name)
	calcium acetate *kal'-see-um*	*capsules:* PhosLo *tablets:* Calphron
	calcium chloride *kal'-see-um*	*injection:* (no longer marketed under trade name)
	calcium gluconate *kal'-see-um*	*injection:* (no longer marketed under trade name) *tablets:* (no longer marketed under trade name)
	magnesium oxide *mag-nee'-zee-um*	*tablets:* MagOx, Phillips' Cramp-Free *capsules:* Uro-Mag, Mag Gel
	magnesium sulfate *mag-nee'-zee-um*	*injection:* (no longer marketed under trade name) *powder:* (no longer marketed under trade name)
	magnesium gluconate *mag-nee'-zee-um*	*tablets:* Mag-G, Magtrate
	magnesium chloride *mag-nee'-zee-um*	*tablets:* Mag-SR *injection:* (no longer marketed under trade name) *delayed-release tablets:* Mag-64
	magnesium lactate *mag-nee'-zee-um*	*extended-release tablets:* Mag-Tab SR
	sodium chloride *sow-dee'-um*	*tablets:* (no longer marketed under trade name) *injection:* (no longer marketed under trade name)

continued

DRUG CLASSIFICATION TABLE (continued)

Classification	Generic Name	Trade Name(s)
Alkalinizing drugs	sodium bicarbonate *sow-dee'-um*	*tablets:* (no longer marketed under trade name)
		effervescent tablets: Alka-Seltzer
		effervescent granules for oral solution: Baros
		injection: Neut
	sodium citrate *sow-dee'-um*	*oral solution:* Oracit, Bicitra, Cytra-Z, Liqui-Dual Citra
	sodium lactate *sow-dee'-um*	*injection:* (no longer marketed under trade name)
	tromethamine *tro-meth'-uh-meen*	*injection:* Tham
Acidifying drugs	acetazolamide *a-set-a-zole'-a-mide*	*tablets:* (no longer marketed under trade name)
		sustained-release capsules: Diamox
		injection: (no longer marketed under trade name)
	ammonium chloride *ah-moe'-nee-uhm*	*injection:* (no longer marketed under trade name)
	ascorbic acid *ass'-kor-bik ass'-id*	*chewable tablets:* (no longer marketed under trade name)
		tablets: (no longer marketed under trade name)
		extended-release tablets: (no longer marketed under trade name)
		extended-release capsules: (no longer marketed under trade name)
		injection: Ascor, Betac
		oral solution: Cecon

CHAPTER 14

Antineoplastic Drugs

CHAPTER OBJECTIVES

- Match brand and generic names of commonly used antineoplastic drugs
- Identify the classification of commonly used antineoplastic drugs
- Identify the route(s) of administration for commonly used antineoplastic drugs
- Describe the mechanism of action for the different classifications of antineoplastic drugs
- Identify the antineoplastic drugs that require storage conditions other than room temperature
- List the most common adverse reactions produced by antineoplastic drugs

KEY TERMS

alkyl sulfonate—a drug that forms covalent bonds with DNA molecules during the process of alkylation

alkylating drugs—antineoplastic drugs that cross-link DNA strands, which stops the ability of DNA to replicate

alkylating-like drugs—drugs that act on the body in the same way as alkylating drugs

alkylation—a chemical reaction that stops DNA molecules from replicating properly

alpha interferons—drugs derived from leukocytes that are used to treat several kinds of cancers

androgens—synthetic derivatives of the naturally occurring male hormone testosterone

antiandrogens—drugs that block the action of androgen, a male hormone

antibiotic antineoplastic drugs—antimicrobial products that bind with DNA to produce tumor-destroying effects

antiestrogens—drugs that bind to estrogen receptors and block the action of estrogen

antimetabolite drugs—cancer-fighting drugs that are similar in chemical structure to DNA base pairs

antineoplastic drugs—drugs used to treat cancer

aromatase—an enzyme involved in the production of estrogen

aromatase inhibitors—drugs that prevent the formation of estrogen by interfering with the action of the enzyme aromatase

asparaginases—cell cycle-specific drugs that are used in treating acute lymphocytic leukemia

beta interferons—drugs derived from connective tissue cells (fibroblasts) that show anticancer activity

bifunctional alkylation—a process in which drug molecules form a bond between two DNA base pairs, which causes cytotoxic effects

folic acid analogues—drugs that interfere with the way the body uses folic acid

gamma interferons—drugs derived from connective tissue cells (fibroblasts) and lymphocytes that can fight cancer cells

gonadotropin-releasing hormone analogues—drugs that lower the testosterone level in the body and are used for palliative treatment of advanced prostate cancer

hormonal antineoplastic drugs—drugs that change the growth of tumors by affecting body hormones

interferons—naturally occurring glycoproteins that can fight cancers

monoclonal antibodies—artificial antibodies designed to target specific substances such as immune cells or cancer cells

monofunctional alkylation—a process in which drug molecules react with one part of a DNA base pair, causing damage to the cell

natural products—antineoplastic agents that are derived from plants or other natural substances

nitrogen mustards—the largest group of alkylating neoplastic drugs

nitrosoureas—alkylating agents that work by preventing cancer cells from multiplying

nonsteroidal inhibitors—inhibitors that have a temporary effect on the enzyme aromatase; also called *type 2 inhibitors*

podophyllotoxins—partially synthetic chemicals that affect tumor cells by acting during the G2 and late S phases of the cell cycle

progestins—hormones that are used for palliative treatment of several different cancers

purine analogues—drugs used in the treatment of leukemias that become part of DNA and affect DNA replication

pyrimidine analogues—drugs that kill cancer cells by interfering with the function of pyrimidine nucleotides (chemicals used in building DNA)

S phase-specific drugs—drugs that act on cells that are in the DNA synthesis phase of replication
steroidal inhibitors—inhibitors that have an irreversible effect on the enzyme aromatase; also called *type 1 inhibitors*

topoisomerase I inhibitors—drugs that block the action of the enzyme topoisomerase, damaging cell DNA
vinca alkaloids—drugs derived from the periwinkle plant that are used to treat several different types of cancer

---

In the 1940s, **antineoplastic drugs** (or chemotherapeutic drugs) were developed to treat cancer. For many of these agents, serious adverse effects were common. Today, many of these toxicities have been reduced, so they aren't as potentially devastating to the patient. With modern chemotherapy, some cancers are considered curable in most patients. These include:

- childhood malignancies, such as acute lymphoblastic leukemia
- adult cancers, such as testicular cancer

If a cancer can't be cured, antineoplastic drugs may control its progress. They can reduce the growth of tumors or slow down the process of metastasis (spreading of cancer to other places in the body). These drugs are also used for palliative therapy to relieve symptoms caused by cancer.

New therapeutic strategies continue to improve the length of time that a patient's cancer remains in remission. Some strategies that you will learn about in this chapter are:

- using monoclonal antibodies
- targeting specific proteins

ALKYLATING DRUGS

Alkylating drugs, alone or with other drugs, act against different malignant neoplasms (tumors). These drugs produce their antineoplastic effects by damaging deoxyribonucleic acid (DNA). Alkylating drugs are cell cycle phase nonspecific. This means that their alkylating actions may take place at any phase in the cell cycle.

Alkylating drugs fall into one of six classes:

- nitrogen mustards
- alkyl sulfonates
- nitrosoureas
- triazines
- ethylenimines
- alkylating-like drugs

Nitrogen Mustards

Nitrogen mustards represent the largest group of alkylating drugs. Because they produce leukopenia, these drugs are effective in treating malignant neoplasms that may have an associated elevated white blood cell count. Examples of these cancers include:

- Hodgkin disease (cancer that causes painless enlargement of the lymph nodes)
- leukemia (cancer of the blood-forming tissues)

Nitrogen mustards have also been effective in fighting:

- malignant lymphoma (cancer of the lymphoid tissue)
- multiple myeloma (cancer of the marrow plasma cells)
- melanoma (a type of skin cancer)
- cancers of the breast, ovaries, uterus, lung, brain, testes, bladder, prostate, and stomach

Nitrogen mustards form covalent bonds, or chemical links, with DNA molecules in a chemical reaction called **alkylation**. The alkylated DNA molecules can't replicate properly. This causes cell death (cytotoxicity).

Chlorambucil

Chlorambucil (Leukeran) is manufactured as oral tablets. It's typically used for short courses of treatment or beginning therapy. It may also be used on an intermittent, biweekly, or once-monthly schedule. This drug must be refrigerated. There are no reported interactions with other drugs. The most common adverse reaction to chlorambucil is bone marrow suppression.

Cyclophosphamide

Cyclophosphamide (Cytoxan) is often used in a treatment regimen with other antineoplastic drugs. It has also been used in treating multiple sclerosis. It's available as oral tablets or as powder for injection solution.

The oral tablets may be dissolved in aromatic elixir to produce an oral solution. This should be stored in a glass container in the refrigerator and used within 14 days.

The parenteral form of cyclophosphamide may be administered by IM, IV, intraperitoneal (abdominal), or intrapleural (around the lungs) injection. The reconstituted solution may be stored for up to six days under refrigeration. It's also stable at room temperature for 24 hours.

 PROCEED WITH CAUTION

Adverse Reactions to Nitrogen Mustards

Many patients experience fatigue during nitrogen mustard therapy.

Other adverse reactions include:

- severe leukopenia and thrombocytopenia
- nausea and vomiting from central nervous system irritation
- stomatitis
- reversible hair loss
- severe skin reactions (with direct contact)

HOW IT WORKS

How Alkylating Drugs Work

Alkylating drugs can attack DNA in two ways, as shown in figure 14-1.

Some drugs become inserted between two base pairs in the DNA chain, forming an irreversible bond between them. This is called **bifunctional alkylation**. It causes cytotoxic effects capable of destroying or poisoning cells.

Other drugs react with just one part of a base pair. They separate the base from its partner, eventually causing it and its attached sugar to break away from the DNA molecule. This is called **monofunctional alkylation**. It leads to permanent cell damage.

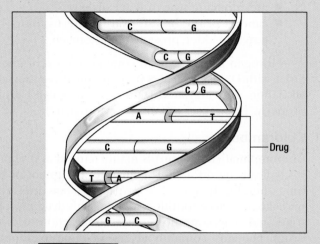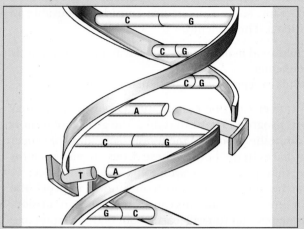

FIGURE 14-1 How alkylating drugs work. (From *Clinical Pharmacology Made Incredibly Easy.* 2nd Ed. Philadelphia, PA: Lippincott Williams & Wilkins; 2005.)

Cyclophosphamide may interact with other medications.

- Taking cyclophosphamide with cardiotoxic drugs produces additive cardiac effects.
- Cyclophosphamide may reduce digoxin levels in the blood.

Estramustine

Estramustine (Emcyt) is used in palliative treatment for metastatic or progressive prostate cancer. It has also been used in treating metastatic renal cell carcinoma (kidney cancer). It's available as capsules, which are normally taken one hour before or two hours after meals. Estramustine should be stored in the refrigerator.

Calcium-containing drugs and foods, such as antacids and dairy products, decrease the body's absorption of estramustine.

Ifosfamide

Ifosfamide (Ifex) is manufactured as powder for injection. It's normally used with other antineoplastic agents. This drug is administered by slow IV infusion over five consecutive days. The powder is mixed with sterile water or sterile bacteriostatic water. The reconstituted solution should be kept in the refrigerator and used within 24 hours.

Ifosfamide may interact with other drugs.

- Corticosteroids reduce the effects of ifosfamide.
- When taken with ifosfamide, allopurinol, barbiturates, chloral hydrate, and phenytoin may increase the risk of ifosfamide toxicity.

Mechlorethamine

Mechlorethamine (Mustargen) was the first nitrogen mustard introduced. This rapid-acting drug comes as a powder for injection. It is administered intravenously in a single dose or divided doses. The injection solution must be prepared immediately before it's used. It should be clear and colorless. Because this drug is corrosive to the skin and eyes, it's important to take proper safety precautions when handling it.

T I P Before handling any antineoplastics, you should be properly trained. This applies especially to injectables, but training is necessary for oral products as well. Improper handling can result in accidental absorption of the antineoplastic product.

Melphalan

Melphalan (Alkeran) is available as oral tablets or as injection powder. Oral tablets may be taken once a day. This drug is normally used for two to three weeks. After this initial treatment, a maintenance dose may be used after a break of up to four weeks. Melphalan should be refrigerated and protected from light.

Other drugs may interact with melphalan.

- Interferon alpha may reduce serum concentration of melphalan.
- The lung toxicity threshold of carmustine may be reduced when taken with melphalan.

Alkyl Sulfonates

Busulfan, an **alkyl sulfonate**, has historically been used to treat several conditions:

- chronic myelogenous leukemia
- polycythemia vera (increased red blood cell mass and increased number of white blood cells and platelets)
- other myeloproliferative disorders (conditions relating to overproductive bone marrow)

It's also used to treat leukemia during bone marrow transplant procedures.

As an alkyl sulfonate, busulfan is a drug that forms covalent bonds with DNA molecules during the process of alkylation. Busulfan mainly affects granulocytes (a type of white blood cell). It also has some effects on platelets. Its action on granulocytes makes busulfan useful in the treatment of chronic myelogenous leukemia and as adjunct therapy in treating leukemia before and after bone marrow transplants.

Busulfan can also be effective in treating polycythemia vera. However, other drugs are usually used because busulfan can cause severe myelosuppression (reduced bone marrow function).

Busulfan is administered as oral tablets (Myleran) or by injection (Busulfex). For oral busulfan, it may take 10 to 15 days to see improvements in the leukocyte count. Leukocyte counts will continue to fall for up to one month after the patient stops taking the drug.

The injectable form of busulfan is used in combination with cyclophosphamide before bone marrow transplantation. It's administered intravenously. This drug should be diluted with normal saline or D5W solution before using. Busulfan ampules should be refrigerated. The diluted solution can be refrigerated for up to 12 hours. At room temperature, the solution is stable for up to eight hours (the infusion must be completed within that time). This form of the drug is normally given as a two-hour IV infusion every six hours for four days. Patients need to take antiemetics throughout treatment.

Busulfan may interact with other medications.

- When taken with anticoagulants or aspirin, there is an increased risk of bleeding.

PROCEED WITH CAUTION

Adverse Reactions to Busulfan

The main adverse reaction to busulfan is bone marrow suppression. This can result in the following:

- severe leukopenia (reduced white blood cells)
- anemia (reduced red blood cells)
- thrombocytopenia (reduced platelets)

However, this reaction is usually dose related and reversible.

- Taking busulfan together with thioguanine may cause liver toxicity, esophageal varices (enlarged, swollen veins in the esophagus), or portal hypertension (increased pressure in the portal vein of the liver).

Nitrosoureas

Nitrosoureas are alkylating agents that work by preventing cancer cells from multiplying. They are used in treating:

- brain tumors
- Hodgkin disease (as a secondary therapy)

During the process called bifunctional alkylation, nitrosoureas interfere with amino acids, purines, and DNA. Because these substances are needed for cancer cells to divide, this process stops the cells from reproducing.

The nitrosoureas are highly fat soluble. This allows them or their metabolites to cross the blood-brain barrier easily. That's good news for patients with brain tumors and meningeal leukemias.

Carmustine

Carmustine is manufactured as a powder for injection (BiCNU) and as an implant in wafer form (Gliadel wafer). It is typically used alone or with other antineoplastic drugs to treat:

- brain tumors
- multiple myeloma
- Hodgkin disease (as a secondary therapy)
- non-Hodgkin lymphomas (as a secondary therapy)

PROCEED WITH CAUTION

Adverse Reactions to Nitrosoureas

Adverse reactions to nitrosoureas may include:

- severe nausea and vomiting
- kidney toxicity
- kidney failure

The injectable form of carmustine may be given as a single dose or divided into daily injections over two days. It's normally given every six weeks as an IV drip. Before use, it must be mixed with the supplied diluent. This reconstituted solution remains stable at room temperature for eight hours. Unopened vials of the drug should be stored in a refrigerator.

The wafer form of carmustine is used as an adjunct to surgery and radiation in the treatment of gliomas. The wafers are used during surgery. After the tumor has been surgically removed, up to eight wafers are implanted in the cavity. The carmustine diffuses into the brain tissues. Double gloves are a necessary precaution when handling wafers. Carmustine can cause severe burning of the skin.

In terms of drug interactions, cimetidine may increase the bone marrow toxicity of carmustine. Adverse reactions to carmustine include:

- bone marrow suppression that begins four to six weeks after treatment and lasts one to two weeks
- reversible liver toxicity (caused by high doses of the drug)
- lung toxicity characterized by lung infiltrates or fibrosis (scarring)

Lomustine

Lomustine (CeeNU) is used alone or with other antineoplastic agents. It's manufactured as oral capsules. It's typically taken as a single oral dose every six weeks. Like carmustine, this drug may cause bone marrow suppression.

Streptozocin

In addition to its effectiveness for treating brain tumors and Hodgkin disease, streptozocin (Zanosar) can also be used to treat metastatic islet cell carcinoma of the pancreas. It's manufactured as a sterile powder for injection. It can be given by IV rapid injection or by IV infusion. A daily or weekly dosage schedule may be used. Streptozocin should be stored in a refrigerator and protected from light.

Streptozocin lengthens the elimination half-life of doxorubicin, prolonging leukopenia and thrombocytopenia.

Triazines

Dacarbazine (DTIC-Dome), a triazine, acts as an alkylating drug after being activated by the liver. It's mainly used to treat patients with malignant melanoma. It's also used with other drugs to treat Hodgkin disease.

First, dacarbazine must be metabolized in the liver to become an alkylating drug. It seems to block RNA and protein synthesis. Like other alkylating drugs, dacarbazine can affect the cell at any phase in the cell cycle.

This drug is manufactured as powder for injection. It must be reconstituted before use with sterile water. It's administered only by IV injection. Treatment typically lasts for five or ten days and may be repeated after a few weeks. The unopened drug should be stored in a refrigerator.

PROCEED WITH CAUTION

Adverse Reactions to Dacarbazine

Dacarbazine may cause some adverse reactions, such as:

- leukopenia
- thrombocytopenia
- nausea and vomiting (beginning one to three hours after administration and lasting up to twelve hours)
- phototoxicity
- flulike symptoms
- hair loss

However, the reconstituted solution may be stored at room temperature for eight hours or refrigerated for up to 72 hours.

No significant drug interactions have been reported with dacarbazine.

Ethylenimines

Thiotepa, an ethylenimine derivative, has several different therapeutic uses. It's used for:

- treatment of bladder cancer
- palliative treatment of lymphomas (cancers that begin in the immune system)
- palliative treatment of breast or ovarian cancers
- treatment of intracavitary effusions (fluid buildup in a body cavity)

Like other alkylating drugs, thiotepa interferes with DNA replication and RNA transcription. It disrupts the work of nucleic acids and causes cell death.

Thiotepa is manufactured as lyophilized powder for injection. It's administered by IV only. The powder must be reconstituted with sterile water before use. This reconstituted solution should be refrigerated and used within eight hours. It must be further diluted with water before use. The solution should be filtered though a 0.22-micrometer filter to eliminate haze.

Thiotepa can be given by rapid IV administration, intracavitary administration, or intravesical administration (inside the bladder). It's absorbed systemically when administered into pleural (around the lungs) or peritoneal (abdominal) spaces, or when instilled into the bladder. The dosing of this drug must be individualized for each patient.

Thiotepa may interact with other drugs.

- Using thiotepa with anticoagulants or aspirin may increase the risk of bleeding.
- Taking thiotepa with neuromuscular-blocking drugs may prolong muscular paralysis.
- Using thiotepa in conjunction with other alkylating drugs or radiation therapy may increase toxicity rather than improve the therapeutic response.

PROCEED WITH CAUTION

Adverse Reactions to Thiotepa

The major adverse reactions to thiotepa are blood related. They include:

- leukopenia
- anemia
- thrombocytopenia
- pancytopenia (deficiency of all cellular elements of the blood)

Other adverse reactions include:

- nausea and vomiting
- stomatitis and ulceration of the intestinal mucosa (especially at bone marrow transplantation doses)
- hives, rash, and pruritus

Alkylating-Like Drugs

Some neoplastic drugs are referred to as **alkylating-like drugs** because they have the same actions on the body as bifunctional alkylating drugs. These drugs are heavy metal complexes that contain platinum. Similar to bifunctional alkylating drugs, they cross-link DNA strands, which stops DNA from reproducing. They are also cell cycle nonspecific, meaning they can affect the cell at any phase in the cell cycle.

Alkylating-like drugs may be used in the treatment of several cancers, including:

- bladder cancer
- lung cancer
- ovarian cancer
- head and neck cancers
- colorectal cancer

The specific use varies for individual alkylating-like drugs.

Alkylating-like drugs interact with a few other drugs. However, administering an alkylating-like drug with an aminoglycoside increases the risk of toxicity to the kidney.

Carboplatin

Carboplatin is mainly used to treat ovarian cancer and lung cancer. It's available as an injection and lyophilized powder for injection. This drug is usually administered as an IV infusion.

Taking carboplatin with bumetanide, ethacrynic acid, or furosemide increases the risk of ototoxicity. Carboplatin may also cause the following adverse reactions:

- bone marrow suppression
- tinnitus and hearing loss

Cisplatin

Cisplatin (Platinol) is used in the treatment of:

- metastatic testicular tumors
- metastatic ovarian tumors
- advanced bladder cancer
- cancers of the head, neck, and lungs
- ovarian cancer

This drug is manufactured as an injection. It's administered by IV infusion over a period of six to eight hours. It should be protected from light.

Cisplatin has the following interactions with other drugs:

- Taking cisplatin with bumetanide, ethacrynic acid, or furosemide increases the risk of ototoxicity.
- Cisplatin may reduce levels of phenytoin in the blood.

In terms of adverse reactions, cisplatin may cause:

- kidney toxicity
- nausea and vomiting
- neurotoxicity
- tinnitus and hearing loss

Oxaliplatin

Oxaliplatin (Eloxatin) is used in combination with other agents to treat colorectal cancer. It's manufactured as an injection solution concentrate and is administered by IV infusion. It must be diluted before use with D5W. This final solution remains stable for six hours at room temperature or up to 24 hours in a refrigerator. It doesn't need to be protected from light after the final dilution.

Oxaliplatin may cause the following adverse reactions:

- anaphylaxis
- anemia
- increased risk of bleeding and infection

Some antineoplastics require refrigeration. It's important to know how the product must be stored in order to retrieve it or check if it's in stock. Table 14-1 indicates which of these drugs should be refrigerated.

ANTIMETABOLITE DRUGS

Antimetabolite drugs are cancer-fighting drugs similar in chemical structure to DNA base pairs. As a result, they may become involved in the synthesis of nucleic acids and proteins. However, they differ enough from the DNA base pairs to interfere with this synthesis. These drugs are cell cycle specific (they affect only a particular phase in the cell cycle). Because they mainly affect cells that are actively synthesizing DNA, they're called **S phase-specific** drugs. These drugs not only affect cancer cells, they can also affect normal cells that are reproducing actively.

TABLE 14-1   Drugs Requiring Refrigeration

Upon Receipt in Pharmacy Unopened	After Reconstitution/Dilution
estramustine	cyclophosphamide tablets (for oral solution)
melphalan	cyclophosphamide injection (for extended stability)
busulfan (injection)	ifosfamide injection
carmustine (injection)	busulfan injection (for extended stability)
streptozocin	dacarbazine injection (for extended stability)
dacarbazine	thiotepa (used within eight hours)
cytarabine liposomal (injection)	oxaliplatin (for extended stability)
cladribine	floxuridine
fludarabine	cladribine (for extended stability)
pentostatin	doxorubicin liposomal injection
daunorubicin	vinblastine
doxorubicin	rituximab
idarubicin (preservative-free injection)	trastuzumab
bleomycin	irinotecan (must be protected from light)
fulvestrant	arsenic trioxide (for extended stability)
leuprolide (depends on trade name)	asparaginase
vinblastine	interferon alfa-2b
vinorelbine (for extended stability)	aldesleukin
etoposide capsules	
teniposide	
alemtuzumab	
rituximab	
trastuzumab	
asparaginase	
pegaspargase	
interferon alfa-2b	
interferon alfa-n3	
aldesleukin	

S phase-specific antimetabolites are grouped into three main types:

- folic acid analogues
- pyrimidine analogues
- purine analogues

Folic Acid Analogues

Folic acid analogues are drugs that interfere with the way the body uses folic acid. Methotrexate is the most common of these drugs. It's especially useful in treating:

- acute lymphoblastic leukemia (abnormal growth of lymphoblasts, the cells that develop into lymphocytes)
- meningeal leukemia
- CNS diseases (given intrathecally, or through the spinal cord)
- choriocarcinoma (cancer that develops from the chorionic portions of the embryo)
- osteogenic sarcoma (bone cancer)
- malignant lymphomas
- cancers of the head, neck, bladder, testis, and breast

Methotrexate may also be prescribed in low doses to treat some disorders that don't respond to standard treatment. These disorders include:

- severe psoriasis
- graft versus host disease
- rheumatoid arthritis

Methotrexate acts by blocking the way folic acid is normally processed in the body. It blocks the action of the enzyme dihydrofolate reductase. This stops the synthesis of DNA and RNA, leading to cell death.

This drug can accumulate in any fluid collection, such as pleural or pericardial effusion (fluid in the space around the lungs or heart). This can result in longer than normal elimination and higher than expected toxicity, especially myelosuppression. The disappearance of methotrexate from plasma typically occurs in three phases:

- rapid distribution
- kidney clearance
- terminal half-life

The last phase, terminal half-life, is three to ten hours for a low dose and eight to fifteen hours for a high dose.

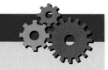

HOW IT WORKS

The Cell Cycle

Body tissues grow through the process of cell division. This complex process is regulated by a number of proteins inside the cell. During cell division, a cell replicates by dividing into two new daughter cells. This process involves a set of ordered steps, referred to as the *cell cycle*.

- During the G1 stage, the cell grows and prepares for replication. This phase is also called Gap 1.
- The S stage, or synthesis, is when the DNA molecule replicates.
- During the G2 stage, the cell is preparing for the M stage. This phase is also called Gap 2.
- During the M stage, mitosis, the chromosomes separate and the material inside the cell (the cytoplasm) divides.

Different cancers may affect different phases in the cell cycle, disrupting normal cell growth.

Methotrexate is manufactured as tablets (Trexall, Rheumatrex), injection solution, and powder for injection. Injectable methotrexate may be given using several different routes:

- intramuscular
- intravenous
- intra-arterial
- intrathecal

The preserved formulation contains benzyl alcohol and shouldn't be used for intrathecal or high-dose therapy. The lyophilized powder should be reconstituted immediately before using. The injection liquids may also be diluted if necessary. All forms of methotrexate are stored at room temperature.

Methotrexate interacts with several other drugs.

- Probenecid decreases methotrexate excretion, increasing the risk of methotrexate toxicity, including fatigue, bone marrow suppression, and stomatitis.
- Salicylates and NSAIDs, especially diclofenac, ketoprofen, indomethacin, and naproxen, also increase methotrexate toxicity.
- Cholestyramine reduces absorption of methotrexate from the GI tract.
- Taking alcohol with methotrexate increases the risk of liver toxicity.
- Cotrimoxazole, when taken with methotrexate, may produce blood cell abnormalities.
- Penicillin decreases the kidneys' secretion of methotrexate, which increases the risk of methotrexate toxicity.

Pyrimidine Analogues

Pyrimidine analogues kill cancer cells by interfering with the natural function of pyrimidine nucleotides (chemicals

! PROCEED WITH CAUTION

Adverse Reactions to Methotrexate

Adverse reactions to methotrexate include:

- bone marrow suppression
- stomatitis
- pulmonary toxicity, shown as pneumonitis (inflammation of lung tissue) or pulmonary fibrosis (scarring of lung tissue)
- skin reactions, such as photosensitivity and hair loss

With high doses, kidney toxicity can also occur. During high-dose therapy, leucovorin (folinic acid) may be used in a technique known as leucovorin rescue to minimize adverse reactions.

Adverse reactions to intrathecal administration may include:

- seizures
- paralysis
- death

Other less severe adverse reactions may also occur, such as:

- headaches
- fever
- neck stiffness
- confusion
- irritability

used in building DNA). These drugs are used to treat many tumors. However, they're mainly used in treatments for:

- acute leukemias (cancers that start in blood-forming tissues such as bone marrow)
- GI tract adenocarcinomas (cancers that develop in the lining of an organ), such as colorectal, pancreatic, esophageal, and stomach adenocarcinomas
- cancers of the breast and ovaries
- malignant lymphomas

No significant drug interactions occur with most of the pyrimidine analogues.

AT THE COUNTER

False Assumptions

A patient drops off a prescription for methotrexate. Can you automatically assume that the patient has cancer and the methotrexate is being prescribed for that purpose?

No. Although methotrexate is useful in treating different types of leukemia and cancer, it's also used to treat psoriasis and rheumatoid arthritis, among other things.

PROCEED WITH CAUTION

Adverse Reactions to Pyrimidine Analogues

Like most antineoplastic drugs, pyrimidine analogues can cause:

- fatigue and lack of energy
- inflammation of the mouth, esophagus, and throat
- bone marrow suppression
- nausea and anorexia

Capecitabine

Capecitabine (Xeloda) is manufactured in tablet form. It's used to treat the following:

- colorectal cancer
- breast cancer
- pancreatic cancer (adjunctive treatment)

Capecitabine is typically administered in three-week cycles. It's given twice a day, morning and evening, for two weeks. This is followed by a one-week rest.

Capecitabine has several possible interactions with other drugs.

- Antacids may increase absorption of capecitabine.
- Capecitabine may increase the effects of warfarin, increasing the risk of bleeding.
- Capecitabine may increase blood levels of phenytoin.

Cytarabine

Cytarabine is administered by injection. It is typically used in treating leukemias in adults and children. It's available as a powder and as a solution. It may be given by SubQ injection, IV infusion, or intrathecally (using the preservative-free preparation). One preparation is specifically for liposomal injection. Reconstituted solutions (with bacteriostatic water and benzyl alcohol) may be stored at controlled room temperature for 48 hours. However, the preparation for liposomal injection must be refrigerated.

In addition to the adverse reactions common to other pyrimidine analogues, cytarabine may cause:

- severe cerebellar neurotoxicity
- chemical conjunctivitis
- diarrhea
- fever
- hand-foot syndrome (a reaction characterized by redness, tenderness, and peeling of the soles of the feet and palms of the hands)
- crab erythema (a type of rash that occurs when high-dose cytarabine is combined with continuous infusions of fluorouracil)

Floxuridine

Floxuridine (FUDR) has been used in the treatment of tumors in the liver, ovaries, or kidneys. Its main use is in treat-

HOW IT WORKS

How Pyrimidine Analogues Work

To understand how pyrimidine analogues work, it's helpful to think about the basic structure of DNA.

DNA looks like a ladder that has been twisted. The rungs of the ladder are made up of pairs of nitrogen-containing bases. These pairs are always the same:

- Adenine always pairs with thymine.
- Guanine always pairs with cytosine.

Cytosine and thymine are pyrimidines. Adenine and guanine are purines.

The basic unit of DNA is the nucleotide. A nucleotide is the building block of nucleic acids. It has three main parts:

- a sugar
- a nitrogen-containing base
- a phosphate group

Pyrimidine analogues do their work on these components.

After pyrimidine analogues are converted into nucleotides, they're incorporated into DNA. Once in DNA, pyrimidine analogues act to block DNA and RNA synthesis. They may also inhibit other metabolic actions needed for proper cell growth.

ing GI adenocarcinoma (cancer that develops in the lining of an organ) that has metastasized to the liver.

This drug is manufactured as lyophilized powder. The powder is reconstituted with sterile water. Once reconstituted, it can be refrigerated for up to two weeks. Administration by continuous arterial infusion is recommended for the hepatic artery (artery in the liver).

Fluorouracil

Typically, fluorouracil is used in palliative treatment of cancers of:

- colon
- rectum
- breast
- stomach
- pancreas

It may also be used in treating ovarian, cervical, bladder, hepatic, prostate, endometrial, esophageal, and head and neck cancers.

Fluorouracil is administered by IV injection (Adrucil). This drug doesn't require dilution. Fluorouracil is also manufactured as a topical cream (Carac, Fluoroplex, Efudex) and topical solution (Efudex) for the treatment of keratoses (skin lesions) of the face and scalp.

The injectable form of fluorouracil may cause the following adverse reactions, in addition to those typical of other pyrimidine analogues:

- diarrhea
- hair loss

Gemcitabine

Gemcitabine (Gemzar) is used in the treatment of cancers of:

- breast
- lungs
- ovary
- pancreas

It's manufactured as lyophilized powder for injection. It should be reconstituted with sodium chloride 0.9 percent. This drug is given only by IV injection and may be administered on an outpatient basis. The reconstituted solution remains stable at room temperature for 24 hours.

Purine Analogues

Purine analogues are used to treat acute and chronic leukemias. They may also be useful in the treatment of lymphomas. Similar to pyrimidine analogues, purine analogues become part of DNA and RNA. They are then able to interfere with the synthesis and replication of nucleic acids.

As with the other antimetabolites, the drugs are first converted through a process called phosphorylation. This allows them to be active at the nucleotide level. The resulting nucleotides are incorporated into DNA. There they inhibit DNA and RNA synthesis, as well as other metabolic reactions needed for cell growth. Purine analogues are cell cycle specific, exerting their effect during the S phase.

Cladribine

Cladribine (Leustatin) is manufactured as a solution for injection. It's mainly used in treating leukemias. The typical course of treatment is a continuous IV infusion for seven consecutive days. The treatment is not repeated. The infusion must be prepared with bacteriostatic NS and filtered. Once diluted, the solution should be given promptly. However, it can be refrigerated for up to eight hours before administration. Unopened vials of cladribine must also be refrigerated.

Fludarabine

Like many other purine analogues, fludarabine (Fludara) preparations are administered intravenously over a period of time. They are manufactured as an injection and as powder for injection. This drug is usually given for five consecutive days, with a break of 28 days between treatments. Fludarabine must be stored in a refrigerator.

Taking fludarabine with pentostatin may cause severe pulmonary toxicity, which can be fatal. In addition to the adverse reactions noted for all purine analogues, fludarabine may cause severe neurological effects when used at high doses, including:

- blindness
- coma
- death

Mercaptopurine

Mercaptopurine (Purinethol) is given orally as tablets. It may be taken once a day. This drug may have delayed action, and dosing may depend on the patient's leukocyte or platelet count. Taking mercaptopurine and allopurinol together may decrease the metabolism of mercaptopurine, resulting in increased bone marrow suppression.

Pentostatin

Pentostatin (Nipent) comes as a powder for IV solution. It's administered by an IV bolus or diluted and given over a period of 20 to 30 minutes. Normally, pentostatin therapy is given once every other week. After six months, the patient's response to treatment should be assessed. Pentostatin is stored in the refrigerator. Diluted or reconstituted pentostatin can be stable at room temperature, but must be used within eight hours.

Pentostatin works differently than other purine analogues. It blocks the action of adenosine deaminase (ADA). This causes an increase in levels of deoxyadenosine triphosphate in cells, leading to cell damage and death. The greatest activity of ADA is in the lymphoid system, especially on malignant T cells.

Pentostatin has several drug interactions that are different from other purine analogue drugs.

- Taking pentostatin with allopurinol may increase the risk of rash.
- Taking pentostatin with vidarabine may enhance the effect of vidarabine and increase the risk of toxicity.

T I P Whereas most drugs ending in the suffix -*statin* are used to reduce cholesterol, it's important to remember that this is not always the rule. You just learned, for example, that pentostatin is used to treat acute and chronic leukemia, not high cholesterol.

Thioguanine

Thioguanine (Tabloid) is often used in combination with other antineoplastic agents. It's manufactured as oral tablets. The entire daily dose may be taken at one time. After four weeks, the patient should be reassessed, and the dosage may be increased.

PROCEED WITH CAUTION

Adverse Reactions to Purine Analogues

Purine analogues can cause:

- bone marrow suppression
- nausea and vomiting
- anorexia
- mild diarrhea
- stomatitis
- a rise in uric acid levels (a result of the breakdown of purine)

ANTIBIOTIC ANTINEOPLASTIC DRUGS

Antibiotic antineoplastic drugs are antimicrobial products that bind with DNA to produce tumor-destroying effects. These drugs block cellular processes in normal and malignant cells. Antibiotic antineoplastic drugs act against many cancers, including:

- acute leukemia
- breast, ovarian, bladder, and lung cancer
- cancers of the GI tract
- choriocarcinoma
- Ewing sarcoma (a malignant tumor that originates in bone marrow, typically in long bones or the pelvis) and other soft-tissue sarcomas
- Hodgkin disease and malignant lymphomas
- melanoma
- osteogenic sarcoma
- rhabdomyosarcoma (malignant neoplasm composed of striated muscle cells)
- squamous cell carcinoma of the head, neck, and cervix
- testicular cancer
- Wilms tumor (a malignant neoplasm of the kidney, occurring in young children)

Sometimes, these drugs may be administered directly into the body cavity being treated.

Antibiotic antineoplastic drugs typically intercalate, or insert themselves, between side-by-side base pairs of a DNA molecule. This causes the base pairs to separate. Then, when the DNA chain replicates, an extra base pair opposes the intercalated antibiotic. This creates a mutant DNA molecule. The overall effect is cell death.

Not surprisingly, these drugs may interact with many other drugs. In particular, combination chemotherapies enhance leukopenia and thrombocytopenia (reduced number of platelets in bloodstream).

Daunorubicin

Daunorubicin is used as part of a treatment regimen with other antineoplastic drugs to induce remission in acute leukemias. It's available as an injection (Cerubidine) and as

PROCEED WITH CAUTION

Adverse Reactions to Antibiotic Antineoplastic Drugs

The main adverse reaction to antibiotic antineoplastic drugs is bone marrow suppression. Other effects include:

- irreversible cardiomyopathy
- acute electrocardiogram changes
- nausea and vomiting

lyophilized powder that must be reconstituted with sterile water for injection (Daunoxome). The reconstituted solution can be stored at room temperature for up to 24 hours. It must be given in a rapidly flowing IV infusion.

Daunorubicin, as a liposomal injection, is used in therapy for advanced HIV-associated Kaposi sarcoma. Administration is intravenous over a one-hour period, once every two weeks. The reconstituted solution can be stored for six hours in a refrigerator. Unopened vials of all forms of the drug must be refrigerated.

> **TIP** Liposomal injections and conventional injections are different formulations. They can't be substituted for one another.

Doxorubicin

Doxorubicin (Adriamycin, Doxil) is manufactured as a lyophilized powder for injection, a preservative-free injection, and as an aqueous injection. It's administered intravenously only. As a single agent, it's commonly administered once every 21 days. Sometimes, it may be given as a topical bladder instillation.

The unopened solution must be refrigerated. The unopened powder, however, is stored at room temperature. Before use, the powdered form should be reconstituted with a sodium chloride injection. This reconstituted solution can be stored for seven days at room temperature.

Doxorubicin is also manufactured as a liposomal injection. This form is used in treating:

- AIDS-related Kaposi sarcoma
- multiple myeloma
- ovarian cancer

Unopened vials of liposomal doxorubicin must be refrigerated. Diluted liposomal doxorubicin must also be stored in a refrigerator. It should be administered within 24 hours.

Doxorubicin may reduce blood levels of digoxin. In addition to the adverse reactions common to all antibiotic antineoplastic drugs, doxorubicin may color urine red.

Idarubicin

Idarubicin (Idamycin PFS) is used in combination with other antineoplastic drugs to treat acute myeloid leukemia in adults. It's manufactured as an injection and must be given as a freely flowing IV infusion. The vials should be reconstituted with water. (Bacteriostatic diluents are not recommended.) The reconstituted solution must be used within 72 hours. It's stable at room temperature and under refrigeration. Unopened idarubicin is stored at room temperature or, in the case of the preservative-free injection, in the refrigerator.

In terms of drug interactions, concurrent therapy with fludarabine isn't recommended because of the risk of fatal lung toxicity.

Bleomycin

Bleomycin (Blenoxane) is considered a palliative treatment. It's used as a single agent or in combination with other antineoplastic drugs to treat:

- squamous cell carcinoma
- lymphomas
- testicular carcinoma

Anaphylactic reactions can occur in patients receiving bleomycin for lymphoma, so test doses should be given first. An antihistamine and an antipyretic should be given before bleomycin is administered to prevent fever and chills.

Bleomycin may be given by IV, IM, or SubQ injection. Solutions of bleomycin are prepared with sterile water, sodium chloride, or sterile bacteriostatic water. When diluted with sodium chloride, the reconstituted solution can be stored at room temperature for 24 hours. The unopened sterile powder should be refrigerated.

Bleomycin may interact with other substances. It may decrease serum levels of digoxin and phenytoin.

Dactinomycin

Dactinomycin (Cosmegen) is often administered as part of a combination therapy with other antineoplastic drugs. It's used in treatment for:

- Wilms tumor
- Ewing sarcoma
- testicular cancer
- solid malignancies

This drug is available as powder for injection. It's administered intravenously, depending on the tolerance of the patient. This drug is highly corrosive to soft tissues and must be handled and administered carefully. Before use, it should be reconstituted with sterile water.

Mitomycin

Mitomycin works differently than other antibiotic antineoplastic drugs. It's activated inside the cell to a bifunctional or even trifunctional alkylating drug. Mitomycin causes single strands of DNA to break. It also cross-links with DNA and blocks DNA synthesis.

Mitomycin is most often used in combination with other chemotherapy agents to treat cancers of the stomach or pancreas. It has also been used in treating the following cancers:

- bladder
- colon and rectum
- breast
- head
- neck
- lung
- cervix

In addition, mitomycin may be used as palliative treatment when other therapies have failed.

This drug comes as a powder that must be reconstituted before injection. It is only administered intravenously. The powder is reconstituted with sterile water. The reconstituted drug must be used within 24 hours. The dry powder should be protected from light.

Mitomycin interacts with vinca alkaloids. Using vinca alkaloids with mitomycin can cause acute respiratory distress.

Mitoxantrone

In combination with other antineoplastic drugs, mitoxantrone (Novantrone) is used in treating acute nonlymphocytic leukemias. Other cancers that may respond to mitoxantrone therapy include the following:

- prostate cancer
- breast cancer
- non-Hodgkin lymphoma

In addition, mitoxantrone may be used in therapy for multiple sclerosis.

This drug is manufactured as an injection. It must be diluted before use with D5W or NS. The diluted drug should be used immediately. Mitoxantrone is administered by IV only. It's given slowly into a freely flowing IV infusion.

In addition to the adverse reactions common to all antibiotic antineoplastic drugs, mitoxantrone may color urine blue-green.

HORMONAL ANTINEOPLASTIC DRUGS AND HORMONE MODULATORS

Hormonal antineoplastic drugs and hormone modulators are prescribed for the following reasons:

- to change the growth of malignant tumors
- to manage and treat the physiological effects of malignant tumors

Hormonal therapies and hormone modulators are effective against hormone-dependent tumors, such as cancers of:

- breast
- prostate
- endometrium (the lining of the uterus)

Lymphomas and leukemias are usually treated with therapies that include corticosteroids. This is due to the drugs' potential for affecting lymphocytes (certain white blood cells).

Aromatase Inhibitors

In postmenopausal women, estrogen is produced through an enzyme called aromatase. Aromatase converts hormone precursors into estrogen. **Aromatase inhibitors** prevent androgen from being converted into estrogen in postmenopausal women. This blocks estrogen's ability to activate cancer cells. Limiting the amount of estrogen means that less estrogen is available to reach cancer cells and make them grow.

 Hormone-dependent (gender-specific) tumors are treated with hormonal therapies. Tumors common to both genders are treated with corticosteroids.

Aromatase inhibitors are mainly used to treat metastatic breast cancer in postmenopausal women. They may be administered alone or with other agents, such as tamoxifen.

Aromatase inhibitors work by lowering the body's production of estrogen. In about half of all patients with breast cancer, the tumors depend on estrogen to grow. Aromatase inhibitors are used only in postmenopausal women because they lower the amount of estrogen produced outside the ovaries (such as in muscle and fat tissue). Because these drugs cause estrogen deprivation, patients may develop bone thinning and osteoporosis over time.

There are two types of aromatase inhibitors: type 1, or steroidal, inhibitors and type 2, or nonsteroidal, inhibitors.

Steroidal Inhibitors

Steroidal inhibitors (or type 1 inhibitors) have an irreversible effect on the enzyme aromatase. That means that once they act on the enzyme, estrogen production is lowered permanently. Exemestane (Aromasin) is a steroidal inhibitor.

In addition to its uses in breast cancer treatment, exemestane has been used to prevent the development of prostate cancer. It's manufactured as tablets. The tablets are usually taken once a day, after a meal.

Nonsteroidal Inhibitors

Nonsteroidal inhibitors are sometimes called type 2 inhibitors. Their effects on the enzyme aromatase are reversible. That means that after treatment, aromatase can return to normal function.

These drugs work by competitively binding to part of the enzyme aromatase. They bind to a portion of the cytochrome P450 (CYP450) enzyme. This leads to decreased estrogen in all body tissues. However, these drugs don't affect the synthesis of adrenocorticoids, aldosterone, or thyroid hormones.

Anastrozole

Anastrozole (Arimidex) is manufactured as tablets for oral administration. It's normally taken once a day.

This drug may cause adverse reactions in addition to those for other aromatase inhibitors. It may elevate both high-density and low-density lipoprotein levels. In terms of drug interactions, certain drugs may decrease anastrozole's effectiveness, including tamoxifen and estrogen-containing drugs.

Letrozole

Letrozole (Femara) is prescribed as tablets, which are taken once a day. Treatment is stopped when tumors relapse. An alternative use for letrozole is to stimulate ovaries and improve the chances of pregnancy for women of childbearing age.

Antiestrogens

Antiestrogens bind to estrogen receptors and block the action of estrogen. These drugs are used to treat breast cancer.

The exact antineoplastic action of these agents isn't known. However, they're known to act as estrogen antagonists. Estrogen receptors, found in the cancer cells of one-half of premenopausal and three-fourths of postmenopausal women with breast cancer, respond to estrogen to induce tumor growth. If the action of estrogen is blocked, this will slow the growth of the tumor cells and block DNA synthesis.

Fulvestrant

Fulvestrant (Faslodex) is a pure estrogen antagonist. It's used in postmenopausal women with receptor-positive metastatic breast cancer that has progressed after treatment with tamoxifen.

This drug is administered as a monthly injection. The injection is given intramuscularly, slowly into the buttock.

 PROCEED WITH CAUTION

Adverse Reactions to Aromatase Inhibitors

Adverse reactions to aromatase inhibitors are rare. They may include:

- dizziness
- mild nausea
- mild muscle and joint aches
- hot flashes

Occasionally, aromatase inhibitors can also affect cholesterol levels.

PROCEED WITH CAUTION

Adverse Reactions to Antiestrogens

The most common adverse reactions to antiestrogens include:

- hot flashes
- nausea
- vomiting

The unopened injection should be refrigerated. Fulvestrant has no known drug interactions. However, it may cause adverse reactions, such as:

- diarrhea
- constipation
- abdominal pain
- headache
- backache
- pharyngitis

These are in addition to the adverse reactions common to all antiestrogens.

Tamoxifen

Tamoxifen (Soltamox) is an estrogen agonist-antagonist. It has several main uses.

- It's used alone and in combination with radiation therapy and surgery *in women* whose breast cancer hasn't spread to the axillary lymph nodes (glands in the armpit).
- It may be used in treating *postmenopausal women* whose cancer has spread from the breast to the axillary lymph nodes.
- It may be used as palliative treatment of advanced or metastatic breast cancer that is estrogen receptor positive.
- It may be used to reduce the likelihood of breast cancer in women who are at high risk.

Tamoxifen is manufactured as tablets and oral solution. It may be taken once or twice a day in divided doses, depending on the size of the dose.

T I P Tamoxifen tablets should be shielded from all sources of light.

Tamoxifen may interact with other drugs.

- Tamoxifen increases the effects of warfarin, increasing the risk of bleeding.
- Bromocriptine increases the effects of tamoxifen.
- Antacids may affect the absorption of tamoxifen in its enteric-coated tablet form.

Adverse effects of tamoxifen include:

- diarrhea
- fluid retention
- leukopenia or thrombocytopenia

Androgens

The therapeutically useful **androgens** are synthetic derivatives of the naturally occurring male hormone testosterone. These Schedule III controlled substances are used for palliative treatment of advanced breast cancer, especially in postmenopausal women with bone metastasis.

Androgens probably act in one or more different ways.

- They may reduce the number of prolactin receptors (receptors for the pituitary hormone prolactin that affects glands in the breast) or may bind competitively to the available prolactin receptors.
- They may block the synthesis of estrogen or competitively bind at estrogen receptors. These actions prevent estrogen from affecting estrogen-sensitive tumors.

Androgens may interact with some other drugs.

- They may alter dosing requirements in patients receiving insulin, antidiabetic drugs, or oral anticoagulants.
- They may increase the risk of liver toxicity when taken with drugs that are toxic to the liver.

Fluoxymesterone

Fluoxymesterone (Androxy) is manufactured as tablets. Normally, this drug is taken as a single daily dose or in divided doses.

Testolactone

Testolactone (Teslac) is available as tablets. It's typically taken four times a day for a minimum of three months.

! PROCEED WITH CAUTION

Adverse Reactions to Androgens

The most common adverse reactions to androgens are:

- nausea
- vomiting
- fluid retention (caused by sodium retention)

Women may develop:

- acne
- clitoral hyptertrophy (abnormal enlargement of the clitoris)
- deeper voice
- increased facial and body hair
- increased sexual desire
- menstrual irregularity

Men may experience several effects as a result of conversion of steroids to female sex hormone metabolites. These include:

- gynecomastia (breast enlargement in the male)
- prostatic hyperplasia (excessive cell growth of the prostate gland)
- testicular atrophy (reduction in testicle size)

Children may develop:

- premature epiphyseal closure (closure of the growth plates in the long bones)
- secondary sex characteristic developments (especially in boys)

Testosterone

Testosterone enanthate (in oil) (Andro LA, Delatestryl) is manufactured as an injection solution. It's administered by deep IM injection into the gluteal muscle. The drug has a long duration of action and doesn't need to be given more often than every two weeks. This injection should be stored at room temperature. If any crystals have formed in the vial, they can be redissolved by warming the vial between the palms of the hands.

Testosterone used as hormone replacement therapy is manufactured in a topical gel (Androgel, Testim), an injection, a transdermal patch (Androderm), a buccal tablet (Striant), and an implant (Testopel Pellet). Another form of testosterone not used in the treatment of cancer is testosterone cypionate (Depo-Testosterone), and it is manufactured as an injection. Testosterone propionate (First-Testosterone MC, First-Testosterone) is available as a topical cream and a topical ointment.

Antiandrogens

Antiandrogens are drugs that block the action of androgen, a male hormone. They're used as an adjunct therapy with gonadotropin-releasing hormone analogues in treating advanced prostate cancer. These drugs either block the uptake of androgen or prevent androgen binding in cell nuclei. Administering antiandrogens with a gonadotropin-releasing hormone analogue helps prevent the disease flare-up that occurs when the gonadotropin-releasing hormone analogue is used alone.

Bicalutamide

Bicalutamide (Casodex) is manufactured as tablets. It's normally taken once a day, with or without food.

In terms of drug interactions, bicalutamide may affect prothrombin time (a test to measure clotting factors) in patients who are taking warfarin.

 PROCEED WITH CAUTION

Adverse Reactions to Antiandrogens

When antiandrogens are used with gonadotropin-releasing hormone analogues, the most common adverse reactions are:

- hot flashes
- decreased sexual desire
- impotence
- diarrhea
- nausea
- vomiting
- breast enlargement

Flutamide

Flutamide is available as capsules. It's typically administered three times a day at eight-hour intervals. Flutamide is dispensed in a light-resistant container.

Like bicalutamide, flutamide may affect prothrombin time in patients who are taking warfarin.

Nilutamide

When being treated with nilutamide (Nilandron), patients take oral tablets. A higher dose is usually prescribed for the first 30 days, and then the dose is reduced. Nilutamide is taken once a day, with or without food. It should be protected from light and stored at a controlled room temperature.

Progestins

Progestins are hormones that are used for palliative treatment of several forms of cancer, including:

- endometrial cancer
- breast cancer
- renal cancer

As you learned in Chapter 12, the term *progestins* also refers to substances that mimic the effects of the naturally occurring hormone progesterone.

The way progestins act to treat tumors isn't completely understood. Researchers think the drugs bind to a specific receptor to act on hormonally sensitive cells. Because they don't exhibit a cytotoxic activity (destroying or poisoning cells), they're considered cytostatic (they keep the cells from multiplying).

Medroxyprogesterone

Medroxyprogesterone is used for adjunctive and palliative therapy of endometrial or renal cancer. It's manufactured as an injection for IM administration (Depo-Provera, Depo-subQ Provera, Depo-Provera Contraceptive). It's also available as tablets (Provera) for treating menstrual irregularities and abnormal uterine bleeding. An unlabeled use of the tablets is for treatment of advanced breast cancer.

 PROCEED WITH CAUTION

Adverse Reactions to Progestins

Mild fluid retention is probably the most common adverse reaction to progestins. Other adverse reactions include:

- thromboemboli (blood clots)
- breakthrough bleeding, spotting, and changes in menstrual flow
- breast tenderness
- liver function abnormalities

Medroxyprogesterone has several interactions with other drugs.

- Aminoglutethimide and rifampin reduce the progestin effects of medroxyprogesterone.
- Medroxyprogesterone may interfere with the effects of bromocriptine, causing menstruation to stop.

In addition to the adverse reactions common to all progestins, reactions to medroxyprogesterone may include:

- drowsiness
- fever
- rash
- weight gain or loss

Megestrol

Megestrol tablets are used for palliative treatment of breast or endometrial cancer. It's also manufactured as an oral suspension (Megace) for use in treating anorexia, cachexia (loss of body weight and muscle mass), and unexplained weight loss in patients with AIDS.

Unlike other progestins, no drug interactions have been identified for megestrol.

Gonadotropin-Releasing Hormone Analogues

Gonadotropin-releasing hormone analogues are used for palliative treatment of advanced prostate cancer. These drugs lower the testosterone level in the body without the adverse psychological effects of castration or the adverse cardiovascular effects of diethylstilbestrol (another drug used to treat inoperable prostate cancer).

Most gonadotropin-releasing hormone analogues work by acting on the male pituitary gland. They increase luteinizing hormone (LH) secretion, which stimulates testosterone production. The peak testosterone level is reached about 72 hours after daily administration.

 PROCEED WITH CAUTION

Adverse Reactions to Gonadotropin-Releasing Hormone Analogues

Commonly reported adverse reactions to gonadotropin-releasing hormone analogues are:

- hot flashes
- impotence
- decreased sexual desire

Other adverse reactions may include:

- peripheral edema
- nausea and vomiting
- constipation
- anorexia

However, with long-term administration, these drugs inhibit LH release from the pituitary gland. This inhibits or blocks the release of testosterone from the testicles. Because prostate tumor cells are stimulated by testosterone, the reduced testosterone level slows their growth.

No drug interactions have been identified for gonadotropin-releasing hormone analogues.

Goserelin

In addition to its use as a palliative treatment for prostate cancer, goserelin (Zoladex) may be used for palliative treatment of advanced breast cancer. Goserelin is manufactured as a monthly or three-month implant. It comes in a sterile, sealed foil pouch containing a desiccant capsule.

Goserelin is administered by SubQ injection on a twenty-eight–day or three-month schedule. For the first eight days of therapy, the drug is absorbed slowly. After eight days, however, it is absorbed rapidly and continuously.

Leuprolide

There are different injectable forms of leuprolide (Lupron Depot, Lupron, Eligard). It's available as an injection, a powder for injection, and as a three-, four-, or six-month depot (microspheres that must be reconstituted with diluent before injection).

Different brands of leuprolide may be administered differently, either by SubQ or IM injection. Because they are released differently, the different forms of leuprolide are not interchangeable.

The leuprolide injection is stored below room temperature. However, different brands of leuprolide depot have different storage requirements. For example, Lupron is stored at room temperature, whereas Eligard must be refrigerated.

Triptorelin

Triptorelin (Trelstar Depot, Trelstar LA) is manufactured as microgranules for injection. The microgranules may be incorporated into a depot formulation and given as a monthly IM injection. The microgranules of triptorelin may also be manufactured as a long-acting formulation. This form is administered every 84 days as an IM injection. Both forms of triptorelin must be reconstituted with sterile water before use.

Triptorelin works differently than other gonadotropin-releasing hormone analogues. It acts to block gonadotropin secretion. After the first dose, levels of LH, follicle-stimulating hormone (FSH), testosterone, and estradiol surge briefly. After long-term continuous administration, LH and FSH secretion steadily drops. Testicular and ovarian production of steroids decrease. In men, testosterone drops to a level normally seen in surgically castrated men. As a result, tissues and functions that depend on these hormones become inactive. The decreased testosterone levels slow tumor growth.

Triptorelin may cause skeletal pain. Less commonly, it may also cause:

- hypertension
- diarrhea
- urine retention

These side effects are in addition to the adverse reactions noted for other gonadotropin-releasing hormone analogues.

NATURAL ANTINEOPLASTIC DRUGS

Some antineoplastic drugs are known as **natural products**. They are derived from natural substances and directly affect cell processes.

Vinca Alkaloids

Vinca alkaloids are nitrogenous bases derived from the periwinkle plant. They are used to treat several different types of cancer, which include:

- metastatic testicular cancer
- breast cancer
- Hodgkin disease

They act to disrupt the normal function of microtubules in cells. Microtubules are structures that are involved in the movement of DNA. Vinca alkaloids disrupt their function by binding to a protein called microtubulin in the microtubules. As a result, the microtubules can't separate chromosomes properly. The chromosomes spread out through the cytoplasm (fluid inside the cell) or form unusual groupings. This stops the mitotic spindle from forming, which is needed for cell division. The cells can't complete the process of mitosis (cell division), and the cells die. This is why vinca alkaloids are said to be cell cycle specific for the M phase.

Disrupting the microtubules may also affect some types of cell movement, phagocytosis (engulfing and destroying microorganisms and cellular debris), and CNS functions.

! PROCEED WITH CAUTION

Adverse Reactions to Vinca Alkaloids

Patients taking vinca alkaloids may experience:

- nausea
- vomiting
- constipation
- stomatitis (sores or inflammation in the mouth)
- neuromuscular abnormalities
- reversible alopecia (hair loss)

Vinblastine

Vinblastine is used for palliative treatment of several different cancers, including:

- metastatic testicular cancer
- lymphomas
- Kaposi sarcoma (the most commonly occurring AIDS-related cancer)
- breast cancer
- neuroblastoma (a highly malignant tumor in the sympathetic nervous system)
- choriocarcinoma

It's manufactured as an injection and as a powder for injection. Administration is by IV only. It's injected into a running IV infusion or directly into a vein over a period of one minute. Bacteriostatic sodium chloride injection must be added to the powder before injection. The reconstituted solution can be refrigerated for 28 days. Unopened vinblastine should also be refrigerated.

Vinblastine may interact with other drugs.

- Erythromycin may increase the toxicity of vinblastine.
- Vinblastine decreases plasma levels of phenytoin.

It also causes adverse reactions in addition to those for all vinca alkaloids.

- Vinblastine may produce intense stinging or burning in the tumor bed one to three minutes after administration. The pain usually lasts 20 minutes to 3 hours.
- Vinblastine suppresses bone marrow function.

Vincristine

Vincristine (Vincasar PFS) is used in combination therapy to treat:

- Hodgkin disease
- non-Hodgkin lymphoma
- Wilms tumor
- cancer in muscle tissues

It's also used in treating acute lymphocytic leukemia.

Vincristine is manufactured as an injection. It's administered by IV only, once a week. Like vinblastine, it's given directly into a vein or into the tubing of a running IV infusion over the course of one minute.

Vincristine has several interactions with other drugs.

- Vincristine reduces the effects of digoxin.
- Asparaginase decreases liver metabolism of vincristine, increasing the risk of toxicity.
- Calcium channel blockers boost vincristine accumulation, increasing the risk of toxicity.

In addition to the adverse reactions common to all vinca alkaloids, vincristine can result in bone marrow suppression.

Vinorelbine

Like other vinca alkaloids, vinorelbine (Navelbine) is administered by IV only. It's manufactured as an injection. This drug is used in treating several conditions, including small-cell lung cancer, metastatic breast cancer, ovarian cancer, and Hodgkin disease. It's usually administered weekly as an IV injection over a period of six to ten minutes. Unopened vinorelbine should be refrigerated and protected from light. However, the unopened vials are stable at temperatures up to 25 degrees C (77 degrees F) for up to 72 hours.

Podophyllotoxins

Podophyllotoxins are semisynthetic glycosides (sugar-containing chemicals that are activated by an enzyme). They are cell cycle specific and act during the G2 and late S phases of the cell cycle.

Although their mechanism of action isn't well understood, podophyllotoxins produce several changes in tumor cells.

- At low concentrations, these drugs block cells at the late S or G2 phase.
- At higher concentrations, they stop cells in the G2 phase.
- Podophyllotoxins can also break one of the strands of the DNA molecule. They block the transport of nucleotides and the process of incorporating them into nucleic acids.

Podophyllotoxins have few significant interactions with other drugs.

⚠ PROCEED WITH CAUTION

Adverse Reactions to Podophyllotoxins

The majority of patients who receive podophyllotoxins experience hair loss. That's because antineoplastic drugs have a systemic effect—they affect all cells in the body, not just cancer cells. Some areas of the body have cells that are growing and dividing at a fast rate, like cancer cells do. These areas of the body, including the mouth and stomach linings and the hair follicles, are especially sensitive.

Hair loss doesn't occur with all antineoplastic drugs. It depends on the drug, the dosage, and the patient.

Other adverse reactions include:

- nausea and vomiting
- anorexia
- stomatitis
- bone marrow suppression, causing leukopenia and, less commonly, thrombocytopenia
- acute hypotension (if a podophyllotoxin is infused intravenously too rapidly)

Etoposide

Etoposide (Toposar, Etopophos) is effective in the treatment of testicular cancer, non-Hodgkin lymphoma, lung cancer, and acute leukemia. It's available as vials or powder for injection. It's also available as capsules. Oral etoposide capsules must be handled with care and dispensed in child-resistant containers. It's important to wear gloves when handling this drug. The capsules are usually taken for four or five days. Etoposide capsules can be stored in a refrigerator for up to 24 months.

The etoposide injection is administered by IV. It may be given in cycles, with a three- to four-week interval between therapy courses. Etoposide should be diluted before use. The solution is typically administered over a 30- to 60-minute period. The diluted injection solution is stable for up to 96 hours at room temperature.

In addition to the adverse reactions common to all podophyllotoxins, etoposide may increase the risk of bleeding in patients taking warfarin.

Teniposide

Teniposide (Vumon) has shown some activity in treating Hodgkin disease, lymphomas, and brain tumors. It's manufactured as an injection and administered intravenously. Unopened ampules of teniposide must be refrigerated.

Teniposide may increase the clearance and intracellular levels of methotrexate.

T I P Undiluted teniposide can soften or crack plastic equipment or devices. Solutions should be prepared in glass or polyolefin plastic.

MONOCLONAL ANTIBODIES

Recombinant DNA technology has led to the development of **monoclonal antibodies**. These artificial antibodies are designed to target specific substances such as other immune cells or cancer cells. They have shown action in treating both tumors and hematologic malignancies, such as:

- non-Hodgkin lymphoma
- chronic lymphocytic leukemia
- acute myeloid leukemia
- breast cancer

Monoclonal antibodies locate and bind to cancer cells or other immune cells wherever they are in the body. They bind to target receptors or cancer cells and cause tumor or cell death in several different ways. They may:

- induce programmed cell death
- recruit other elements of the immune system to attack the cancer cell
- deliver a dose of a toxic chemotherapy drug or radiation to the tumor site

Adverse Reactions to Monoclonal Antibodies

All monoclonal antibodies are associated with infusion-related reactions that have occasionally been fatal. These include:

- fever
- chills
- shortness of breath
- low blood pressure
- anaphylaxis

Alemtuzumab

Alemtuzumab (Campath) is manufactured as a concentrate for an injection solution. It's administered by IV infusion over two hours. The dose is gradually increased to the maximum dosage in three to seven days. The patient should be premedicated with diphenhydramine and acetaminophen before the first infusion and before each dose escalation. Alemtuzumab should be used within eight hours of dilution. Diluted alemtuzumab can be stored at room temperature or refrigerated. Undiluted alemtuzumab, however, must be refrigerated.

Adverse reactions related to alemtuzumab include:

- myelosuppression
- increased risk of opportunistic infections, such as pneumocystitis, pneumonia, and fungal and viral infections

These are in addition to the adverse reactions common to all monoclonal antibodies.

Gemtuzumab Ozogamicin

Gemtuzumab ozogamicin (Mylotarg) is manufactured as a powder for injection. After reconstitution, it's normally administered by IV infusion over a two-hour period. It must be reconstituted with sterile water and then diluted prior to use. It should only be diluted with sodium chloride 0.9 percent solution. The reconstituted solution can be stored for less than two hours at room temperature or under refrigeration. However, after dilution, it may be stored for up to 16 hours at room temperature.

In addition to the adverse reactions common to other monoclonal antibodies, gemtuzumab ozogamicin may cause:

- significant myelosuppression
- liver toxicity

Ibritumomab Tiuxetan

Ibritumomab tiuxetan (Zevalin) comes as an injection in a kit with sodium acetate, a formulation buffer vial, a reaction vial, and identification labels. The therapy regimen is given in two steps. The first step is a single infusion of rituximab (not included in the kit) and then a fixed dose of In-111 ibritumomab tiuxetan administered as a ten-minute IV push. The second step occurs seven to nine days later. It's a second infusion of rituximab, followed by Y-90 ibritumomab tiuxetan given as a ten-minute IV push. Ibritumomab tiuxetan is prepared differently in its two different forms, so it's important to follow the exact instructions. Both forms of ibritumomab tiuxetan should be refrigerated.

Ibritumomab tiuxetan may interfere with the actions of other drugs such as:

- warfarin
- aspirin
- clopidogrel
- ticlopidine
- NSAIDs
- azathioprine
- cyclosporine
- corticosteroids

This drug is associated with increased myelosuppression.

Rituximab

Rituximab (Rituxan) is typically used as part of a treatment regimen with other antineoplastic drugs. It may also be used in the treatment of rheumatoid arthritis. This drug is administered by IV infusion. Rituximab should be stored in the refrigerator and protected from direct sunlight. Because the solution doesn't contain a preservative, diluted rituximab solutions must be refrigerated.

Trastuzumab

Trastuzumab (Herceptin) is given on its own or with other chemotherapy drugs to treat breast cancer. It's manufactured as a powder for injection. The drug is typically administered by IV infusion once a week. The first infusion should take 90 minutes. If well tolerated by the patient, other infusions can be 30 minutes. Trastuzumab shouldn't be given through an IV line that has been used for dextrose solutions.

Storage of trastuzumab and trastuzumab solution should be in the refrigerator. The reconstituted solution can be stored for 28 days. Once the solution is diluted, it should be used within 24 hours.

Trastuzumab increases the cardiac toxicity related to anthracycline administration.

TOPOISOMERASE I INHIBITORS

Topoisomerase I inhibitors are derivatives of camptothecin, a nitrogen-containing chemical (alkaloid).

These drugs block the action of the enzyme topoisomerase, which damages cell DNA. They can be used to fight solid tumors and hematologic malignancies such as:

- colorectal cancer
- small-cell lung cancer
- ovarian cancer
- acute myeloid leukemia

The topoisomerase enzyme normally allows supercoiled DNA to relax. Topoisomerase I inhibitors work by binding to the DNA topoisomerase I complex. They prevent the DNA from resealing and cause the DNA strands to break. This ruins DNA synthesis.

TIP Topoisomerase I inhibitors are derived from the Chinese tree *Camptotheca acuminata*.

Irinotecan

Irinotecan (Camptosar) is given as part of a therapy regimen with other drugs (5-fluorouracil and leucovorin) in the treatment of colon or rectal cancer. It may also be used in the treatment of lung cancer. This drug is manufactured as an injection. It's given as an IV infusion over 90 minutes. It may be given weekly or once every three weeks, depending on the treatment regimen. Irinotecan must be diluted before use. The diluted solution can be refrigerated for 48 hours if protected from light.

Irinotecan may interact with several other drugs.

- Ketoconazole significantly increases blood levels of SN-38, increasing the risk of toxicities related to the use of irinotecan.

PROCEED WITH CAUTION

Adverse Reactions to Topoisomerase I Inhibitors

The more common reactions to topoisomerase I inhibitors include:

- diarrhea
- abdominal cramps
- hair loss or thinning
- increased sweating and production of saliva
- nausea, vomiting, and loss of appetite
- tiredness
- watery eyes

Occasionally, these other reactions may occur:

- mouth sores and ulcers
- muscle cramps
- rashes, which may be itchy
- significant myelosuppression (rare)
- temporary effects on liver function test results

- Taking diuretics with irinotecan may worsen the dehydration caused by irinotecan-induced diarrhea.
- Laxatives taken with irinotecan can induce diarrhea.
- When prochlorperazine is given with irinotecan, there is an increased likelihood of extrapyramidal toxicities.

Topotecan

Topotecan (Hycamtin) is manufactured as powder for injection. The injection is given as part of treatment for cervical, ovarian, or small-cell lung cancer. The powder should be reconstituted with sterile water and administered by IV infusion over 30 minutes. The reconstituted solution is stable for 24 hours at room temperature.

TARGETED THERAPIES

A groundbreaking approach to anticancer therapies involves drugs that target different proteins. These proteins cause the growth of specific types of cancer.

Patients should avoid becoming pregnant while taking targeted therapy drugs, because these drugs caused fetal harm and death in animal studies. There are also adverse reactions specific to each therapy.

Bortezomib

Bortezomib (Velcade) is used to treat multiple myeloma that has relapsed after standard chemotherapy. It works by blocking proteosomes, the protein complexes that are involved in key cell-cycle functions and also promote tumor growth. Bortezomib disrupts normal cell processes and leads to cell death through proteolysis (the process of breaking up proteins).

Bortezomib isn't absorbed orally and must be given by IV. It's manufactured as a powder for injection. The powder must be reconstituted before use. After reconstitution, the drug may be stored up to eight hours in a syringe at room temperature. Unopened bortezomib should be stored at controlled room temperature and protected from light.

Bortezomib may interact with some other drugs.

- When taken with drugs that affect certain CYP450 enzymes (such as amiodarone, carbamazepine, cimetidine, erythromycin, diltiazem, fluoxetine, nevirapine, phenobarbital, phenytoin, rifampin, verapamil, zafirlukast, and zileuton), bortezomib could cause either toxicity or reduced effectiveness of these drugs.
- Taking bortezomib with oral hypoglycemics could cause hypoglycemia and hyperglycemia in patients with diabetes.

The most common adverse reactions to bortezomib include:

- fatigue, malaise, or weakness
- nausea and vomiting

- diarrhea or constipation
- appetite loss
- fever

Less common reactions include:

- peripheral neuropathy
- headache
- low blood pressure
- liver toxicity
- cardiac toxicity, such as arrhythmias, heart failure, myocardial ischemia and infarction, pulmonary edema, and pericardial effusion

Gefitinib

Gefitinib (Iressa) is used as a single agent for patients with non–small-cell lung cancer that hasn't responded to two standard chemotherapy regimens. It's available as oral tablets. One tablet is taken daily, with or without food. This drug should be stored at controlled room temperature.

Gefitinib works by blocking the epidermal growth factor receptor-1 tyrosine kinase. This substance is overexpressed in some cancers, such as non–small-cell lung cancer.

The following drug interactions may occur with gefitinib:

- Plasma levels of gefitinib are decreased when this drug is given with carbamazepine, dexamethasone, phenobarbital, phenytoin, rifampin, or St. John's wort.
- Taking gefitinib in conjunction with high doses of ranitidine with sodium bicarbonate reduces levels of gefitinib.
- Administration of gefinitib with warfarin increases the risk of bleeding.

Adverse reactions to gefitinib include:

- rash
- diarrhea
- abnormal eyelash growth
- lung and liver damage

Imatinib

Imatinib (Gleevec) is used to treat chronic myeloid leukemia, acute lymphoid leukemia, and GI stromal tumors. It's manufactured as oral tablets. The tablets are taken with a meal and a large glass of water. They are taken once or twice a day, depending on the dosage. For patients who can't swallow the tablets, they may be dissolved in water or apple juice.

In patients with chronic myeloid leukemia, a protein called BCR-ABL stimulates other tyrosine kinase proteins. This causes abnormally high levels of white blood cells to be produced. Imatinib binds to places where adenosine triphosphate normally binds to the BCR-ABL protein.

This shuts down the abnormal production of white blood cells.

Imatinib is known to cause several drug interactions:

- Like gefitinib, plasma levels of imatinib are decreased when this drug is given with carbamazepine, dexamethasone, phenobarbital, phenytoin, rifampin, or St. John's wort.
- Also similar to gefinitib, administering imatinib with warfarin increases the risk of bleeding.
- Taking imatinib with warfarin increases the risk of bleeding.
- When taken with imatinib, drugs such as clarithromycin, erythromycin, itraconazole, and ketoconazole may increase plasma levels of imatinib.
- When given with simvastatin, imatinib increases simvastatin levels about threefold.
- Imatinib increases plasma levels of other CYP450-metabolized drugs, such as triazolo-benzodiazepines, dihydropyridine calcium channel blockers, and certain HMG-CoA reductase inhibitors.

Taking imatinib can result in several adverse reactions, such as:

- periorbital and lower limb edema, possibly resulting in pulmonary edema, effusions, and heart or renal failure
- nausea
- vomiting
- liver function abnormalities
- myelosuppression (especially neutropenia and thrombocytopenia)

UNCLASSIFIABLE ANTINEOPLASTIC DRUGS

Many other antineoplastic drugs can't be included in existing classifications. These drugs have different uses and effects on the body. Drug interactions and adverse reactions are specific to each drug.

Arsenic Trioxide

Arsenic trioxide (Trisenox) is a commercially available treatment for patients with acute promyelocytic leukemia (a rare form of acute myeloid leukemia). This drug works by causing DNA to break up or fragment. It's indicated when standard therapy has failed.

Arsenic trioxide is manufactured as an injection. It's administered by IV. Before administration, it must be diluted. The diluted drug can be stored at room temperature for 24 hours or refrigerated for up to 48 hours.

Giving arsenic trioxide with other drugs known to prolong the QT interval may increase the risk of cardiac arrhythmias.

PROCEED WITH CAUTION

Adverse Reactions to Arsenic Trioxide

Arsenic trioxide can cause electrocardiogram abnormalities. These could progress to life-threatening cardiac arrhythmias. Other possible adverse reactions include:

- anxiety
- dizziness
- headache
- hypocalcemia
- insomnia
- liver damage
- muscle and bone aches
- nausea and vomiting
- rash
- tremor

In addition, arsenic trioxide can produce a unique toxicity called APL differentiation syndrome, which is characterized by an increasing white blood cell count with respiratory distress. This syndrome may be fatal if not treated immediately with corticosteroids.

Asparaginases

Asparaginases are used in treating acute lymphocytic leukemia. They are cell cycle-specific drugs that act during the G1 phase.

Most normal cells can synthesize asparagine, an amino acid found in proteins. However, some tumor cells depend on other sources of asparagines for survival. Asparaginase drugs help degrade asparagines to aspartic acid and ammonia. When they are deprived of their supply of asparagine, tumor cells die.

Asparaginase drugs may interact with other drugs.

- Asparaginase drugs may reduce the effectiveness of methotrexate.
- Taking asparaginase drugs with prednisone or vincristine increases the risk of toxicity.

Asparaginase

Asparaginase (Elspar) is mainly used in combination with standard chemotherapy to induce remission in patients with acute lymphocytic leukemia. It's manufactured as a powder for injection. The powder is reconstituted and given either by IM or IV injection. When given intravenously, this drug is normally introduced into an already running infusion. Asparaginase does not contain any preservatives, so it must be stored under refrigeration. Before use, the reconstituted solution should be refrigerated. It's discarded after eight hours or if the solution becomes cloudy.

PROCEED WITH CAUTION

Adverse Reactions to Asparaginase Drugs

Many patients receiving asparaginase drugs develop nausea and vomiting. Other adverse reactions include:

- fever
- headache
- abdominal pain
- pancreatitis
- coagulopathy
- liver toxicity

These drugs can also cause anaphylaxis. This is more likely to occur with intermittent IV dosing than with daily IV dosing or IM injections. The risk of a reaction rises with each successive treatment. In addition, hypersensitivity reactions may occur.

Pegaspargase

Pegaspargase (Oncaspar) is used to treat acute lymphocytic leukemia in patients who are allergic to the native form of asparaginase. It comes as an injection. Like asparaginase, this drug may be given IV or by IM injection. It should be stored in a refrigerator. Unused portions of the drug must be discarded. The drug shouldn't be administered if it has been shaken vigorously, frozen, or stored at room temperature for more than 48 hours. If the drug is cloudy or has a precipitate, it should be discarded.

Procarbazine

Procarbazine (Matulane) is used to treat Hodgkin disease and primary and metastatic brain tumors. This drug is a methylhydrazine derivative with MAOI properties. It's cell cycle specific and acts on the S phase.

Procarbazine must be activated metabolically in the liver before it can produce changes in cells. It can:

- damage chromosomes
- suppress mitosis
- block the synthesis of DNA, RNA, and proteins

Procarbazine is manufactured as oral capsules. It can have significant interactions with other substances.

- When taken with CNS depressants, procarbazine produces an additive effect.
- Taking procarbazine with meperidine may result in severe hypotension and death.
- Because of procarbazine's MAOI properties, hypertensive reactions may occur when it's administered with sympathomimetics, antidepressants, and tyramine-rich foods (such as wine, yogurt, ripe cheese, and bananas).

PROCEED WITH CAUTION

Adverse Reactions to Procarbazine

Initially, taking procarbazine may lead to flulike symptoms such as:

- fever
- chills
- sweating
- lethargy
- muscle pain

Late-onset bone marrow suppression is the most common toxicity related to procarbazine. This effect is dose related. Other adverse reactions may include:

- interstitial pneumonitis (lung inflammation)
- pulmonary fibrosis (scarring)
- nausea
- vomiting
- stomatitis
- diarrhea

Hydroxyurea

Hydroxyurea (Droxia, Hydrea) is used most commonly for patients with chronic myelogenous leukemia. In addition, it may lead to temporary remission in some patients with metastatic malignant melanomas. It's also used in combination therapy with radiation to treat solid tumors and cancers of the head, neck, and lungs.

Hydroxyurea blocks the enzyme ribonucleotide reductase. Because this enzyme is needed for DNA synthesis, the drug affects the cell cycle. It kills cells in the S phase of the cell cycle and holds other cells in the G1 phase, at which they're most susceptible to irradiation.

Hydroxyurea is manufactured as oral capsules of different strengths. It may interact with other drugs. The following will enhance the toxic effects of hydroxyurea:

- cytotoxic drugs
- radiation therapy

PROCEED WITH CAUTION

Adverse Reactions to Hydroxyurea

Treatment with hydroxyurea leads to few adverse reactions. Those that do occur include:

- bone marrow suppression
- drowsiness
- headache
- nausea and vomiting
- anorexia
- elevated uric acid levels (this may require some patients to take allopurinol to prevent kidney damage)

Interferons

A family of naturally occurring glycoproteins called **interferons** can fight cancers. There are three main types of interferons.

- **Alpha interferons** are derived from leukocytes.
- **Beta interferons** are derived from connective tissue cells called fibroblasts.
- **Gamma interferons** are derived from fibroblasts and lymphocytes.

Alpha interferons have shown their most promising activity in treating blood malignancies, including:

- hairy cell leukemia
- AIDS-related Kaposi sarcoma
- condylomata acuminata (genital warts)

These drugs have also demonstrated some activity against chronic myelogenous leukemia, malignant lymphoma, multiple myeloma, melanoma, and renal cell carcinoma.

Although their exact mechanism of action isn't known, alfa interferons seem to bind to specific membrane receptors on the cell surface. After binding, they start a sequence of events within the cell that affects certain enzymes. This process may be the reason why interferons are able to:

- block viral replication
- suppress cell growth
- enhance the activity of macrophages (cells that surround and destroy invading organisms)
- increase the cytotoxicity of lymphocytes for target cells

Interferons interact with other drugs.

- Interferons may enhance the effects of CNS depressants. They substantially increase the half-life of methylxanthines (including theophylline and aminophylline).
- Concurrent use of interferons with a live virus vaccine may stimulate replication of the virus, increasing adverse reactions to the vaccine and decreasing the patient's antibody response.
- Taking interferons while undergoing radiation therapy or also taking a drug that causes blood abnormalities may increase bone marrow suppression.
- Alfa interferons increase the risk of kidney failure.

Interferon Alfa-2b

Interferon alfa-2b (Intron A) is available as a powder for solution and as an injection solution in multidose pens or vials. In addition to its uses in the treatment of cancer, it's used to treat chronic hepatitis B and chronic hepatitis C. The powder must be reconstituted with sterile water before injection or IV infusion. The injection solution isn't recommended for IV administration. The reconstituted powder should be used immediately but, if necessary, may be stored for up to 24 hours under refrigeration.

! PROCEED WITH CAUTION

Adverse Reactions to Interferons

The most common adverse reaction to alfa interferons is the development of flulike symptoms such as:

- fever
- fatigue
- muscle pain
- headache
- chills
- joint pain

Blood toxicity occurs in up to one-half of patients taking interferons. It may produce:

- leukopenia
- neutropenia
- thrombocytopenia
- anemia

Adverse GI reactions include:

- anorexia
- nausea
- diarrhea

Other adverse reactions associated with interferon therapy are:

- coughing
- breathing difficulties
- hypotension
- edema
- chest pain
- heart failure

Interferon Alfa-n3

Alfa-n3 (Alferon N) is manufactured as an injection. It's typically used for treatment of condylomata acuminata. It must be refrigerated.

Aldesleukin

Aldesleukin (Proleukin) is produced through a process of human recombinant DNA. It's derived from interleukin-2, a natural protein that stimulates the growth of certain white blood cells. Aldesleukin is used to fight metastatic renal cell carcinoma. It's also used in the treatment of metastatic melanoma and Kaposi sarcoma.

Aldesleukin is manufactured as a powder for injection. It's administered by a 15-minute IV infusion every eight hours. There are normally two five-day treatment cycles separated by a rest period of at least seven days. The drug needs to be stored in a refrigerator and protected from light. Reconstituted or diluted aldesleukin is stable for up to 48 hours in the refrigerator.

AT THE COUNTER

Being Informed About Interferon

A patient drops off a prescription at the pharmacy for interferon. Where in the pharmacy would you find the interferon?

Interferon is kept in the refrigerator.

What needs to be dispensed with the interferon for administration purposes?

Syringes and needles will be needed to administer the interferon. Interferon is administered by IM or SubQ injection. It's your responsibility to make sure that the patient has syringes and needles if the product does not come with them or they aren't prefilled.

The patient's prescription is for interferon alfa. What would you expect to be the patient's most common adverse reaction?

Common adverse reactions to interferon alfa are flulike symptoms, which may include fever, fatigue, muscle pain, headache, chills, and joint pain.

T I P Many antineoplastic drugs must be protected from light.

The exact mechanism for how aldesleukin works isn't clear. It's thought that the drug stimulates an immunologic reaction against the tumor.

Aldesleukin will interact with other drugs.

- Taking aldesleukin with drugs that have psychotropic properties (such as opioids, analgesics, antiemetics, sedatives, and tranquilizers) may produce additive CNS effects.
- Glucocorticoids may reduce the antitumor effects of aldesleukin.
- Antihypertensive drugs can increase the hypotensive effects of aldesleukin.
- Taking aldesleukin with drugs that are toxic to the kidneys (such as aminoglycosides), bone marrow (such as cytotoxic chemotherapy drugs), heart (such as doxorubicin), or liver (such as methotrexate or asparaginase) may increase these drugs' toxicity to these organs.

Altretamine

Altretamine (Hexalen) is a synthetic cytotoxic antineoplastic drug, which means it's a man-made chemotherapy drug for attacking tumor cells. It's used as palliative treatment for patients with ovarian cancer.

Altretamine is manufactured as capsules. It's usually given for 14 or 21 consecutive days in a 28-day cycle. The total daily dose is given as four divided doses after meals and at bedtime.

PROCEED WITH CAUTION

Adverse Reactions to Aldesleukin

During clinical trials, more than 15 percent of patients developed adverse reactions to aldesleukin. These include:

- pulmonary congestion and difficulty breathing
- anemia, thrombocytopenia, and leukopenia
- elevated bilirubin, transaminase, and alkaline phosphate levels
- hypomagnesemia (low blood levels of magnesium) and acidosis
- reduced or absent urinary output
- elevated serum creatinine level
- stomatitis
- nausea and vomiting

The way altretamine works isn't known. However, it breaks down into alkylating drugs. Altretamine has a few significant interactions with other drugs.

- Taking altretamine with cimetidine may increase the toxicity of altretamine.
- MAOIs taken with altretamine may cause severe orthostatic hypotension (a drop in blood pressure when rising).

Paclitaxel

Paclitaxel (Onxol, Taxol, Abraxane) is a taxane used to treat metastatic ovarian and breast cancer after chemotherapy has failed. It may also be used in treating head and neck cancers, prostate cancer, and non–small-cell lung cancer.

The drug works by disrupting the microtubule network needed for mitosis and other vital cellular functions.

Paclitaxel is manufactured as a powder for injection. It's administered intravenously. Gloves should be worn when handling the drug. The drug must be diluted before use. The diluted solution remains stable for up to 27 hours at room temperature.

Paclitaxel may interact with other drugs.

- Taking paclitaxel with cisplatin may cause additive bone marrow suppression effects.

PROCEED WITH CAUTION

Adverse Reactions to Altretamine

More than ten percent of patients using altretamine in clinical trials experienced adverse reactions, such as:

- nausea and vomiting
- neurotoxicity and peripheral neuropathy
- anemia

Bone marrow suppression is also common.

PROCEED WITH CAUTION

Adverse Reactions to Paclitaxel

During clinical trials, 25 percent or more patients experienced these adverse reactions:

- bone marrow suppression
- hypersensitivity reactions
- abnormal EEG tracings
- peripheral neuropathy
- muscle pain and joint pain
- nausea, vomiting, and diarrhea
- mucous membrane inflammation
- hair loss

- Phenytoin may decrease blood serum levels of paclitaxel, leading to a reduced effect of the drug.
- Quinupristin/dalfopristin may increase the blood levels of paclitaxel, increasing the risk of toxicity.

Docetaxel

Like paclitaxel, docetaxel (Taxotere) is a taxane drug. It's used to treat metastatic breast cancer. It may also be used for treatment of head and neck cancers, non–small-cell lung cancer, and prostate cancer. It's administered as a one-hour IV infusion. A typical treatment course may be once every three weeks. The diluted drug should be stored in glass bottles or polypropylene bottles or bags. Plasticized equipment isn't recommended. Unopened docetaxel can be stored between 2 degrees and 25 degrees C (36 degrees and 77 degrees F). It should be allowed to stand at room temperature for five minutes before mixing with the diluent. The diluted solution can be stored at room temperature for up to eight hours, and the infusion remains stable for four hours.

In terms of drug interactions, cyclosporine, ketoconazole, erythromycin, and troleandomycin may change the metabolism of docetaxel.

Clinical trials of docetaxel in Japanese and American patients with breast cancer revealed significant differences in the incidence of adverse reactions between the two cultures.

Japanese women were more likely to develop thrombocytopenia—14.4 percent versus 5.5 percent. However, the Japanese women in this study were less likely than the American patients (6 percent versus 29.1 percent) to develop many of the other adverse reactions, such as hypersensitivity reactions.

Other results showed fewer incidences of fluid retention, neurosensory effects, muscle pain, infection, and development of anemia in the Japanese patients. The study also indicated that Japanese patients are more likely to develop fatigue and weakness than are American women.

The results are important to consider when providing docetaxel to patients. These findings also provide clues for knowing what adverse reactions to expect.

PROCEED WITH CAUTION

Adverse Reactions to Docetaxel

Adverse reactions to docetaxel include:

- hypersensitivity reactions
- fluid retention
- leukopenia, neutropenia, or thrombocytopenia
- hair loss
- stomatitis
- numbness and tingling
- pain
- weakness and fatigue

QUICK QUIZ

Answer the following multiple-choice questions.

1. Why are nitrogen mustards effective in treating tumors that raise a person's white blood cell count?
   a. because they produce leukopenia
   b. because they interact with many other drugs
   c. because they are S phase specific
   d. none of the above
2. Which of the following drug groups contains drugs that are S phase specific?
   a. antimetabolite drugs
   b. alkylating-like drugs
   c. nitrosoureas
   d. ethylenimines
3. Which of the following drugs is *not* available in an oral form?
   a. mercaptopurine
   b. doxorubicin
   c. capecitabine
   d. gefitinib
4. Which of the following is *not* an effect of alfa interferons?
   a. blocking viral suppression
   b. damage to hearing and balance organs
   c. suppressing cell growth
   d. enhancing the effects of CNS depressants
5. What are the most common adverse reactions to antineoplastic drugs?
   a. nausea and vomiting
   b. hair loss

c. bone marrow suppression
d. all of the above

Please answer each of the following questions in one to three sentences.

1. What is the difference between S phase-specific and cell cycle-nonspecific drugs?

   _____

   _____

2. How do pyrimidine analogue drugs work?

   _____

   _____

3. How do monoclonal antibodies differ from antibiotic antineoplastics?

   _____

   _____

4. Describe two uses of tamoxifen.

   _____

   _____

5. What is the difference between steroidal and nonsteroidal aromatase inhibitors?

   _____

   _____

Answer the following questions as either true or false.

1. ___ All cancers affect the same stage in the cell cycle—the S phase.
2. ___ An analogue is a drug that is structurally similar to another substance.
3. ___ Methotrexate is especially useful in treating acute lymphoblastic leukemia.
4. ___ Hormone-dependent (gender-specific) tumors are treated with corticosteroids.
5. ___ Vinca alkaloids work by disrupting the process of mitosis, causing death of tumor cells.

Match the generic name of each drug in the left column with the correct trade name from the right column.

1. busulfan	a. Proleukin
2. triptorelin	b. Myleran
3. bortezomib	c. Trexall
4. methotrexate	d. Velcade
5. aldesleukin	e. Trelstar

DRUG CLASSIFICATION TABLE

Classification	Generic Name	Trade Name(s)
Nitrogen mustards	chlorambucil *klor-am'-byoo-sill*	*tablets:* Leukeran
	cyclophosphamide *sye-klo-foss'-fam-ide*	*tablets:* Cytoxan *injection:* Cytoxan
	estramustine *ess-tra-muss'-teen*	*capsules:* Emcyt
	ifosfamide *eye-fos'-fam-ide*	*injection:* Ifex
	mechlorethamine *me-klor-eth'-a-meen*	*injection:* Mustargen
	melphalan *mel'-fa-lan*	*tablets:* Alkeran *injection:* Alkeran
Alkyl sulfonates	busulfan *byoo-sul'-fan*	*tablets:* Myleran *injection:* Busulfex
Nitrosoureas	carmustine *car'-mus-teen*	*injection:* BiCNU *implant:* Gliadel Wafer
	lomustine *ioe-mus'-teen*	*capsules:* CeeNU
	streptozocin *strep'-toe-zoe'-sin*	*injection:* Zanosar
Triazines	dacarbazine *da-kar'-ba-zeen*	*injection:* DTIC-Dome
Ethylenimines	thiotepa *thye-oh-tep'-a*	*injection:* (no longer marketed under trade name)
Alkylating-like drugs	carboplatin *kar-boe-pla-tin*	*injection:* (no longer marketed under trade name)
	cisplatin *sis-pla'-tin*	*injection:* Platinol AQ
	oxaliplatin *ox-al'-i-plah-tin*	*injection:* Eloxatin
Folic acid analogues	methotrexate *meth-oh-trek'-sate*	*tablets:* Trexall, Rheumatrex *injection:* (no longer marketed under trade name)
Pyrimidine analogues	capecitabine *kap-ah-seat'-ah-bean*	*tablets:* Xeloda
	cytarabine *sye'-tare-uh-bene*	*injection:* (no longer marketed under trade name) *injection (liposomal):* (no longer marketed under trade name)
	floxuridine *flox-yoor'-i-deen*	*injection:* FUDR
	fluorouracil *flure'-oh-yoor'-a-sill*	*injection:* Adrucil *topical cream:* Carac, Fluoroplex, Efudex *topical solution:* Efudex
	gemcitabine *jem-site'-ah-ben*	*injection:* Gemzar
Purine analogues	cladribine *kla'-dri'been*	*injection:* Leustatin
	fludarabine *floo-dar'-a-bean*	*injection:* Fludara
	mercaptopurine *mer-kap'-toe-pyoor'-een*	*tablets:* Purinethol
	pentostatin *pen'-toe-stat-in*	*injection:* Nipent
	thioguanine *thye'-oh-gwon'-een*	*tablets:* Tabloid
Antibiotic antineoplastic drugs	daunorubicin *daw-noe-roo'-bi-sin*	*injection:* Cerubidine *injection (liposomal):* Daunoxome
	doxorubicin *dox-oh-roo'-bi-sin*	*injection:* Adriamycin *injection (liposomal):* Doxil

continued

DRUG CLASSIFICATION TABLE (continued)

Classification	Generic Name	Trade Name(s)
Antibiotic antineoplastic drugs (continued)	idarubicin *eye-duh-roo'-bi-sin*	*injection:* Idamycin PFS
	bleomycin *blee-oh-my'-sin*	*injection:* Blenoxane
	dactinomycin *dak'-ti-no-my'-sin*	*injection:* Cosmegen
	mitomycin *mye-toe-mye'-sin*	*injection:* (no longer marketed under trade name)
Aromatase inhibitors	mitoxantrone *mye-toe-zan'-trone*	*injection:* Novantrone
	exemestane *ex-ah-mess'-tane*	*tablets:* Aromasin
	anastrozole *an-ass'-troe-zole*	*tablets:* Arimidex
	letrozole *le'-tro-zol*	*tablets:* Femara
Antiestrogens	fulvestrant *fool-ves'-trant*	*injection:* Faslodex
	tamoxifen *ta-mox'-i-fen*	*tablets:* (no longer marketed under trade name) *oral solution:* Soltamox
Androgens	fluoxymesterone *floo-ox-i-mes'-te-rone*	*tablets:* Androxy
	testolactone *tes'-toe-lak'-tone*	*tablets:* Teslac
	testosterone enanthate *tess-toss'-ter-ohn*	*injection:* Andro LA, Delatestryl
	testosterone propionate *tess-toss'-ter-ohn*	*topical cream:* First-Testosterone MC *topical ointment:* First-Testosterone
	testosterone *tess-toss'-ter-ohn*	*topical gel:* Androgel, Testim *injection:* (no longer marketed under trade name) *transdermal patch:* Androderm *buccal tablet:* Striant *implant:* Testopel Pellet
	testosterone cypionate *tess-toss'-ter-ohn*	*injection:* Depo-Testosterone
Antiandrogens	bicalutamide *bye-cal-loo'-ta-mide*	*tablets:* Casodex
	flutamide *flu'-ta-mide*	*capsules:* (no longer marketed under trade name)
	nilutamide *nah-loo'-ta-mide*	*tablets:* Nilandron
Progestins	medroxyprogesterone *me-drox'-ee-proe-jess'-te-rone*	*injection (malignancy):* Depo-Provera *injection (contraception):* Depo-subQ Provera, Depo-Provera Contraceptive *tablets:* Provera
	megestrol *me-jess'-trole*	*tablets:* (no longer marketed under trade name) *oral suspension:* Megace
Gonadotropin-releasing hormone analogues	goserelin *goe'-se-rel-in*	*implant:* Zoladex
	leuprolide *loo-proe'-lide*	*injection:* Lupron Depot *injection:* Lupron, Eligard
	triptorelin *trip-toe-rell'-in*	*injection (depot):* Trelstar Depot *injection (long-acting):* Trelstar LA
Vinca alkaloids	vinblastine *vin-blas'-teen*	*injection:* (no longer marketed under trade name)
	vincristine *vin-kris'-teen*	*injection:* Vincasar PFS
	vinorelbine *vin-nor'-el-bean*	*injection:* Navelbine

continued

DRUG CLASSIFICATION TABLE *(continued)*

Classification	Generic Name	Trade Name(s)
Podophyllotoxins	etoposide *e'-toe-poe'-side*	*capsules:* (no longer marketed under trade name) *injection:* Toposar, Etopophos
	teniposide *teh'-nip-oh'-side*	*injection:* Vumon
Monoclonal antibodies	alemtuzumab *ay'-lem-tuh'-zoo-mab*	*injection:* Campath
	gemtuzumab ozogamicin *gem-too'-zoo-mab oh-zoh-gam-ih'-sin*	*injection:* Mylotarg
	ibritumomab tiuxetan *ib-ri-tu'moe-mab tie-ux-eh'tan*	*injection:* Zevalin
	rituximab *ri-tux'-i-mab*	*injection:* Rituxan
	trastuzumab *trass-to-zoo'-mab*	*injection:* Herceptin
Topoisomerase I inhibitors	irinotecan *eh-rin-oh'-te-kan*	*injection:* Camptosar
	topotecan *toe'-poh-te'-kan*	*injection:* Hycamtin
Targeted therapies	bortezomib *bor-tez'-oh-mib*	*injection:* Velcade
	gefitinib *geh-fit'-in-ib*	*tablets:* Iressa
	imatinib *im-a'-ti-nib*	*tablets:* Gleevec
Unclassifiable antineoplastic drugs	arsenic trioxide *are'-seh-nick*	*injection:* Trisenox
	asparaginase *ass-par'-ah-jin-ase*	*injection:* Elspar
	pegaspargase *peg-as-par-jase*	*injection:* Oncaspar
	procarbazine *pro-kar'-ba-zeen*	*capsules:* Matulane
	hydroxyurea *hye-drox-ee-yoor-ee'-a*	*capsules:* Droxia, Hydrea
	interferon alfa-2b *in'-ter-feer'-on al'fa*	*injection:* Intron A
	interferon alfa-n3 *in'-ter-feer'-on al'fa*	*injection:* Alferon N
	aldesleukin *al-dess-loo'-kin*	*injection:* Proleukin
	altretamine *al-tret'-a-meen*	*capsules:* Hexalen
	paclitaxel *pak'-li-tax-el*	*injection:* Onxol, Taxol *injection (albumin-bound):* Abraxane
	docetaxel *doe'-se-tax'-el*	*injection:* Taxotere

Answers to Quick Quiz Questions

Chapter 1

Answer the following multiple-choice questions.

1. a.
2. c.
3. d.
4. c.
5. a.

Please answer each of the following questions in one to three sentences.

1. Drug tolerance occurs when a patient develops a decreased response to a drug over time, requiring larger doses to produce the same response. Drug dependence is when a patient displays a physical or psychological need for the drug. Drug dependence often leads to withdrawal symptoms when the patient stops taking the drug.
2. Possible answers may include any four of the following: additive effects, potentiation, antagonistic effects, decreased or increased absorption, and decreased or increased metabolism and excretion.
3. Pharmacokinetics involves the absorption, distribution, metabolism, and excretion of a drug.
4. A competitive antagonist competes with the agonist for receptor sites. Administering larger doses of an agonist can overcome the antagonist's effects. A noncompetitive antagonist binds to receptor sites and blocks the effects of the agonist. Administering larger doses of the agonist can't reverse the antagonist's action.
5. Possible answers may include the following: An allergic reaction occurs when a patient's immune system identifies a drug as a dangerous foreign substance that must be neutralized or destroyed. An allergic reaction can be an immediate, life-threatening reaction or a mild reaction with a rash and itching. An adverse reaction results from the known pharmacologic effects of a drug and is typically dose related. It is not caused by patient sensitivity and can be controlled by adjusting the dose of the drug.

Answer the following questions as either true or false.

1. True
2. True
3. False
4. False
5. True

Match the description in the left column with the correct route of administration from the right column.

1. c
2. a
3. b
4. e
5. d

Chapter 2

Answer the following multiple-choice questions.

1. b.
2. d.
3. c.
4. b.
5. c.

Please answer each of the following questions in one to three sentences.

1. Anticholinesterase drugs are commonly used to treat mild to moderate dementia, diagnose myasthenia gravis, increase muscle contraction in patients with myasthenia gravis, and counteract the effects of anticholinergic drugs.
2. Possible answers may include the following drugs: acetylcholine, bethanechol, carbachol, cevimeline, pilocarpine.
3. Possible answers may include: reduced blood pressure, reduced heart rate, decreased force of heart's contractions, constriction of bronchioles, constriction of peripheral blood vessels.
4. Direct-acting adrenergics act directly on the organ or tissue in which the nerve is stimulated, whereas indirect-acting adrenergics stimulate the release of a neurotransmitter. Dual-acting adrenergics, however, can work both ways.
5. Cholinergic agonists directly arouse cholinergic receptors. These drugs imitate the action of the neurotransmitter acetylcholine.

Answer the following questions as either true or false.

1. True
2. False
3. False
4. True
5. True

Match the generic name of each drug in the left column with the correct trade name from the right column.

1. c
2. d
3. e
4. b
5. a

Chapter 3

Answer the following multiple-choice questions.

1. b.
2. c.
3. d.
4. a.
5. d.

Please answer each of the following questions in one to three sentences.

1. Baclofen produces less sedation than diazepam and less peripheral muscle weakness than dantrolene.
2. Nondepolarizing blocking drugs block acetylcholine's action at the cholinergic receptor sites of the skeletal muscle membrane, which prevents the muscle from contracting. Depolarizing blocking drugs act like acetylcholine, but are metabolized at a slower rate. They remain attached to the receptor sites for a longer time, which prevents repolarization of the motor end plate and results in muscle paralysis.
3. Carbidopa isn't metabolized as quickly or as extensively as levodopa. It enhances levodopa's effectiveness by blocking levodopa's metabolism outside the brain. This permits increased levels of levodopa to reach the brain.
4. Anticonvulsant drugs are used for (1) long-term management of the recurring seizures of chronic epilepsy; (2) short-term management of isolated acute seizures not caused by epilepsy; and (3) emergency treatment of status epilepticus, a continuous seizure state.
5. Ischemic heart disease or coronary artery disease (or having risk factors for these conditions) generally contraindicates the use of a triptan. So does a history of stroke, TIAs, or peripheral vascular disease.

Answer the following questions as either true or false.

1. True
2. True
3. False
4. False
5. True

Match the generic name of each anticonvulsant drug in the left column with its classification from the right column.

1. d
2. b
3. e
4. c
5. a

Chapter 4

Answer the following multiple-choice questions.

1. c.
2. c.
3. d.
4. c.
5. b.

Please answer each of the following questions in one to three sentences.

1. Selective NSAIDs block only COX-2 enzymes, whereas nonselective NSAIDs block COX-1 and COX-2 enzymes. Nonselective NSAIDs are more likely to irritate the stomach lining.
2. Opiates bind to opiate receptors and mimic the effects of natural endorphins. These drugs stop the release of substances that cause the body's pain response.
3. The antagonist fills up the receptor sites so that the opioid can't bind with them (competitive inhibition).
4. Possible answers may include: General anesthesia—patient is unconscious and feels no pain or sensations over entire body; local anesthesia—loss of sensation in body part, administered by injection; topical anesthesia—loss of sensation in specific area of body, administered through skin or mucosal tissue.
5. Possible answers may include at least three of the following: relieve or prevent pain, especially minor burn pain; relieve itching and irritation; anesthetize an area sore throat or mouth pain when used in a spray or solution.before an injection is given; numb mucosal surfaces before insertion of a tube; relieve

Answer the following questions as either true or false.

1. False
2. True
3. True
4. False
5. True

Match the generic name of each drug in the left column with the correct trade name from the right column.

1. c
2. e
3. d
4. a
5. b

Chapter 5

Answer the following multiple-choice questions.

1. a
2. b
3. d
4. c
5. a

Please answer each of the following questions in one to three sentences.

1. It dilates the veins, arteries, and arterioles, reducing resistance to pumping blood and thereby reducing the workload and oxygen requirements of the heart.
2. Class IA alters the myocardial cell membrane. Class IB blocks the rapid influx of sodium ions. Class IC slows conduction.
3. Bile-sequestering drugs lower levels of bile acids, which triggers the liver to produce more bile acids from cholesterol, thereby lowering cholesterol levels in the blood. Statins lower cholesterol levels by interfering with the liver's production of cholesterol.
4. Both are used in treating heart failure. ACE inhibitors are also antihypertensives.
5. Antihypertensive drugs work in different ways, and because hypertension can have several causes, a single drug might not be sufficient.

Answer the following questions as either true or false.

1. True
2. True
3. False
4. False
5. True

Match each brand name drug in the left column with its use in the right column.

1. a
2. c
3. e
4. b
5. d

Chapter 6

Answer the following multiple-choice questions.

1. b
2. c
3. b
4. c
5. d

Please answer each of the following questions in one to three sentences.

1. The amount of iron absorbed depends on how much is already stored in the body.

2. Pregnant women are advised to take folic acid supplements to prevent neural tube defects (for example, spina bifida) in their developing babies.
3. Warfarin may be used to treat thromboembolism, to prevent DVT, for patients with prosthetic heart valves or diseases of the mitral valves, to decrease the risk of arterial clotting, or in combination with an antiplatelet drug.
4. Warfarin dosages are highly dependent on individual patient response. The prescribing physician needs to monitor results of PT and INR in determining dosage, and the dosage schedule may vary from day to day.
5. Anticoagulant drugs can reduce the ability of the blood to clot, whereas thrombolytic drugs can lyse or dissolve existing clots.

Answer the following questions as either true or false.

1. True
2. False
3. True
4. False
5. False

Match each brand name drug in the left column with its use in the right column.

1. a
2. d
3. b
4. c
5. e

Chapter 7

Answer the following multiple-choice questions.

1. a
2. b
3. d
4. b
5. c

Please answer each of the following questions in one to three sentences.

1. Short-acting beta$_2$-adrenergic agonists are generally used when needed for fast relief from asthma attacks. Long-acting beta$_2$-adrenergic agonists are used to control and prevent such attacks and are thus administered on a set schedule.
2. Leukotriene modifiers inhibit the body's formation of leukotrienes or the absorption of leukotrienes at receptor sites. Mast cell stabilizers stabilize the mast cell membrane and block the release of histamines from mast cells.
3. Smoking cigarettes or marijuana, eating charbroiled meats, and taking supplements containing St. John's wort can reduce the effectiveness of theophylline. Drinking caffeinated beverages and eating high-fat foods can

increase theophylline's concentration, possibly resulting in toxicity.
4. Expectorants are intended to loosen mucus so that it can be expelled from the body. This usually happens through coughing. An antitussive will suppress coughing, which would lessen the effectiveness of the expectorant.
5. Inhaled and topical forms usually have only local effects. Systemic drugs, which are processed in the liver or GI tract, are absorbed into the bloodstream and circulate throughout the body.

Answer the following questions as either true or false.

1. false
2. true
3. true
4. true
5. false

Match each generic drug in the left column with its classification in the right column.

1. b
2. a
3. d
4. e
5. c

Chapter 8

Answer the following multiple-choice questions.

1. c
2. b
3. d
4. a
5. a

Please answer each of the following questions in one to three sentences.

1. For a patient with an *H. pylori* infection, triple or quadruple therapy may be required. Triple therapy consists of two antibiotics and a proton pump inhibitor, whereas quadruple therapy consists of two antibiotics, a proton pump inhibitor or H_2 receptor antagonist, plus bismuth subsalicylate.
2. H_2 receptor antagonists work by binding with H_2 receptors and blocking the action of histamine, reducing the secretion of gastric acid. Proton pump inhibitors combine with hydrogen, potassium, and adenosine triphosphate in the parietal cells of the stomach. By blocking the "acid pump," they halt the final step in acid production and reduce the secretion of gastric acid.
3. Aluminum causes constipation. Magnesium causes diarrhea. By combining the two in a single product, the result is generally no change in bowel function.
4. Hyperosmolar laxatives draw water into the stool, stimulating peristalsis; stimulant laxatives act directly on the intestinal mucosa.

5. Answers may include two of the following: to treat nausea and vomiting following surgery; to treat nausea and vomiting related to chemotherapy; to treat severe nausea and vomiting associated with a virus.

Answer the following questions as either true or false.

1. true
2. false
3. true
4. false
5. true

Match the generic name of each drug in the left column with the correct trade name from the right column.

1. e
2. a
3. d
4. b
5. c

Chapter 9

Answer the following multiple-choice questions.

1. b
2. a
3. c
4. d
5. c

Please answer each of the following questions in one to three sentences.

1. Some antimicrobial drugs have been prescribed when they did not need to be. This unnecessary exposure of some microbes to these drugs has caused those microbes to evolve and develop strains that are resistant to the overprescribed drug.
2. The recommended regimen is isoniazid, rifampin, pyrazinamide, and ethambutol or streptomycin. It should be modified by adding a fifth and sixth drug if testing shows resistance to one or more of the first-line drugs.
3. Answers will vary but should show recognition that antiretroviral drugs are used in combination in a multidrug regimen.
4. Tetracyclines have many interactions with other drugs and food. They should be taken on an empty stomach and with no iron, dairy products, or antacids.
5. To prevent formation of stones and crystals in the kidneys, patients must have adequate fluid intake when taking a sulfonamide. Each dose should be taken with 8 oz of water, and patients should drink 2 to 3 L of fluid per day.

Answer the following questions as either true or false.

1. False
2. True

3. True
4. True
5. False

Match each antifungal drug in the left column with the fungal infection it treats in the right column.

1. e
2. a
3. b
4. d
5. c

Chapter 10

Answer the following multiple-choice questions.

1. c
2. d
3. b
4. c
5. a

Please answer each of the following questions in one to three sentences.

1. Nonsedating antihistamines don't cross the blood-brain barrier, so they don't affect the CNS as much as sedating antihistamines do. Sedating antihistamines may be attracted to receptor sites in the brain.
2. They block symptoms related to the inflammatory response such as redness, edema, heat, and tenderness. They stop immune responses in cells, reduce levels of white blood cells, stop immunoglobins from binding and identifying invading cells, and stop the body from making interleukin.
3. They suppress hypersensitivity reactions; they reduce immune system responses and stop white blood cells from attacking the transplanted organ.
4. Uricosurics can't be used during acute gouty attacks; other antigout drugs such as allopurinol and colchicine can be used to treat gouty attacks.
5. Antihistamines work by competing with histamine for binding to H_1-receptor sites. They stop histamine from producing its effects. Mast cell stabilizers act on the mast cells to stop them from releasing histamine.

Answer the following questions as either true or false.

1. false
2. true
3. true
4. true
5. true

Match each generic drug in the left column with its classification in the right column.

1. e
2. c
3. a

4. b
5. d

Chapter 11

Answer the following multiple-choice questions.

1. d
2. c
3. a
4. d
5. a

Please answer each of the following questions in one to three sentences.

1. Sedatives reduce anxiety or excitement. Hypnotics induce sleep.
2. An injectable would be used for quick relief of agitation and other behaviors produced by the symptoms of psychosis. Oral administration is for prevention of such symptoms.
3. TCAs and SSRIs work by blocking the reuptake of certain neurotransmitters. MAOIs work by blocking the metabolism of neurotransmitters. In each case, the drugs' action makes more neurotransmitters available for relieving depression.
4. Antipsychotics are prescribed to treat delusions, hallucinations, and other thought disorders associated with various psychoses. Antidepressants are mood elevators that are prescribed to treat depression.
5. Tardive dyskinesia, which is characterized by a number of potentially irreversible involuntary muscle movements, may occur.

Answer the following questions as either true or false.

1. true
2. true
3. true
4. true
5. false

Match each generic drug in the left column with its classification in the right column.

1. a
2. c
3. e
4. d
5. b

Chapter 12

Answer the following multiple-choice questions.

1. c
2. d
3. b
4. a
5. c

Please answer each of the following questions in one to three sentences.

1. The amount of insulin taken depends on the results of blood sugar tests.

    Different amounts of insulin are prescribed by a physician for different ranges of glucose levels.
2. Possible answer: In type 1 diabetes, patients are unable to produce insulin. In type 2 diabetes, patients can produce small amounts of insulin, but the amount isn't enough to control their blood glucose levels.
3. Possible answers include: regulating the menstrual cycle and decreasing blood loss; decreasing the chance of iron deficiency anemia; reducing dysmenorrhea; decreasing the chance of ovarian cysts and ectopic pregnancies; reducing the likelihood of fibrocystic breast disease, pelvic inflammatory disease, endometrial cancer, and ovarian cancer; helping maintain bone density; reducing symptoms of endometriosis]
4. Possible answers include: Advantages of HRT are reduced risk of osteoporosis and reduced symptoms of menopause, including hot flashes and flushing, vaginal dryness, burning, and itching. Disadvantages include increased risks for endometrial cancer and heart disease.
5. Possible answers include: Monophasic means that the levels of estrogen and progestins stay constant throughout the cycle. For biphasic and triphasic contraceptives however, levels of progestins and/or estrogens change in phases. Biphasic formulations have two phases, whereas triphasic forms have three phases.

Answer the following questions as either true or false.

1. false
2. true
3. false
4. true
5. true

Match each generic drug in the left column with its classification in the right column.

1. e
2. c
3. a
4. d
5. b

Chapter 13

Answer the following multiple-choice questions.

1. d
2. b
3. a
4. a
5. d

Please answer each of the following questions in one to three sentences.

1. Some potassium dosages are much lower and are measured in milliequivalent units rather than in milligrams, like other drugs. These potassium drugs (such as potassium chloride) can cause cardiac arrest if an overdose is taken.
2. It's important to having strong bones and teeth and to maintain normal heart, kidney, and lung function.
3. It stimulates parathyroid hormone secretion, which regulates ICF calcium levels. It also aids in the movement of sodium and potassium across cell membranes.
4. It maintains the osmotic pressure and concentration of ECF and the body's acid-base and water balance. It also contributes to nerve conduction and neuromuscular function and plays a role in glandular secretion.
5. Potassium is an essential element for proper function of many types of cells, including heart and all other muscle cells and all nerve cells. This makes it important to the transmission of nerve impulses and to muscle contraction. It's also essential for tissue growth and repair and for maintaining the body's acid-base balance.

Answer the following questions as either true or false.

1. True
2. False
3. True
4. False
5. False

Match each drug in the left column with the condition it treats in the right column.

1. e
2. a
3. b
4. d
5. c

Chapter 14

Answer the following multiple-choice questions.

1. a
2. a
3. b
4. b
5. d

Please answer each of the following questions in one to three sentences.

1. Drugs that are cell cycle nonspecific act on cells in any phase of the cell cycle. Drugs that are S phase specific only affect cells that are in the S phase, or synthesis phase, of the cell cycle.
2. They interfere with the synthesis of DNA by acting like nucleotides, They become incorporated into the DNA strands and stop DNA synthesis.

3. Monoclonal antibodies are artificial antibodies designed to target specific substances such as immune cells or cancer cells, and antibiotic antineoplastics are antimicrobial products.
4. Tamoxifen may be used alone and as adjunct therapy in women with breast cancer that hasn't spread to the axillary lymph nodes. It may be used in treatment of postmenopausal women whose cancer has spread to the axillary lymph nodes. It may also be used as palliative treatment of breast cancer. In addition, tamoxifen reduces the likelihood of breast cancer in women who are at high risk.
5. Nonsteroidal aromatase inhibitors have temporary or reversible effects on the enzyme aromatase, whereas the effects of steroidal inhibitors are not reversible.

Answer the following questions as either true or false.

1. false
2. false
3. true
4. false
5. true

Match the generic name of each drug in the left column with the correct trade name from the right column.

1. b
2. e
3. d
4. c
5. a

Index

Page numbers followed by f indicate figures and t tables.